P9-BZM-513

Handbook of Behavioral Assessment *edited by Anthony R. Ciminero, Karen S. Calhoun, and Henry E. Adams*

Counseling and Psychotherapy: A Behavioral Approach *by E. Lakin Phillips*

Dimensions of Personality *edited by Harvey London and John E. Exner, Jr.*

The Mental Health Industry: A Cultural Phenomenon *by Peter A. Magaro, Robert Gripp, David McDowell, and Ivan W. Miller III*

Nonverbal Communication: The State of the Art *by Robert G. Harper, Arthur N. Weins, and Joseph D. Matarazzo*

Alcoholism and Treatment *by David J. Armor, J. Michael Polich, and Harriet B. Stambul*

A Biodevelopmental Approach to Clinical Child Psychology: Cognitive Controls and Cognitive Control Theory *by Sebastiano Santostefano*

Handbook of Infant Development *edited by Joy D. Osofsky*

Understanding the Rape Victim: A Synthesis of Research Findings *by Sedelle Katz and Mary Ann Mazur*

Childhood Pathology and Later Adjustment: The Question of Prediction *by Loretta K. Cass and Carolyn B. Thomas*

Intelligent Testing with the WISC-R *by Alan S. Kaufman*

Adaptation in Schizophrenia: The Theory of Segmental Set *by David Shakow*

Psychotherapy: An Eclectic Approach *by Sol L. Garfield*

Handbook of Minimal Brain Dysfunctions *edited by Herbert E. Rie and Ellen D. Rie*

Handbook of Behavioral Interventions: A Clinical Guide *edited by Alan Goldstein and Edna B. Foa*

Art Psychotherapy *by Harriet Wadeson*

Handbook of Adolescent Psychology *edited by Joseph Adelson*

Psychotherapy Supervision: Theory, Research and Practice *edited by Allen K. Hess*

Psychology and Psychiatry in Courts and Corrections: Controversy and Change *by Ellsworth A. Fersch, Jr.*

Restricted Environmental Stimulation: Research and Clinical Applications *by Peter Suedfeld*

Personal Construct Psychology: Psychotherapy and Personality *edited by Alvin W. Landfield and Larry M. Leitner*

Mothers, Grandmothers, and Daughters: Personality and Child Care in Three-Generation Families *by Bertram J. Cohler and Henry U. Grunebaum*

Further Explorations in Personality *edited by A.I. Rabin, Joel Aronoff, Andrew M. Barclay, and Robert A. Zucker*

Hypnosis and Relaxation: Modern Verification of an Old Equation *by William E. Edmonston, Jr.*

Handbook of Clinical Behavior Therapy *edited by Samuel M. Turner, Karen S. Calhoun, and Henry E. Adams*

Handbook of Clinical Neuropsychology *edited by Susan B. Filskov and Thomas J. Boll*

The Course of Alcoholism: Four Years After Treatment *by J. Michael Polich, David J. Armor, and Harriet B. Braiker*

Handbook of Innovative Psychotherapies *edited by Raymond J. Corsini*

The Role of the Father in Child Development (Second Edition) *edited by Michael E. Lamb*

Behavioral Medicine: Clinical Applications *by Susan S. Pinkerton, Howard Hughes, and W.W. Wenrich*

Handbook for the Practice of Pediatric Psychology *edited by June M. Tuma*

Change Through Interaction: Social Psychological Processes of Counseling and Psychotherapy *by Stanley R. Strong and Charles D. Claiborn*

Drugs and Behavior (Second Edition) *by Fred Leavitt*

(*continued on back*)

ADVANCES IN ART THERAPY

Advances in Art Therapy

Edited by

HARRIET WADESON
JEAN DURKIN
DORINE PERACH

WILEY

A WILEY-INTERSCIENCE PUBLICATION

JOHN WILEY & SONS

New York • Chichester • Brisbane • Toronto • Singapore

This publication is designed to provide accurate and
authoritative information in regard to the subject
matter covered. It is sold with the understanding that
the publisher is not engaged in rendering legal, accounting,
or other professional service. If legal advice or other
expert assistance is required, the services of a competent
professional person should be sought. *From a Declaration
of Principles jointly adopted by a Committee of the
American Bar Association and a Committee of Publishers.*

Library of Congress Cataloging-in-Publication Data:

Advances in art therapy.

Bibliography: p.
1. Art therapy.   I. Wadeson, Harriet, 1931–
II. Durkin, Jean.   III. Perach, Dorine.
RC489.A7A38   1989   615.8'5156   88-17350
ISBN 0-471-62894-8

Printed in the United States of America

10 9 8 7 6 5 4 3 2

Contributors

Robert E. Ault, MFA, ATR, HLM, is an art therapist and psychotherapist at the Menninger Foundation in Topeka, Kansas, and an assistant professor in the Division of Psychology and Special Education at Emporia State University, where he directs a Master of Science in Art Therapy program. In 1978, he opened a private art school, Ault's Academy of Art, where he teaches studio art. He is a frequent presenter of papers on art therapy and has published a number of articles in the art therapy literature. He is a past president of the American Art Therapy Association and in 1986 was presented with its Honorary Life Membership award.

Penny H. Baron, MPS, is an art therapist in private practice in Ithaca, New York, and author of *Journeying Towards Health Through Creativity: A Workbook Experience.* In 1985, she won a media award from the American Cancer Society for a series of articles entitled "Healing Cancer: Can the Mind Influence the Body?" She regularly runs groups and workshops for the lay public and professionals on changing attitudes towards cancer and creatively coping with stress and has recorded a series of relaxation cassettes entitled: "Journeying Towards Health Through Imagery."

Susan Buchalter-Katz, MA, ATR, is affiliated with Princeton House, the psychiatric and substance abuse unit of Princeton Medical Center, Princeton, New Jersey, where she works with depressed, schizophrenic, alcoholic, and manic-depressive individuals. She consults at St. Lawrence Rehabilitation Center, Lawrenceville, New Jersey, has taught at Trenton State College, and is the co-founder, past vice-president, and present corresponding secretary of the Garden State Art Therapy Association. She maintains a small private practice and has previously published in *Art Psychotherapy.*

Mary Cairns, MA, is an art therapist at Fred Hutchinson Cancer Research Center in Seattle, Washington, working with children who have leukemia. Previously she conducted art therapy with psychotic patients at Illinois State Psychiatric Institute.

Devorah Samet Canter, MA, works as a consultant for the Vivarium Project, an Apple Computer educational research project, and is co-owner of MacroMind, Inc., a Macintosh software and publishing company that designs animation, music, and graphics software for the Macintosh computer. She has published previously in *Art Therapy* and *HyperAge Magazine*.

Elizabeth Johns Clark, PhD, is an associate professor in the Department of Health Professions at Montclair State College, New Jersey. A member of the Academy of Certified Social Workers, she has published a variety of articles on death and dying, grief, and social oncology.

Irene E. Corbit, PhD, ATR, LPC, is an art therapist in private practice in Houston, Texas. She is an adjunct faculty member at the University of Houston—Clear Lake, a faculty member of the Jung Education Center in Houston, a member of the Editorial Board for *The Arts in Psychotherapy*, consultant to schools in Houston and Spring Branch, Texas, and on staff at three local hospitals.

Carol Thayer Cox, MA, ATR, is an art therapist with severely learning disabled and emotionally disturbed children and adolescents at Accotink Academy, Springfield, Virginia. She is also clinical instructor for the Graduate Art Therapy Program, the George Washington University, Washington, D.C. Previously she worked with sexually abused children and as a family therapist.

Elizabeth Strait Day, MA, has worked with art therapy clients at Chicago's Cermak Jail and at Wyler Hospital with seriously ill children.

Jean Durkin, MA, is the creative arts coordinator for Deborah's Place serving homeless women in Chicago. She is also on the staff of *Hotwire, A Journal of Women's Music and Culture* and a collective member of Mountain Moving Coffeehouse, a showcase for women musicians. She has presented her work at professional conferences and workshops.

Leigh Files, MEd, MA, ATR, is executive director of the Northwest Institute for the Creative Arts Therapies, Eugene, Oregon, which offers a Graduate Certificate Program in Art Therapy. She is adjunct instructor, Department of Leisure Studies and Services, University of Oregon, Eugene, and Department of Counseling Psychology, Oregon State University, Corvallis. She also maintains a private practice.

Barbara Fish, MA, ATR, has worked with hospitalized adults and is currently working at Allendale School as an art therapist with behaviorally disturbed, emotionally disturbed, and substance-abusing children and adolescents in a residential and day treatment setting. She has presented her work with countertransference as well as her work with substance-abusing children at state and national conferences. She is adjunct assistant professor at the University of Illinois and current president of the Illinois Art Therapy Association.

Mari Marks Fleming, MA, ATR, MFCC, is an art therapist in private practice in Berkeley, California. She is a lecturer at the College of Notre Dame, Belmont, California, and at California State University in Sacramento and consultant to the Eating Disorder Unit, Marshal Hale Hospital, San Francisco. She has published extensively in art therapy.

Jerry L. Fryrear, PhD, ATR, is a clinical psychologist and art therapist. He is professor of psychology at the University of Houston–Clear Lake, is co-author of *The Arts in Therapy* and co-editor of *Videotherapy in Mental Health* and *Phototherapy in Mental Health.* He has published 27 articles and chapters on the expressive therapies, and has presented numerous workshops nationally and internationally. He maintains a private practice in Houston.

Deborah Golub, EdD, ATR, assistant professor of art therapy at Wright State University, Dayton, Ohio, is a 1988 visiting professor of psychology at Beijing Normal University, People's Republic of China. She has published and presented her work in cross-cultural counseling of survivors of trauma.

Marge Heegaard, MA, is an art therapist and grief counselor at Lakeland Counseling Center in Minneapolis. She is author of a workbook for bereaved children, vice-president of the Minnesota Art Therapy Association, vice-president of the Minnesota Coalition for Terminal Care, and Co-chair of its Childhood Bereavement Committee. She also facilitates grief support groups for children and adults at Colonial Church of Edina and leads grief facilitator training workshops, conference workshops, school faculty inservice, and bereavement art therapy seminars in churches and schools.

David Henley is associate professor and chair of the Department of Art Education and Art Therapy at the School of the Art Institute of Chicago. He worked as an art therapist at the Katzenbach School for the Deaf in West Trenton, New Jersey, for 15 years. His most recent clinical experiences were at the Center for Deafness in Des Plaines, Illinois, the New Jersey School for the Deaf, West Trenton, New Jersey, and the Guild School for the Blind in New York City. He is consultant to the Art for the Handicapped Council in New Jersey. He was awarded the 1987 Research Award from the American Art Therapy Association for his work on artistic giftedness and the multiply handicapped. His current work as an artist is in high bas-relief on plaster, paper, and canvas.

Rosemary Lagorio, MA, is founder of Creative Communication Systems, a consulting firm for organizational development using nonverbal, symbol-making techniques. Previously she established an art therapy program at the Evanston Shelter for Battered Women and Children, Evanston, Illinois.

Gregory Thomas Onorato is a doctoral candidate at the Illinois School of Professional Psychology and for 8 years has specialized in forensic psychology. In 1984 he addressed the National Sheriff's Association on Suicide Prevention in a Correctional Setting.

Dorine Perach, MA, art therapist, has worked with both the elderly and the chronically mentally ill and has presented their work in two Chicago-area art shows. Her holistic approach to healing is reflected in her workshops that focus on physical well-being in relation to mental well-being. She has worked as a program assistant to the University of Illinois's Art Therapy Program and to its Summer Art Therapy Institute in Lake Geneva, Wisconsin. Now living in Israel, she works privately with immigrants, both adults and children, as they adjust to their new surroundings.

Jean Peterson, ACSW, ATR, TEP, is co-director of RiverCenter, Inc. She is former director of creative arts therapies at the Institute for Sociotherapy, where she directed a graduate-level training program for art therapists. She is a certified trainer, educator, and practitioner in psychodrama, sociometry, and group psychotherapy. She is on the art therapy faculty of the Expressive Therapies Program, Lesley College Graduate School, Cambridge, Massachusetts, and is a practicing psychotherapist.

Joanne Ramseyer, MA, is a staff therapist at Chicago's Edgewater Uptown Community Mental Health Center, where she implemented an art therapy program and currently supervises art therapy graduate students. She has organized several client art exhibits, which have been shown in the community. She is also an adjunct assistant professor at the University of Illinois at Chicago and conducts a private practice in art therapy.

Julie S. Serrano, MA, works in a community mental health center in New Hampshire as an emergency services therapist and in private practice. She has presented lectures on the use of the arts in therapy with sexually abused clients to mental health agency clinicians and to students and professionals at the University of New Hampshire. She has used her own artwork in lectures on college and university campuses, and has exhibited on campuses and in several northeastern cities.

Ellen Sontag, MSW, MA, ATR, is currently the school social worker for Aptikistic-Tripp District 102, Illinois, and was the art therapist at Illinois State Psychiatric Institute and adjunct assistant professor in the University of Illinois Art Therapy Program. She lectures locally and nationally about various aspects of art therapy.

Lenore Steinhardt, MA, ATR, works at the Rakefet Children's Therapy Center in Ramat Hasharon, Israel, and teaches a practicum course for the

Arts Institute Project in Israel in association with Lesley College. She has published previously in *Art Therapy*. A member of the Israeli Artists Union, she is a painter who exhibits in group shows.

Shirley Thrasher, MSW, ACSW, is adjunct lecturer at Hunter School of Social Work, Hunter College; doctoral candidate at Hunter School of Social Work; and former director of the East Brooklyn Prevention Program. She has made a film *The Affordable Choice* and has presented her work at professional conferences and in social work journals. She is recipient of the 1986–1988 Council of Social Work Education Minority Doctoral Fellowship Award in Research.

Harriet Wadeson, PhD, ATR, is associate professor and coordinator of the art therapy graduate program she developed at the University of Illinois at Chicago and former director of the art therapy graduate program at the University of Houston—Clear Lake. She is author of *Art Psychotherapy* and *The Dynamics of Art Psychotherapy,* numerous chapters in psychology texts, and more than 40 articles in professional journals. A worldwide guest lecturer, she also maintains a private practice in psychotherapy and art therapy in Chicago. She serves on the Executive Board of the American Art Therapy Association as research chair and was past publications chair. She has received that association's First Prize for Research as well as the American Psychiatric Association's Benjamin Rush Award for Scientific Exhibit.

Judith Wald, MS, ATR, is visiting instructor in art therapy at Concordia University, Montreal, Canada, and instructor of art therapy, University of Bridgeport, Bridgeport, Connecticut. She has previously published in *The American Journal of Art Therapy, The Arts in Psychotherapy, Clinical Gerontolgist,* and *Art Therapy.*

Evelyn Yee, MPS, ATR, is art therapist and caseworker for the East Brooklyn Prevention Program of the Catholic Guardian Society, providing services to West Indian families. She has presented her work with West Indian families at professional conferences.

Sarah Zahnstecher, MFA, MPS, is art therapist and caseworker for the East Brooklyn Prevention Program of the Catholic Guardian Society, providing services to West Indian families. She has conducted workshops for local agencies.

Grace C. Zambelli, MA, ATR, is a consultant to The Hospice, Inc., in Montclair, New Jersey. She has developed bereavement support programs for children for a number of hospitals and agencies in New Jersey. She also has lectured and published several articles on the use of art therapy with bereaved children.

Series Preface

This series of books is addressed to behavioral scientists interested in the nature of human personality. Its scope should prove pertinent to personality theorists and researchers as well as to clinicians concerned with applying an understanding of personality processes to the amelioration of emotional difficulties in living. To this end, the series provides a scholarly integration of theoretical formulations, empirical data, and practical recommendations.

Six major aspects of studying and learning about human personality can be designated: personality theory, personality structure and dynamics, personality development, personality assessment, personality change, and personality adjustment. In exploring these aspects of personality, the books in the series discuss a number of distinct but related subject areas: the nature and implications of various theories of personality; personality characteristics that account for consistencies and variations in human behavior; the emergence of personality processes in children and adolescents; the use of interviewing and testing procedures to evaluate individual differences in personality; efforts to modify personality styles through psychotherapy, counseling, behavior therapy, and other methods of influence; and patterns of abnormal personality functioning that impair individual competence.

IRVING B. WEINER

Fairleigh Dickinson University
Rutherford, New Jersey

Preface

Art therapy is truly an interdisciplinary profession, encompassing as it does the realms of art, psychology, and therapy. Often it enters the fields of education and social services as well. Each one of these areas is complex and varied. Therefore, it is to be expected that art therapy is a richly diverse field. As such, the profession continues to grow and develop, reaching new populations and challenging art therapists to create new ways of utilizing art for human understanding, treatment, and growth.

It is that challenge this book hopes to address. At the heart of art therapy is creativity, the encouragement to create imagery for healing and growth. By the nature of their work, therefore, art therapists are creative people. But beyond the creativity in work with individual clients and groups, art therapists are creative in evolving their profession. It is this latter creativity that is the subject of this book.

As a young profession, art therapy has evolved considerably since it was established only a few decades ago. As a distinct profession art therapy was developed by Margaret Naumburg and Edith Kramer in New York. It began to achieve wider recognition through their publications in the 1950s. Although there are many and ancient precursors to their work (reaching all the way back to prehistoric cave paintings), these two pioneers, more than any others, created the *discipline* of art therapy. Their work was firmly rooted in psychoanalytic theory, with Naumburg placing emphasis on the free-associative process of that approach and Kramer focusing on another psychoanalytic constituent, sublimation, as it may be achieved through art making. Both women continued to publish as art therapy attracted others to its ranks during the next several decades.

In its early period of rapid growth in the 1960s and 1970s, much of the material published by new art therapists was descriptive in nature, illustrating how art therapy "works." As the profession proliferated, it expanded beyond the psychoanalytic tradition and treatment settings in which Naumburg and Kramer worked. Art therapists were being hired by geriatric centers, by substance abuse programs, by rehabilitation facilities. New challenges were addressed. Art therapists began to see their work in a much broader perspective. From its beginnings as a treatment modality for the mentally ill or emotionally disturbed, art therapy began to be transformed into a more diverse profession whose foundations are buttressed by many disciplines and whose applications extend into many settings.

Advances in Art Therapy has several foci. The first, "New Populations" (Part I), describes work with populations that have been described very little or not at all in the art therapy literature heretofore. The expansion of art therapy beyond its earlier applications in psychiatric treatment settings and schools for the emotionally disturbed or mentally handicapped has broadened the profession significantly. In many ways, art therapy's advances into new areas of work have paralleled the broader recognitions of groups in need of human services, such as refugees, battered women, incest victims, bereaved children, and others. Each of the identified populations described in this section has its own special needs. As a result, it has been necessary for art therapists to become knowledgeable in special areas (such as brain injury, Alzheimer's disease, incarceration) and to develop innovative ways of designing art therapy to address the particular problems of these new populations.

A related area of concern is "New Methods" (Part 2). As art therapists have ventured into new settings, they have encountered new problems to be addressed through art therapy. These have stimulated the development of new ways of working. Additionally, the creative possibilities inherent in the work itself have challenged art therapists to be innovative in developing new ways of facilitating the enabling power of art to further human growth. In doing so, some art therapists have utilized that important constituent of creativity, synthesis. Several of the chapters of this section describe the development of a new process formed from merging art therapy with another mode of expression, such as computer animation, photography, or psychodrama. In other instances old methods are used in new ways or for new purposes. The refinement of the art-therapeutic process is one of the richest realms of art therapy, spurring the profession toward its greatest creative potential.

Finally, as the profession broadens through work with new populations and the development of new methods, so must "Art Therapy Training" (Part 3) evolve to prepare the art therapist to understand the field's expanding frontiers. The chapters of this section, unlike the others in the book, however, address not particular client populations or methods of working, but rather the professional personhood of the art therapist. Embodied in all the chapters of this book by its many and varied authors is the manifestation of the art therapist's essential creative and reflective resources. The final section of the book presents training developments that encourage the sort of responsibility that will further the field's evolution.

HARRIET WADESON

Chicago
November 1988

Contents

PART 1

New Populations

HARRIET WADESON

Although the profession of art therapy is both small and young, it is extraordinarily broad. From its early roots in the traditional psychiatric settings of hospitals, clinics, and schools for the emotionally disturbed, it has branched out into rehabilitation, custodial, medical, educational, and other human services. Art therapy has also entered the arena of personal growth workshops, where enhanced living, rather than treatment, is the goal. In this section of the book, we are provided with examples of still broader horizons in art therapy.

It is noteworthy that the "New Populations" section of this book comprises over half its chapters. Art therapy's greatest movement appears to be horizontal at this time. We are still a young profession, sufficiently unformed to be able to adapt art therapy's essential potential for enhancing self-expression, understanding, and creativity to the varying needs of widely diverse populations who can benefit from its services. Some of the chapters in this section might also be grouped in the "New Methods" part of the book, as their authors have developed innovative methods of working to suit the needs of these new populations. They are placed here, however, because their thrust is a focus on the very special needs and circumstances of these groups, of which the art therapist must be especially aware and sensitive.

For example, art therapy is just beginning to reach the refugee populations of this country, populations that often face enormous difficulties. The book begins with Deborah Golub's moving account of her work with adolescent Cambodian refugees in her chapter "Cross-Cultural Dimensions of Art Psychotherapy: Cambodian Survivors of War Trauma." She pointedly alerts art therapists to the significant problems in attempting to apply a western clinical approach to peoples from other cultures and highlights the necessity for therapist values clarification and understanding of the client's culture. In addition to cultural differences between client and therapist, for this population there is the further difference that few American clinicians have experienced the extensive trauma that survivors of the Pol Pot regime have endured. Since there are often no words to convey the suffering, imagery

1

can serve as a useful aid to communication and integration of the experience. Golub's suggestions apply to work with victims of other severe traumas as well as to work with other refugees.

Shirley Thrasher, Evelyn Yee, and Sarah Zahnstecher also highlight the need for cross-cultural awareness in their chapter entitled "West Indian Children and Their Families: Art Therapy with New Immigrants." The cultural conditions of this population are different from those of the Cambodians, as are their problems. Although adjustment to a new culture is paramount for both, the family situations are quite different. The Cambodian adolescents with whom Golub worked are "unaccompanied minors" who are being integrated into American families, having lost their natural families and been taken in by foster parents of the host culture. West Indian families, on the other hand, often immigrate in a piecemeal way so that years may separate the migrations of family members to the United States. In both populations there may be severe family adjustment problems in addition to immigration problems. These first two chapters delineate the difficulties refugees face, difficulties that art therapy can help to allieviate. These authors show us how.

Separation in the family is an issue for bereaved children, another group of children who have recently been identified as a specific population in need of human services. As bereavement counseling is becoming recognized as an important service to those suffering a death in the family, particular attention is needed for the confusion, guilt, and fear children may bear when a parent or sibling dies. The editors have combined material submitted by Marge Heegaard, about special groups she established for bereaved children at an elementary school, with reports of the work with children by Grace C. Zambelli and Elizabeth Johns Clark at a hospice. This chapter, "Art Therapy for Bereaved Children," provides a discussion of the special needs and developmental issues facing children suffering a family death, followed by case illustrations from both the elementary school and hospice. Art therapy appears to aid in the integration of the loss, and, it is hoped, helps to prevent further emotional difficulties for individuals who have suffered the death of a family member in their childhood. Few programs such as those established by these authors have been described in the literature heretofore.

Family issues are also a focus for the troubled women for whom Mary Cairns and Rosemary Lagorio developed art therapy programs. As a mother of a young child herself, Cairns became interested in the plight of psychotic women with recurrent hospitalizations who were repeatedly separated from their children and had to relinquish their mothering responsibilities to others. The needs of this particular group have hardly been identified and have not been addressed in the art therapy literature at all heretofore. In her chapter, "A Mothers' Art Therapy Group in a Short-Term Psychiatric Setting," Cairns discusses how group art therapy was beneficial to these mothers in providing them support around their feelings about the circumstances of their mothering. She found that a prominent issue for these women was their struggle with their own mothers.

In addition to work with victims of political violence (Cambodian), this section presents several chapters on work with victims of domestic violence. Although battered women have been identified as a segment of the population needing human services, to date there have been no reports in the literature of art therapy programs for this population. Rosemary Lagorio, in her chapter "Art Therapy for Battered Women," describes her work at a shelter where she designed innovative art therapy activities to help the women recognize the elements of the "fit" between themselves as victims and their abusers. Through the art they also became aware of their often unacknowledged anger. The end result was that the women left the shelter feeling more empowered and confident in directing their own lives.

Work with other victims of family abuse, in the chapter "The Arts in Therapy with Survivors of Incest," is described by Julie Serrano. Here, the author presents various techniques of art making, body work, and guided imagery through the stages of a group's growth in which its members moved from incest "victims" to "survivors." Dealing with their many feelings in this way, group members progressed from fragmentation toward integration.

Moving from victims of illegal perpetration to alleged offenders, the chapter by Elizabeth Strait Day and Gregory Thomas Onorato, "Making Art in a Jail Setting," provides us an inside view of incarceration, a perspective from which most of us are shielded. The authors describe the substantial challenges this setting imposes and the ways that both individual and group art therapy addressed these problems, often in spite of overwhelming odds.

Additional new populations that are responding to art therapy are individuals with severe medical conditions. Moving beyond their traditional positions on hospital psychiatric floors, art therapists have found that other medical patient populations can benefit significantly from art therapy. Particularly in realms of self-image, problem solving, and cognitive functioning, art therapy plays a major role.

Penny H. Baron's "Fighting Cancer with Images" and Mari Marks Fleming and Carol Thayer Cox's "Engaging the Somatic Patient in Healing Through Art" explore the exciting possibilities of influencing life changes through modifying imagery. Rather than simply understanding the art expression diagnostically as a reflection of the patient's life situation, these art therapists encourage their patients to modify their imagery in a healing or soothing way. Although art therapists have encouraged emotional change wrought by the art-making and reflection process, Baron and Fleming and Cox encourage modification of the art for the purpose of effecting positive physical as well as emotional change. It is exciting indeed to anticipate the possibilities suggested in these two chapters for further developments in which visualization and its concrete manifestations in art expression can profoundly shape the course of physical and emotional change.

Further interventions in the medical realm are presented in two chapters by Judith Wald, "Severe Head Injury and Its Stages of Recovery Explored Through Art Therapy," and "Art Therapy for Patients with Alzheimer's Disease and Related Disorders." In both populations the limitations imposed by the injury or the disease are extensive, severely altering the self-perception of the patient. The challenges to the art therapist working with these individuals are considerable. They require an understanding of the physical processes of these conditions and their progressions, necessitating much attention to the logistics and appropriateness of particular art activities. A challenge to the art therapist, as well, is the encouragement of optimism in the patients and oneself in the light of the hopelessness such extreme physical and mental limitations can engender. Wald shows us how art therapy can assess and monitor progress, aid in emotional needs, and even provide an uplifting experience for these patients.

Art therapists are true interdisciplinarians. Much of the discussion presented here focuses on our work as clinicians. But in the chapters by Robert E. Ault and David Henley, our position in the world of art is emphasized as well. Although art therapy traditionally serves a "patient" population, Robert Ault has discovered that those who seek therapy through art do not always identify themselves as patients, nor do they necessarily approach treatment facilities. His chapter, "Art Therapy with the Unidentified Patient," presents an account that illustrates the sensitivity and flexibility of an art therapist–artist in responding to needs of "nonpatients" in an art school setting.

Henley's poetic descriptions of both the art-making process and the resultant products in his chapter "Artistic Giftedness in the Multiply Handicapped" are indeed eye opening to those of us unfamiliar with this very special population. Henley strongly identifies himself as an artist aligned with the art world, and we can see in his art therapy his sensitive encouragement (or noninterference) with artistic development. The chapter concludes with challenging questions regarding both aesthetics and art criticism of "outsider" art as well as ethical considerations for art therapists regarding the exploitation of multiply handicapped "savants."

Taken as a whole, the "New Populations" section of the book shows art therapists on the move, advancing the frontiers of the profession into territories where art therapy had not yet been established. The various characteristics of these diverse new populations of all ages challenge the art therapist to respond creatively to the special problems these groups face.

CHAPTER 1

Cross-Cultural Dimensions of Art Psychotherapy

Cambodian Survivors of War Trauma

DEBORAH GOLUB

> *My sick hungry friend lay beside me.*
> *His lips and eyes turned white.*
> *His hands and mouth closing tight.*
>
> *Same time I heard a machine gun,*
> *People started to run.*
> *I tried hard to carry my friend,*
> *But neither he nor I could stand.*
> *My ears filled of devil sound,*
> *My friend begged me to go alone!*
> *I looked at my sadness friend at last,*
> *And I took off very fast!*
>
> FROM "ESCAPE (TRUELY STORY)"
> BY A CAMBODIAN "UNACCOMPANIED
> MINOR"

Everyday I always have one deep question asks myself, how will I be able to help my foster parents and my country when I will be older, because every thing seems very hard to me . . . now. . . . I can't answer my deep question, I think next year I will be able to answer it.

FROM THE "LIFE BOOK" OF A CAMBODIAN ADOLESCENT

An emergency art therapy session is requested by the American foster parents of a 14-year-old Cambodian refugee who recently arrived in the United States. The night before, in an apparent rage, he swept through the house overturning furniture and uprooting plants. Then he fled. You arrive at the home early the following morning. The boy seems to glare through you from behind strands of hair that fall over his eyes. His English is minimal; your Khmer is nonexistent. How do you interpret his behavior? What do you do? How do you communicate? How do you achieve trust?

5

A Romany child has "heard voices" and comes to the large city medical center accompanied by an encampment of gypsies from his tribe. He draws crucifixes and tapes them around his hospital room to protect him from the "ghosts." Another boy, quite suddenly unable to move his legs, describes his terror at watching dogs run around his West Indian island with the head of a goat in their mouth. During art therapy sessions he draws in uncanny detail other traumas that are occurring in another location during the very moment he represents them and about which the world will learn only on the 11 o'clock news. Do you treat psychosis and conversion disorder, respectively?

Art therapy as a profession is rooted in western psychological constructs of understanding human behavior. Clinicians, including art therapists, tend to understand the diagnosis, etiology, and treatment of psychopathology according to definitions set forth by the "dominant" society within that western cultural framework. Art therapy curricula appropriately prepare students to converse in the standard theoretical language that will enhance their credibility among colleagues. But what happens when two sets of world-views intersect in the therapeutic relationship—when the client and therapist do not share assumptions about the nature of the problem, goals, and strategies of treatment?

Many clients in the United States whose cultural worldview is likely to differ from that of the therapist are immigrants or refugees. Their psychological stress of relating to a western-oriented healer may be exacerbated by entry into an unfamiliar society with little hope of returning home, as well as by possible placement in transit camps, which isolates them from the receiving society, and subsequent scattering throughout the country, which isolates them from each other.

Therapy, like refugee resettlement, is a political act. An institution tends to evaluate its consumers according to definitions of normality that reflect its own status quo. In some cases, successful psychological and social integration of clients from culturally diverse communities is measured in terms of their adaptation to criteria that the prevailing psychiatric community itself establishes and represents. There is an imbalance in the power relationship when the client is assessed according to criteria and rules about which the therapist is fully cognizant and the client is only partially aware.

The act of naming exerts enormous power over the named. The process can be therapeutic or exploitative depending upon who labels and for what purpose. One effect of naming when practiced by society is that it can neutralize the power of the stranger, incorporate that person into or separate him or her from the local community, and protect the status quo. At the same time, it can precipitate a self-fulfilling prophecy. Outsiders might internalize characteristics of the label until they too use it as a self-description. Xenophobic institutions consequently have reason to feel assured of their diagnostic accuracy and continue treating patients according to their now realized label.

If the client is to become empowered rather than merely be "helped," the clinician must at least for the moment relinquish his or her usual constructs of thinking in order to reevaluate their relevance to a client's needs. This means not simply revising and adapting theories and methods of treatment, but reconsidering the basic premises upon which he or she will relate to the individual who arrives with a problem. It means relating to a person and not to a diagnostic category or to a representative of a culture.

Shared culture need not be a prerequisite for effective therapy. If the clinician transcends differences of everyday perception, he or she can rediscover those universals of human experience and symbolizing that are the common ground on which client and therapist can communicate. It is quite possible that true healing occurs in this transpersonal realm of experiencing commonality rather than difference.

It is not enough to focus on common denominators, however. Individual identity often is tied to a sense of group belonging and the need for cultural referents. In other words, the client may wish to maintain separation between his or her home world and that represented by the therapist. The therapist might not and, if the client and his or her community consider it inappropriate, should not be privy to certain secret knowledge or be a participant in traditional healing rituals. Misunderstanding can be averted if the therapist has clarified feelings about his or her own cultural identity and has understood any needs or expectations he or she has of the client.

Another feature in the history of some immigrant or refugee clients can make therapeutic interaction even more complex and obstacles to communication more likely. In addition to the variable of culture, probably it is the client alone who has experienced catastrophic stress, often related to war or political strife in the home country. In this case, not only are the cultural lenses through which therapist and client perceive and assess the world different and their spoken languages dissimilar, but even if the therapist and client could speak the same idiom, no vocabulary has been invented to describe adequately the experience. Words by their very nature are delimiting and therefore desecrate the pain. Only silence is infinite enough to contain the horror. Yet the indelible images persist in the form of dreams, recurrent or intrusive waking thoughts, and, on rare occasions, dissociative flashbacks.

There is an additional problem particularly when working with Cambodian refugees. The horrors committed during Pol Pot's regime were among the most massive and hideous in human history. Worse, they were self-inflicted—acts of autogenocide initiated by a Cambodian against his own people. It is difficult for those of us who have never witnessed such reality to absorb that scale of inhumanity. We do not want to believe that such things really happen and, in order to protect our own psyche and the familiar constructs by which we make sense of the world, we may close ourselves off from the client who has been victim, witness, and in some cases agent of extreme violence.

Is it therefore possible to treat a client effectively when the therapist has never experienced a similar extreme trauma? Again the answer must be affirmative. For this to happen, however, therapists have to be willing to consider the horror, the potential for inhumanity, the annihilation that is within themselves; they must in their own way have "looked over the edge" and confronted death.

At some point in their careers art therapists might treat survivors of extreme trauma whose cultural orientations differ from their own. They are assisted by the fact that nonverbal artistic expression is a powerful catalyst for bridging both culture and silence. Imagery, after all, is a logical vehicle for communicating with individuals whose encoding of the catastrophe and whose subsequent symptomatology involve images of the event. However, in order to understand better the catastrophic experience and to avoid the ethnocentric danger of proceeding clinically as if the principles and methods of art therapy were directly transferable in all settings, it may be useful for the western-oriented therapist to explore eight aspects of cross-cultural art psychotherapy (see the Appendix to this chapter).

These areas include the nature and history of the *traumatic stressor,* ways that the client and the client's community name the problem (*diagnosis*), what they view as the source of illness (*etiology*), and, given their perception of causality, what they consider the appropriate *goals* and *forms of treatment.* In addition, the clinician might consider whom the client regards as the most appropriate *healer* given the particular complaint, as well as how both western and traditional communities view the intricate *relationship* between healer, client, and society. Finally, and of paramount concern to the art therapist, is the *role of the arts* in the healing practices to which the client subscribes.

This chapter attempts to address two separate concerns of the art therapist: culture and trauma. It draws upon the author's clinical work with child victims of rape and incest and survivors of war and combat, as well as her consultations involving both non–English-speaking patients from various countries and survivors of traumatic violence in Africa, the Middle East, Asia, and Latin America. Ideas also evolve from the author's experience over 20 years of living and working in diverse communities: a remote Pacific island pineapple plantation, towns in the Andes and the Pampas, European cities, northeastern United States inner-city neighborhoods, Chicano farm worker communities in California, American Indian reservations and Yaqui villages, and university-sponsored cross-cultural training groups.

Within the context of the eight areas of cross-cultural art therapy, one specific community with whom the author worked is highlighted—Cambodian unaccompanied minors who survived the Pol Pot regime, Vietnamese invasion, refugee camps in Thailand, and resettlement in the United States. A brief review outlines contributions to the literature on cross-cultural applications of art therapy in general and art therapy with survivors of war in Southeast Asia in particular.

Details of traumas experienced by Cambodian children provide a historical context for understanding artwork, clinical issues, and modifications that were necessary such that art therapy effectively would address those clinical issues within a Cambodian Buddhist worldview. Case material provides concrete examples of theories presented. Finally, implications for art therapy research and training are outlined.

THE LITERATURE

The fields of anthropology, mythology, and ethnopsychiatry have contributed to our understanding of the universal and culturally specific meanings of symbols as they relate to sickness and healing (Billig & Burton-Bradley, 1978; Boas, 1972; Campbell, 1973; Eliade, 1961, 1964; Jung, von Franz, Henderson, Jacobi & Jaffé, 1964; Kiev, 1972, 1974; Róheim, 1970; Torrey, 1973). Professionals other than art therapists have discussed symbolic productions of survivors of extreme human-induced trauma such as kidnapping (Terr, 1981, 1983) and natural disasters such as floods (Newman, 1976). Some of the traumas that they describe are war related and have taken place within diverse cultural contexts. Allied professionals have elucidated the visual imagery of victims or survivors of torture throughout the world (Bloch & Møller, 1986) and of Nazi concentration camps (Costanza, 1982; Volavková, 1964), the bombings of Hiroshima (Japan Broadcasting Corp., 1977; Lifton, 1969), racial strife in South African townships (Open School, 1986), and war in El Salvador (Silverstein, Eth, & Arroyo, 1986; Vornberger, 1986), Israel (Kovner, 1971; Lieblich, 1978), Uganda (Hilsum, 1986), and Southeast Asia (Boothby, 1983; Branfman, 1972; Brett & Mangine, 1985; Brett & Ostroff, 1985; International Rescue Committee, 1982; Langford, 1980).

Until now, articles concerning cross-cultural dimensions of art therapy generally have had one of two foci; either they address theoretical issues without detailing pragmatic application, or they describe a specific population such that it is difficult for readers to generalize to their own clientele. Art therapists are only beginning to discuss cross-cultural aspects of art therapy theory, practice, and training (Garcia, 1975; Gardano, 1986; Lofgren, 1981; McConeghey, 1986; McNiff, 1979, 1981, 1984, 1986; Moreno & Wadeson, 1986; Steinhardt, 1986; Wong-Valle, 1981) and to describe clinical work with survivors or witnesses of catastrophic traumas like rape (Abbenante, 1982; Garrett & Ireland, 1979; Malchiodi, 1986; Spring, 1980), incest and abuse (Cohen and Phelps, 1985; Levinson, 1986; Stember, 1977, 1980; Wohl & Kaufman, 1985), terrorist acts (Silverstein, 1984, 1986), and air disasters (Di Maria, 1986).

A minority of art therapists work in the area where cross-cultural issues intersect with stressors of war (Grossman, 1981; Landgarten, 1981; Schwarcz, 1982; Steinhardt, 1986). Corbit (1985) noted a correlation between transformations in graphic representations of dreams among a group of American combat veterans and men's working through of trauma. Golub (1985) described recurring stylistic features in creative process and products of Vietnam combat vets including a fracturing of self-representation reflected as polarities in their imagery.

Although western clinicians have discussed cultural implications of psychiatric interventions with Southeast Asian refugees (Fong, 1983; Langford, 1980; Kinzie, 1981; Kinzie, Fredrickson, Ben, Fleck, & Karls, 1984; Kinzie, Tran, Breckenridge, & Bloom, 1980; Sabatier, 1984; Tobin & Friedman, 1983; Williams & Westermeyer, 1983), these clients have received scant attention in the art therapy literature. References mostly pertain to Vietnamese refugees in the United States (Burch & Powell, 1980; Carlin, 1979; Harding & Looney, 1977; McHammond, 1985; Rahe, Looney, Ward, Tung, & Liu, 1978; Salant, 1976). Two art therapists (Golub, 1984; McHammond, 1985) independently observed a cleavage in the way Cambodian adolescents represented history and the relationship between internal and external worlds. McHammond compared polarities in the art of Cambodian and Vietnamese refugees. Whereas Cambodian children divided history into halves, before and after Pol Pot, and struggled with personal identity as it related to "good and evil," Vietnamese clients tended to experience the split as confusion about their identification with eastern versus western culture. She hypothesized that differences related to whether or not the child had experienced war for his or her entire life.

THE HISTORICAL SETTING

Official statistics are controversial. Eyewitness accounts of Cambodians with whom the author worked are difficult to refute, however. In order to appreciate clinical issues, artwork, and art interventions in the adolescents' treatment, it is essential to know something about the traumatic stressors that they endured.

Cambodia, 1975–1979: During Pol Pot's Communist regime and the subsequent Vietnamese invasion, an estimated one to three million Cambodians died or were killed by the Khmer Rouge—in other words, possibly up to half of Cambodia's population of seven million people. Cities were outlawed, their citizens evacuated on marches to the countryside. Some people with known connections to the Lon Nol government were taken away soon after the Khmer Rogue entered Phnom Penh and, according to anecdotal reports, a number were disposed of quickly from the open doors of captured helicopters. Children as young as 6 or 7 were separated from parents and forced to work in labor camps. They dug ditches and hauled earth for 16 hours a day, all night long when the moon was full, sustained by a couple of spoonsful of rice gruel.

Executed: teachers, artists, doctors, intellectuals, the wealthy, former army personnel, monks, ethnic minorities, city dwellers, anyone with formal education, those heard speaking French or using the polite form of speech, people who wore eyeglasses or those who merely had marks on their noses suggesting eyeglass use, individuals with dental repairs, children who showed emotion when forced to watch living parents have their livers cut out or parents when required to witness their infants being tossed between soldiers' bayonets.

Memories: sloshing through bloody streets of Phnom Penh, seeing Khmer Rouge soldiers waiting for a woman to give birth by the side of the road before killing both mother and infant, saving a friend from fatal dehydration by suspending a coconut and dripping its fresh milk through bamboo into her veins, being forced in the work camps to decapitate with portable guillotines other young friends whom the Khmer Rouge considered lazy, hearing the dying words of parents as to how they might avenge this all—by becoming the best person they possibly could be. And witnessing all of this between the ages of 4 and 11.

When the Vietnamese invaded Cambodia in 1979 children took advantage of the confusion in their work camps to escape the Khmer Rouge. Most returned to their homes seeking parents and relatives, but, unable to locate them, decided to flee to the border. They found protectors along the way: an old man, soldiers, a group of traders, fellow refugees. Some children traveled alone behind bands of monkeys and scavenged food remnants tossed aside by the messy eaters. A few boys became guerrilla soldiers and left booby traps for the advancing Vietnamese. All of the children walked and walked hundreds of miles through jungles filled with mines, dangerous animals, and frightening spirits. Many arrived at the border with malaria, malnourished, or unconscious.

The camps brought a sense of security but also different sources of stress. There were the soldiers, Thai this time. There were life decisions to be made about third-country resettlement. Children became adept at learning the "correct" answers and behaviors during interviews with representatives of potential host governments. Suspended between past and future, they waited for news of family and for news of a sponsor. In this limbo of uncertain duration they formed bonds with international relief workers, teachers, friends, and houseparents at the children's center. But the new attachments inevitably were followed by more separations as friends departed for countries all over the world.

The journey to a busy northeastern United States airport was arduous, and when they landed most children, adolescents by now, appeared exhausted, glassy-eyed, confused, and scared. They arrived with only the clothes they wore, the ubiquitous plastic bag containing immigration documents, and perhaps some photographs or schoolbooks purchased with earnings from a private vegetable garden in the camps. The awkward moment of meeting new "parents" was the first of many adjustments, to food, climate, language, school, relationships, styles of expression, and the absence of life-threatening situations. It was in this context that adolescents began art therapy.

In summary, children were victims, witnesses, and sometimes agents of human-induced catastrophe that was not a single event but rather persisted over years. They survived precipitous separations at an early age from parents and from all aspects of a familiar life. They endured harsh living conditions that included starvation, disease, and exhaustion from forced labor. Children repeatedly witnessed violent death that they had to observe passively so as not to die themselves. They constantly feared for their own lives and made decisions over and over that affected their very survival. After catastrophic threats to life ended, their stress continued as adolescents adjusted to a new culture and dealt with old losses.

THE CLINICAL SETTING

Twenty-two Cambodians between the "official" (sometimes different from actual) ages of 12 and 17 attended art therapy groups and individual sessions during the first year following their arrival in the United States. It had been 7 to 8 years since the Khmer Rouge entered Phnom Penh and 3 to 4 years since they arrived in the Thai refugee camps. All came as unaccompanied minors—their parents had died from disease or starvation, been killed, or their fate was unknown—and were placed with American foster families in the event of family reunification at a later date.

The refugee resettlement program under whose auspices the author worked as family therapist/art therapist was a community-based church-related voluntary organization, one of two agencies contracted by state and federal governments to assist Cambodian children arriving alone. The local agency subscribed to a holistic approach to healing in which expressive–arts therapy was considered part of and dependent upon the success of an entire program: a family support network for American foster parents, respite care and mentor systems provided by local Khmer families, Khmer social and religious gatherings and cultural institutes, and education of school personnel and host communities about their new citizens. Expressive modalities were regarded as particularly useful among individuals whose command of English was minimal as they encountered the difficult process of resettlement in a new culture.

None of the adolescents arrived with or later received a psychiatric diagnosis of post-traumatic stress disorder. Staff recognized the inevitability of some psychological traumatization given their experience; nevertheless weekly meetings in which art was included were viewed as support rather than therapy groups. Those adolescents referred for individual sessions in order to hasten developmental gains or because of specific behavioral problems attended art therapy. Adolescents participated in one of two weekly groups, and the girls came to an additional group. Those adolescents seen individually met with the art therapist once a week, more often at the client's request or if an emergency arose. The art therapist also held family sessions on request or as deemed necessary by staff.

Groups lasted 2½ hours and were facilitated by the art therapist, the program's American coordinator, and a Cambodian interpreter. The art therapist worked alone during individual and family art sessions and with the girls' group but the Cambodian interpreter was on call or available by telephone if needed.

THE CLINICAL ISSUES

Clinical issues related to trauma and resettlement appeared in adolescents' behavior and artwork and suggested treatment approaches. Issues affecting treatment also surfaced in adjustment responses of American foster families and in countertransference reactions of the art therapist. A holistic approach to healing requires that the responses of all members of the client's intimate community be considered. Paragraphs below outline psychological factors experienced by some adolescents, families, and staff in the aftermath of trauma. They are followed by discussions about the influence of clinical issues on both art phenomenology and clinical response.

Client Issues

Guilt

Numerous acts of commission or omission during and after Pol Pot triggered children's guilt. Some felt guilty that they had not returned, perhaps out of fear or lack of food, to seek families when the Vietnamese invaded. Many felt responsible for "abandoning" people in Cambodia as they purposefully fled to the border. In order to aid chances of obtaining unaccompanied minor status and thus increase the possibility of leaving camps, children had to deny further that they might have living family. Later they felt guilty about leaving behind friends in the camps and about choosing third-country resettlement instead of repatriation, although this would have meant certain death. Many wondered why they survived when others died and made an emotional commitment to "study hard" in order one day to return and help friends and country. In reality, they would remain functionally powerless for years.

Loss and Unresolved Grief

Adolescents were unable to complete the mourning process or resolve separations when they did not know their parents' fate, nor could they feel tranquil knowing that dead parents had not received proper burial and thus their spirits were not at rest. Some clients were unable to remember parents' names and had memory lapses about extended portions of their social history. All longed for the peaceful past, and privately a number of adolescents sought the nurturance from foster parents that they had missed for years.

Trust

During Pol Pot times one trusted few people. Intelligence, discrimination, manipulation, and caution saved children's lives. In the United States most adolescents continued to find it difficult to trust and to abandon those survival attitudes and habits that, although currently dysfunctional, once had kept them alive. Many tested foster parents until they believed that the new family understood the depth of their suffering and would not desert them.

Initially, some adolescents displayed paranoid or hostile behavior when they felt that they were being discussed in English. Lack of trust, apprehensiveness, and habit often led to physical or emotional withdrawal; experience had taught them that flight was a more effective way to survive.

Expression of Affect

Cultural proscriptions discouraged showing "negative" emotions such as anger or sadness because these make the listener uncomfortable. Smiles and humor sometimes accompanied descriptions of painful social history. The expression of emotion during Pol Pot times directly threatened survival. Adolescents needed to trust before they privately would reveal anger, fear, depression, or sorrow in the United States.

Adolescents felt unaccustomed to the facile display in public of innermost feelings, and uncomfortable and threatened by the American style of verbal confrontation as a mode of problem solving. Their preference was to flee. Headaches and earaches sometimes were associated with "not wanting things to come out." In an attempt to bridge two worlds, the Cambodian interpreter urged adolescents to deal with problems by talking; keeping them inside would make them "sick." At the same time, western families and therapists had to restrain themselves from probing with direct questions. Their close attendance more likely was interpreted as nosiness. Polite disinterest usually evoked more disclosure from adolescents.

Anger

Traditionally it is rude to display anger especially toward parents. A person ought to wait a day or so and then quietly explain why one thinks he or she is correct. Adolescents had difficulty verbally expressing anger toward American foster parents who had opened their homes when there was nowhere else to go. The newcomers were unfamiliar with American styles of confrontation and uncomfortable with the loud voices that accompany anger.

Beneath normative anger concerning daily problems was rage about the extremity of children's victimization and loss. During Pol Pot's regime rage got one killed. In the United States older boys privately expressed their hatred of the Khmer Rouge and desire for vengeance. Some Cambodian girls, although not those in our program, hinted about one particular source of anger and pain. The author heard reports that Pol Pot soldiers kidnapped certain young girls and forced them to be their "wives." Others intimated sexual misuse during flight or in the camps. Girls were very reluctant to discuss past sexual issues. It probably is not by chance that fewer girls than boys arrived unaccompanied in the camps. More had remained with families or friends, lacking the resources to flee or survive on their own.

Relationships

Adolescents' relationships in the United States were influenced largely by prior experiences of separation and abandonment. Many felt abandoned by parents and caretakers who disappeared in Cambodia. They considered that they themselves had left families of origin, country, and friends in the camps. Adolescents feared abandonment by American foster parents at the same time that they could not make an emotional commitment to them. For those whose parents' fate was unknown, a commitment to "new" parents meant further renunciation of the old. Divided loyalties led to frustration in the new family system. Adolescents struggled with issues about how to relate to the two sets of parents and how to fit foster parents into their construct of lost family. At the same time, they had no problem immediately calling American parents "mother" and "father." Unfortunately, these traditional forms of address determined by age and social status sometimes were misconstrued by Americans as signs of emotional connection.

A honeymoon period in the United States characterized by mutual "enchantment" (Fong, 1983, p. 2) was followed by emerging problems in some foster families. Adolescents who had survived alone in Cambodia and had not been scrutinized in the camps suddenly were expected to follow rules and obtain permissions. They now had to assume the role of child, and the older ones resented the felt infantilization.

A number of adolescents had difficulties with each other. Some who functioned well in Cambodia or Thailand were not as successful in the new society because their skills were not necessarily appropriate in the United States. Others carried prejudices with them, not fully accepting peers who were from ethnic minorities or mixed marriages or who had acquired a "reputation" in the camps. Staff speculated that the ease of adjustment among some adolescents related to strong nurturance in early life as well as to not being marginal in terms of ego identity.

Identity

Adolescents searched for their role in a new culture. Some appeared confused about their identity as Cambodian, Vietnamese, American, Buddhist, or that religious orientation represented by relief workers in Thailand or by foster families. Ambivalence about whether they could be bicultural was tied in part to the uncertain future of Cambodia. Adolescents struggled with their cultural pride on one hand and shame about their history on the other. At large gatherings of Cambodians, it took adolescents time to feel that it was all right to be Cambodian again. In some cases, behavioral regression accompanied their transition back into the majority society.

Family Issues

American foster families had different motivations and expectations in requesting that an adolescent live with them and different degrees of understanding about the catastrophic experience. Many imagined that the newcomer about whom they had little specific information beyond a name would fit into an established household and there would be an open expression of intimacy by all. Illusions of a happy and loving new family in which parents were mentors began to dissolve as the difficult process of mutual adjustment became apparent.

Some parents did not understand certain initial behaviors: running away, hiding under bed covers, being reticent about sharing feelings. Parents became angry if an adolescent gave an answer that seemed incorrect, not realizing that according to a Cambodian perspective subjective reality and people's feelings are more important than objective truth. What adolescents perceived as respect, some foster parents interpreted as lying.

Parents found it more difficult to deal with acting-out behavior on the part of a few foster children after the initial novelty wore off. They desired to return to normal routine at a time when adolescents were confronting realities of resettlement and were beginning to express feelings.

Difficulties emerged in some families when siblings became jealous of a parent's attention to the newcomer. A few Cambodians acted out when a second refugee adolescent later joined the family. Some parents felt that they competed with an invisible and idealized Cambodian family. They had to deal with the possible reappearance of a foster child's relatives and the ambivalence those rare occasions triggered.

Therapist Issues

Clinicians probably do not "select" a population by chance. Rather, it is possible that personal issues connect somehow to the client's experience. Therapeutic process is affected as much by the the clinician's experience and personality as by the client's. In the author's case, issues of war and death related to the Holocaust, Vietnam, and a long-term life-threatening illness that later was cured. These confrontations with death in her personal and family history surely influenced her work with a traumatized population.

The author's overwhelming sense upon meeting the Cambodian adolescents was of their gentleness, love, and lack of bitterness despite the hardships and losses that they endured. Their attitude seemed to reflect a wisdom such that the author began to view the children as her teachers. While this may have been gratifying initially for the therapist, it can be dangerous and burdensome for clients. Idealization of clients either because of a therapist's extraordinary respect for their survival or because of an attraction to the "exoticness" of their culture may make the therapist less flexible in seeing clients as individuals or in giving them room to be human.

The author's impression after working with survivors of various traumatic stressors is that at times clients and therapist collude in treatment. The magnitude and irrevocability of extreme trauma leave the therapist feeling extremely helpless. Unable to erase the past or provide clients with an existential meaning to their pain, the therapist can only try to help individuals find a way to live with the memories. A sense of inadequacy makes a therapist question the very meaning of his or her work and professional identity. It is difficult to tolerate this felt helplessness and so the therapist sometimes deludes both himself or herself and the client with gestures of assistance or trite reassurances.

Clients also are in a bind. They want help, want to believe that the pain is curable, and are angry if the clinician has no answers. Yet they also know that there are no answers. Any attempt on the therapist's part to offer simplistic palliatives is considered counterfeit and jeopardizes trust.

Therapists face another risk in working with survivors of catastrophe in general. Post-traumatic symptomatology such as memory impairment, exaggerated startle response, depression, and a sense of being disconnected from ordinary society is transmitted easily to those in close contact with the survivor. The art therapist noted in herself one particular response that may be connected to her intense interaction with clients' imagery. She found that she incorporated their imagery into her own dreams. That is, she dreamed aspects of the traumatic experiences reported by clients. Overidentification with the client threatens both client and therapist as much as does potential affective numbing of a clinician who is unable to tolerate emotionally the descriptions of intense traumatic content.

Society regards differently the healers of those who experience diverse catastrophes. When the disaster is of natural origin such as an earthquake or flood, rescue workers are viewed as heroes (Benedek, 1984). Clinicians dealing with survivors of human-induced disaster may feel more isolated by society because the trauma assumes a moral dimension. Yet therapists working with "victims" of human-induced catastrophe often are accepted more easily than those treating "perpetrators" or clients who engaged in reactive violence beyond that required for survival. In the latter case there is a sense that society fears contamination via the therapist. The work of these clinicians receives little overt acknowledgment or sanction except from clients. Furthermore, the clinicians must come to terms with their own potential for violence and with acts of atrocity reported to them by some clients.

Burnout rates are high. At times clients assume the role of therapist to the clinician. They are torn between wanting to repay those individuals who have helped them and feeling guilty for "causing" the therapist's burnout.

Clearly it becomes the clinician's responsibility to monitor countertransference, seek balance and nurturance elsewhere in his or her life, and determine when job stress becomes counterproductive to all involved.

THE CLINICAL RESPONSES

Cultural factors pertaining to adolescents' concepts of diagnosis, etiology, treatment, and healer required that art therapy function integrally within the community. Adolescents felt a stigma attached to western psychotherapy. They were used to problem solving with the extended family and not with an outside practitioner. According to them, one saw a western healer in pre–Pol Pot Cambodia only as a last resort, when truly "crazy." Great resistance and shame accompanied the thought of western therapy in the United States, and adolescents did not want peers to learn that they had been referred.

In two cases of more serious behavioral problems adolescents saw an American psychologist. Program staff preferred to use other available resources that might be less threatening. Some teenagers having difficulty in their American families, for example, were placed for temporary respite in the home of a Cambodian family. Traditionally it was rare to send children to nonrelatives. The rationale in this case was to connect clients who had lost their own social network with an alternative and familiar kind of support system.

Adolescents also were encouraged to speak with members of the Cambodian community who could be their honorary elder sister, aunt, or grandmother, for instance, and whose advice they might seek because of this traditional relationship. The Cambodian interpreter was invaluable in assessing adolescents' needs for specific types of healing. He was considered by them as either father, uncle, or elder brother depending on the child's age and gender, and in his appropriate role provided them with endless hours of counseling.

In cases where adolescents acted out or felt themselves "possessed," staff drove them some distance to visit or to reside temporarily at the Cambodian Buddhist temple. A beloved monk whom the adolescents respected counseled them, led them in prayers, or performed ceremonies to exorcise the spirits. He often encouraged them to be studious, independent, and proud of their cultural identity.

On occasion *Kroue Khmers,* traditional healers who use various herbs, were sought. Coining was the appropriate treatment for common somatic complaints such as headaches, stiff necks, stomachaches, and dizziness, which the adolescents attributed to "bad airs" inside the body. Coining is a system not requiring a specialist in which the smooth edge of a coinlike object is rubbed with oil along designated meridian lines of the body related to the specific complaint. The process is very painful and leaves temporary bruises, and there are prohibitions against particular activities such as bathing or intravenous injections for some hours after.

Some of the older adolescents knew how to coin. Peers came to them for treatment in the United States. The art therapist learned fundamentals of coining from these adolescents as a way of understanding concepts of healing better. Her interest and respect for traditional healing practices seemed important to the clients, who in many cases felt that they had to hide traditional beliefs from Americans in order to be accepted.

Another form of healing became evident to the art therapist after clients began to trust her and report their dreams. It was common that missing parents came to their children in dreams and gave advice about current problems. Usually adolescents projected a great sense of reassurance and security after such encounters. The art therapist began to view these dream spirits as the clients' primary therapists to whom she and the clients listened as guides for treatment.

The program sought other resources in the Cambodian community that might prove healing for adolescents. A Khmer institute was held twice a year in which surviving Khmer artists, musicians, dramatists, dancers, writers, and historians taught intensive courses. Unaccompanied minors from a broad geographic area attended, thus allowing reunions with friends whom they had not seen since Thailand. American staff participated as co-learners with the children or as assistants to the teachers. On the request of the Cambodian organizers of the institute, the art therapist also provided an open group for children and adolescents to engage in the spontaneous use of art materials. A Cambodian monk came to the institute, giving individual counsel and leading daily prayers.

One feature that contributed to the success of the agency's overall program was the mutual respect between Americans and Cambodians involved in treatment and their acceptance of each other's methods. Americans readily made referrals to appropriate healers in the Cambodian community. The art therapist realized that not being a Cambodian Buddhist she was unable to provide certain prerequisite care. The monk could offer in 5 minutes what it would take the westerner months to achieve, if ever.

At the same time, the monk appreciated and supported efforts of American staff. His counsel to adolescents helped alleviate the teenagers' sense of being divided within. When, for example, many voiced to him their dilemma of being asked by American foster parents to attend Christian church while they wished to retain a Buddhist identification, the monk advised them that they need not feel disloyal to their Buddhist identity; one feels torn only if one views life dualistically. When there are no polarities there are no contradictions. Children could be both Christian and Buddhist.

Clinical response involved not only the Cambodian community. Visits or telephone calls from American relief workers who had known the children in Thailand provided a consistency of relationship as the adolescents struggled to form new bonds. Care was taken to assist bonding from the moment of arrival. Adolescents were met at the airport by a group of Cambodian peers. Foster parents greeted the teenager first, and the initial physical contact by "mother" seemed to represent for both child and mother a kind of birthing.

The agency functioned according to a "cluster" policy of resettlement based on the belief that the mental health of refugees depends in great part on the mutual support allowed by geographic proximity. Three communities within a 10-mile radius were selected on the basis of available services and probable openness to diversity among their citizens. Public presentations by Cambodians and American staff about Cambodian history and culture were well attended. Private sessions for American foster parents provided them additional training and a place to discuss feelings and issues arising in the homes. While working with American and Cambodian family members together, the art therapist had to pay special attention that the adolescent did not feel excluded or unsupported simply because parents and therapist shared language and culture.

THE ART

The following description of selected aspects of phenomenology and their assessment evolved from impressionistic observations by the art therapist and her clients during art sessions. Statements are to be viewed as speculative and in process since it is impossible to generalize about post-trauma imagery of Cambodian adolescents or of survivors in general on the basis of such a limited sample. Readers should be cautioned against hasty institutionalization of observations into diagnostic "certainties." It does seem likely in the case of these particular adolescents that relationships existed between clinical issues arising from the trauma and their artistic response. The following discussion refers to some aspects of traumatic history that may relate to artistic phenomenology.

Media

When offered various materials including wood-carving tools, clay, markers, oil and water pastels, colored pencils, inks, charcoal, tempera, and watercolor with bamboo pens and assorted brushes, adolescents usually selected watercolor with fine brushes. Most first engaged in short-lived experimentation with media that were unfamiliar. Art supplies had been limited in Thailand. When presented with the array of new media in the United States some clients tried every material in a superficial rather than studied manner. This usually gave way to serious efforts with a single medium such as marker, pastel, or watercolor. Clients seemed to be much more comfortable and facile with watercolor than their American counterparts and sensitively applied layers of subtle colors to one painting a session with sustained concentration.

Small paper often was chosen, and some adolescents preferred to work in miniatures such as those they may have seen in traditional Cambodian art. Generally the entire paper space was filled. Many adolescents spontaneously added their own Khmer poetry to drawings, using highly descriptive forms of expression that were unavailable in the English language. They generally avoided clay, associating it with childishness. This medium was more acceptable to girls working separately if they felt that its use was utilitarian.

Color

Adolescents employed a wide palette from the beginning. This contrasted with American veterans of combat in Vietnam, who usually started therapy with achromatic materials and progressed in stages through red and shades of green before arriving at a chromatic range (Golub, 1985). Cambodians' drawings of catastrophic events, like the veterans', often incorporated red. Also, like the veterans, they rarely used charcoal. Few employed black exclusively with the notable exception of one client who manifested behavioral problems and who used black alone to depict ghostlike figures that appeared to make him anxious. Black may have had toxic connotations for the children, because the Khmer Rouge wore black. Often they became frightened by American police officers in black uniforms. The art therapist had to be sensitive to the use of black in her dress and in the therapeutic environment.

Elaboration and Repetition

Representational drawings of landscapes or traumatic scenes were characterized by a great deal of detail. In pastoral landscapes this involved intricate cloud formations, foliage, and water surfaces (see Fig. 1.1). When traumatic memories were produced the enemy usually possessed more detail than the victim (see Fig. 1.2). This took the form of additional color, shading, and details of weapons and paraphernalia. The author's impression of this selective elaboration is that it was through assiduous observation of the enemy that children knew in an instant whether to stay or flee. Few stick figures appeared in adolescents' art in contrast to human figure representations of other adult survivors of war early in their therapy (Golub, 1985).

Repetitions were noted in the depiction of red dots for flowers and planted fields. It might be more appropriate to view this in the light of traditional stylization rather than defensive perseveration.

Manifest Content

Upon their arrival in the camps of Thailand sensitive relief workers provided Cambodian children with art materials and opportunities to express their unspoken images on paper. Soon they burst forth with what has been called

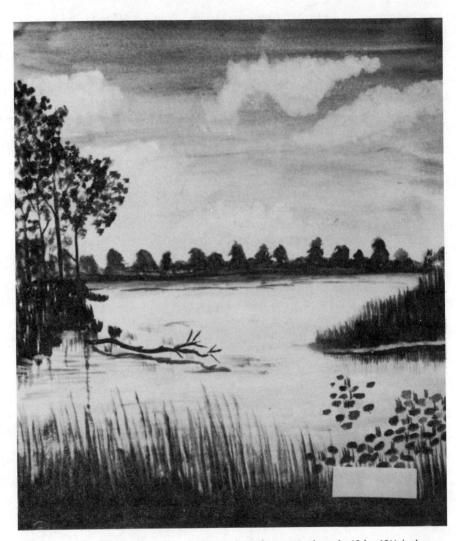

Figure 1.1. Pre–Pol Pot nostalgic scene, a watercolor; approximately 12 by 13½ inches.

catastrophic art, detailed replications of witnessed scenes. Although the western staff encouraged this type of expression, Cambodian houseparents urged children to draw "pretty" pictures, which they believed would ingratiate the children to prospective sponsors more easily than would scenes of disaster. Too much depended on children being accepted for refugee status.

The art therapist had anticipated in children's artwork of the trauma a paucity of detail and integration. Quite the opposite seemed true; rich and integrated content in most cases suggested that perhaps children had retained strong ego integrity despite the excruciating content they depicted. This may

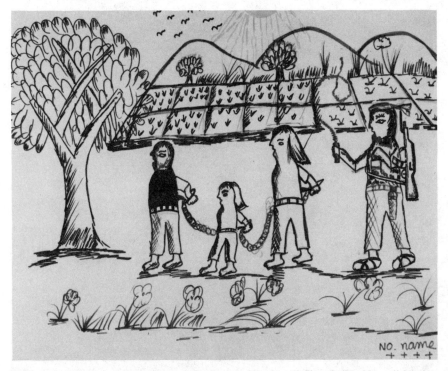

Figure 1.2. "Students and Teachers Being Led to Slaughter." Signed "No Name." Victims are black. The Khmer Rouge soldier contains red, blue, green, and purple. Felt-tip pen; 11 by 14 inches.

be connected to their earlier life of stability and nurturance by family, community, and tradition.

Catastrophic scenes drawn in the camps were quite individualized and based on personal memory; common themes reappeared, however. Drawings often included either queues of victims awaiting slaughter or solitary figures running. Sometimes, as is the case in one drawing by a late adolescent housed in a refugee camp in Thailand, paper seems unable to contain the explosive imagery, hurling movement, and screams (see Fig. 1.3). Artwork shows piles of human bones and individuals being eviscerated against trees whose branches often are reminiscent of those same bones. Figure 1.4, depicting one such "liver torture," was completed in the camps by a young teenager who had been partially blinded and had lost an arm.

Human figures in drawings commonly sustain blows to the head. In Cambodian culture one's spirit is believed to reside in the head; it is impolite to touch this part of the body. Beatings to the skull and decapitation were reported by children, and perhaps not coincidentally many of them manifested headaches in the United States. It is common in catastrophic art to see anthropomorphized suns from whose eyes red tears fall toward earth.

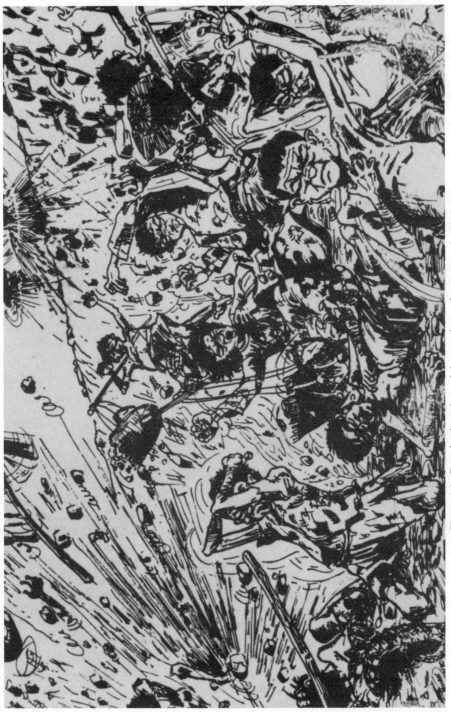

Figure 1.3. Drawing by a late adolescent in a refugee camp in Thailand.

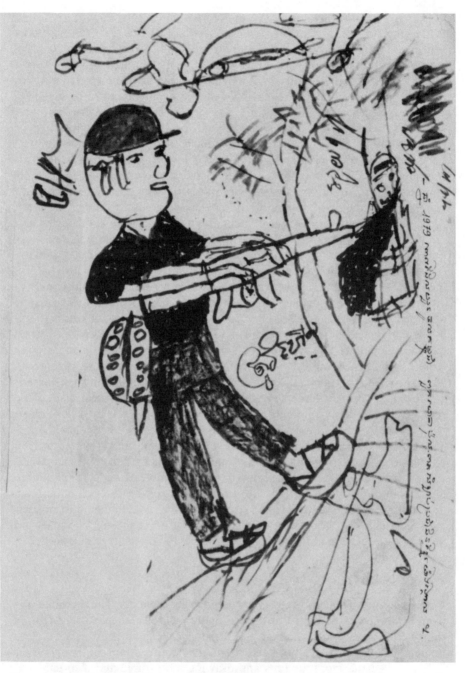

Figure 1.4. Catastrophic drawing completed in a Thai refugee camp depicting a "liver torture." The artist had received traumatic physical injuries. Mixed media.

This may relate to the fact that in the Khmer language the word for "sun" is the same as the word for "nation" or "people." More importantly, it may reflect children's ability to allow nature to weep for them when direct expression of emotion during the trauma would have meant death.

An explosive release of traumatic imagery often characterized initial productions in the United States. However, these quickly were replaced by nostalgic scenes of pre–Pol Pot life, flowers, or the beloved Angkor Wat, symbol of past glory of Cambodia. Typically drawings contained two or three mountains, a rising or setting red sun without tears, a bamboo hut at lower left, and road or river traversing diagonally to upper right banked by red flowers. Individual expression manifested as the infusion of highly personal style into traditional artistic structures. Figure 1.5, for example, excludes any evidence of human life other than planted rice fields. The artist in fact came from the most rural background of any of the adolescents and continued to be somewhat isolated from his peers in the United States. Less overt individuality of content appeared in nostalgic art than in traumatic scenes. One possible explanation is that, as was not the case for pastoral landscapes, no traditional prescriptions existed for rendering catastrophe.

It is possible to speculate about the emergence of pre–Pol Pot scenes after arrival in the United States. Adolescents looked forward with hope to a "new life" and desperately wanted to be liked. Perhaps they felt as had their houseparents that pictures that did not arouse anxiety in the viewer would assist acceptance. Perhaps catastrophic scenes in art represented a stage in mastery of trauma through which the adolescents already had passed.

Nostalgic art may have served another function—that of assisting the refugees during their long and powerless wait until adulthood when, as so many expressed, they wished to return to help restore a "Free Cambodia." These clients had lost everything: family, country, language, revered artists. Perhaps the representations of fond memories within the security of a familiar artistic structure helped adolescents as they attempted to adjust in an alien land. Continuing identification with Cambodian culture through adherence to traditional structure in a group setting seemed crucial in the midst of such monumental loss. The art therapist supported group cohesion and made no attempt to intervene in the repeated thematic and stylistic productions.

Latent Content

Occasionally ghostlike presences appeared in art products. These ambiguous forms emerged as revisions of human figures. Circles encapsulated figures that were verbally identified by the artist and became their new faceless bodies. Adolescents did not talk about the modifications, although their behavior became more anxious and drawing more rapid and disorganized. The author's impression is that this might relate to the existence for many children of numerous spirits of the enemy, the forest, and the dead for whom they could not provide proper burial. Buddhism protects people from spirits. In the forests there were no people and therefore no protective Buddhism.

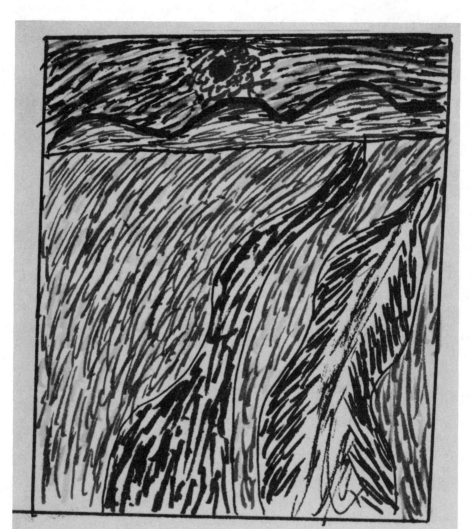

Figure 1.5. "Rice Fields." The artist, who came from a very rural province of Cambodia, wrote, "I had 6 brothers and sisters but now I don't have anybody but me." The fields are green and yellow; the sun is red. Felt-tip pen; 6½-by-7½-inch ruled frame on 11-by-14-inch paper.

Contrasts appeared in art as transformations of personal identity and discrepancies in the amount of detail between victim and agent of disaster. Content usually showed child as victim. There seemed to be an internal consistency or integrity in portraits of victims with whom they identified, perhaps because in most cases the locus of chaos for them rested in the external world rather than the self. Some transformations suggested identity confusion. One adolescent's self-portrait evolved into a "Vietnamese Christian'' before terminating as a blond American. The creator of Figure 1.6 began drawing "Me When I Wake Up in the Morning." This became a ghostlike enemy soldier with a weapon before it was crossed out and the drawing crumpled.

The theme of contrast also manifested as differences between the natural and human world. Idyllic scenes of warm sun and ordered fields sometimes appeared as a backdrop to scenes of horror (see Fig. 1.2). This incongruity may relate to the absolute incomprehensibility for children that a Cambodian like themselves could murder his own people—that such scenes of auto-genocide and chaos could occur in their once predictable world.

Process

During early sessions adolescents adhered to a familiar artistic process as well as to traditional content and composition. To be a "good" artist meant copying the masters and following designated form. Often a frame was ruled out within the boundaries of the paper space and a picture executed in pencil. Paint was applied sequentially from the background or top of the paper toward the foreground. This process was reinforced during the Khmer institute where adolescents relearned the traditional drawing process from some of the few surviving Cambodian artists.

Transformations in the artistic depictions of disaster suggested movement toward mastery of trauma. Initially scenes replicated specific remembered events. In time, traumatic events became generalized to other contexts. Decapitation, for example, now took place in an American historical setting wherein an Indian is represented killing women with hatchet blows to the neck while Pilgrim husbands passively watch (see Fig. 1.7). The artist of this particular etching, which was completed in school, signed his pictures in the direct line of fire of the various weapons, suggesting that an unconscious identification with the victims remained.

In time adolescents added snowcapped mountains to their tropical nostalgic scenes. Their Cambodian school took on American flagpoles, and Phnom Penh homes were landscaped with North American evergreens. Perhaps the incorporation of both Cambodian and American worlds into a single composition was an unconscious attempt through symbolization to master trauma and to reintegrate identity.

Art therapy responded within the context of values placed on community cohesion and extended family and social relationships. The development of trust and confidence depended on the author relating to adolescents not as therapist but as elder sister, mother, or aunt. Soon after meeting her, girls privately asked the author's age and marital status in order to determine the proper form of address. Many weeks were required to cultivate this relationship. With the girls, for example, it involved activities like cooking, shopping, taking short walks, practicing traditional dances, combing each other's hair. After a while the girls began to express their fears, anger,

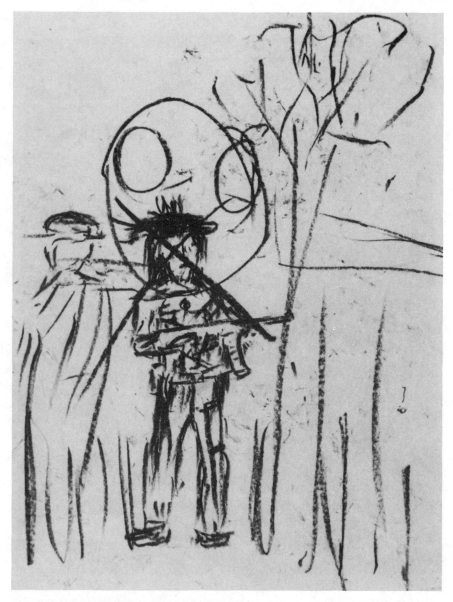

Figure 1.6. "Me When I Wake Up in the Morning" transformed into a Khmer Rouge soldier. Black craypas; 8½ by 11 inches.

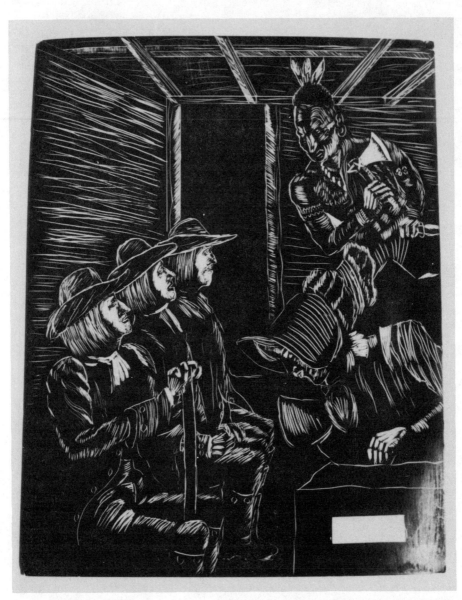

Figure 1.7. Decapitation in an American historical context. Reproduction in black India ink and scratchboard.

sadness, and questions about sexuality in an American high school setting.

Individual art sessions took place at the adolescent's home. Spontaneous interaction with available materials seemed more significant to the clients in dealing with issues such as anger, trust, and fear. The following case examples from work with two clients demonstrate cross-cultural applications of art therapy where clinical issues relate to the trauma of war and resettlement.

CASE EXAMPLE 1

An early adolescent and her foster parents had worked hard to establish a trusting relationship. The teenager was beginning to express her tremendous anger that had grown during years of pain and abandonment. A caring and consistent approach by the parents allowed her a secure context in which to work through feelings. The art therapist was contacted for an unscheduled morning session following an intense family argument while preparing dinner the night before. She arrived to find the teenager completely under her bed covers in a fetal position and clutching the housekey.

The therapist mentioned to the girl that she had brought a new art material and explained the circumstances of her coming that day. She said that when she was her age she, too, had had some "big" fights with her mother. The girl peeked out from the blankets to look inquisitively at the therapist. As the teenager listened intently, the therapist continued by saying that it is all right to be angry. She then modeled one way of talking to one's mother when upset.

The girl turned toward the new block of clay and spoke her first words. "What's that? Like earth?" She mentioned that she had used clay in the past to "make people." "Good idea! Would you like to make people?" She jumped out of bed. As client and therapist worked together, the teenager gave the author instructions about what to do with the author's figure: "Make her fat!" "Put stick through her head!" The art therapist complied.

The girl simultaneously fashioned a kitchen scene including rice cooker, wok, hot-sauce jar, dishes, table, stools, and a smaller human figure. "Here. Baby. This her daughter." Spontaneous enactment with the pieces followed. Finally the teenager placed the child in the mother's lap, asked to keep all the figures, and went to the kitchen to prepare real food. The art therapist's impression was that the adolescent used clay in an attempt to reconstruct and transform events of the previous evening from the moment just before the crisis occurred. Spontaneous play allowed her to try out the ending she may have desired.

Later in therapy spontaneous play again reflected a growing alliance with her foster mother. One sunny day the client led the author to sit with her on the lawn. She made positive comments about her foster mother. As client and therapist spoke the girl began playing with some twigs, leaves, and grass, and she suddenly began construction of a "house." The client taught the art therapist how to plant stakes, bind beams, weave the roof and walls, and tie them down. Mutual effort was necessary in order to protect the structure from a breeze. Finally the completed house stood intact. "What a good house! Strong house! We do good," she exclaimed. Perhaps the "strong house" represented the growing security that she felt both in her own living situation and in the therapeutic alliance.

CASE EXAMPLE 2

A boy, here called Sovann, was discovered alone on the edge of a Thai refugee camp malnourished, covered with sores, and protecting a small cache of food with animallike sounds and gestures. Native speakers of Khmer had great difficulty comprehending the boy's speech. Some camp physicians considered him to be developmentally delayed; others offered the diagnosis of minimal brain damage with psychosocial retardation. His chronological age was estimated at 11 or 12.

Nobody knew what the boy had experienced. More confusing was how he had survived. Descriptions of the traditional Khmer response to mental retardation indicate that unless individuals have a relative to care for them they often are left to fend for themselves. The staff and foster family began to hypothesize about one possible survival strategy that had saved Sovann's life during the flight to Thailand; Sovann made people laugh by his impersonations. In the camps he mimicked politicians. In his American home he mimed humorous caricatures of television actors with uncanny accuracy. Sovann seemed to have extraordinary abilities of observation and enactment which allowed him to abstract the essence of a person or experience. Was it possible that he had procured gifts of food from other fleeing Cambodians by using this ability to make them laugh?

Early drawings from the camps contained disorganized scribbles and some cephalopods. Although Sovann spent much of his time at the camps engaged in solitary wandering and scavenging, he did begin to establish some relationships with female caretakers. As this occurred his human figure representations developed hands and feet; however, faces still included a multitude of undifferentiated dots. After 1½ years, a body trunk began to appear together with a differentiated single eye and intimations of gesture, primarily that of running. Indeed, the experience of running and hiding must have been paramount in his life. Approximately 2 years after his arrival in the camps rather sophisticated animals emerged in Sovann's art, monkeys and birds in motion and with facial features drawn with greater clarity than those of his human figures.

Sovann arrived in the United States a year later. Individual art therapy was recommended in order to enhance the development of social relationships, to provide him a vehicle for expression, and to prepare him to enter school by fostering English language skills. He spoke no English and was barely verbal in Khmer. The art therapist's Khmer consisted of a handful of words. Art sessions, she realized, would depend largely on nonverbal communication—gesture, enactment, intonation, touch, eye contact, facial and body expression, art materials, and creative process. It also seemed that

Sovann probably could communicate his story and feelings although words were unavailable to him. Therapist and client needed to discover a common "vocabulary."

The therapist went to his home. It was the territory with which Sovann was most familiar and where he felt most in control. Knowing the importance of flowers in Cambodian culture, she brought a carnation to his first session. Excitedly Sovann accepted the gift, placed it in water, and began bowing toward the vase. This to him was an offering to Buddha, and the ritual became a prerequisite to subsequent art therapy sessions.

Sovann led the therapist to his room, where he hastily explored her large bag of art materials selecting markers, paint, and the largest pad of paper. During the session he completed 17 drawings before indicating quite clearly that he was tired and the meeting was terminated.

Sovann began by spontaneously leafing through a picture dictionary and painting a copy of a uniformed mailman. Abandoning the book he drew his wristwatch, a recent gift from his foster mother. Often during art sessions he attracted the therapist's attention to his watch with what seemed to be excitement mixed with anxiety. In fact, during Pol Pot times only Khmer Rouge soldiers owned watches.

Sovann chose a smaller piece of paper to draw one of the most expressive portraits the therapist had ever seen—one that she perceived to be full of bewilderment and terror (see Fig. 1.8). This was not a schematic drawing of a face. Detailed beard and scar over the left eyebrow made this a particular person. Sovann was becoming increasingly agitated but seemed consumed with representing an inner vision.

A helicopter soon followed; he must have seen some. Line pressure increased. Sovann drew rapidly and anxiously, punctuating his work with chopper sounds. The therapist continued to supply art materials as he raced through a pad of newsprint. Airplanes were followed by tanks. One tank became encapsulated in a circle which in turn transformed into the belly of a man. A wristwatch reappeared on the man's right arm. Sovann jumped up, drew an imaginary gun from his belt, and plowed down an imaginary crowd of people with a barrage of gunfire rounds and chopper sounds.

At that very instant a helicopter happened to fly over the house where we were working. Sovann gazed toward the ceiling in terror. His entire body became rigid. He froze. The therapist touched his shoulder, looked steadily into his eyes, and spoke calmly. Although Sovann did not understand the words he locked into her eyes until his body relaxed and his eyes softened.

With great care Sovann picked up a red craypas and drew the carnation she had brought him. She drew a picture of him; he made one of her. Finally Sovann completed a self-portrait with eyes and ears pronounced and mouth omitted. Although he could not express himself verbally he could use art to recount his life, relate his fear, and form human relationships. Within the sanction of a setting made sacred by his blessing to Buddha, art could become a vehicle for interpersonal and cross-cultural communication and bonding in this incomprehensible new environment.

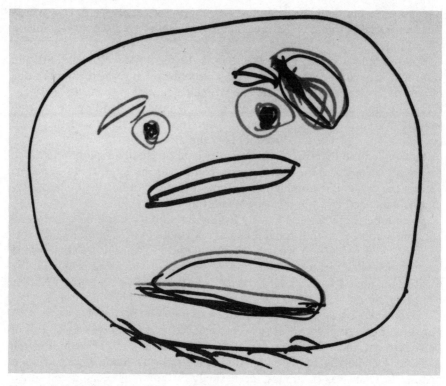

Figure 1.8. Portrait of a man with scar and beard by a "developmentally delayed" adolescent. Green and black felt-tip pen; 7-by-8-inch image on 11-by-14-inch paper.

CONCLUSIONS

The experience of Cambodian adolescent war survivors in art therapy provides a framework for thinking about applications of art in therapeutic settings where client and therapist represent different value systems or life experiences. This wider clientele of survivors of normative or catastrophic stress is as diverse as to include victims of sexual abuse or witnesses of violence, patients hospitalized with life-threatening illness, the homeless, "dependent" children in overseas schools, incarcerated individuals from the nondominant culture, and elderly immigrants in nursing homes.

It is possible to make a few general statements regarding cross-cultural dimensions of art psychotherapy:

1. Therapists can minimize the dangers of ethnocentrism, overinterpretation, and imposition of a status quo paradigm upon their clients through a process of personal values clarification and through a clearer understanding of the client's worldview.

2. Art therapy across cultures probably will be more effective when it evolves from an understanding of the client's perspective of the world rather than direct imposition of the western therapist's theories and methods. Clinicians need to be willing to retrain their thinking about the meaning and purpose of therapy, their role in the therapeutic relationship, and the appropriate context for healing.

3. Art therapy training that meets needs for cultural sensitivity might consist of the following: cross-cultural communications and *training*, including values clarification, workshops on sexism, racism, and ageism, role plays, simulations, critical incidents, case studies, and immersion experiences; *coursework* on culture and personality, culture and cognition, interviewing, projective testing and art evaluation across cultures, medical anthropology, ethnopsychiatry, psychiatric epidemiology, culture of institutions, critical pedagogy, mythology, art across cultures, and nonverbal communication; and *clinical experiences* such as international internships and student or instructor exchanges.

IMPLICATIONS FOR FUTURE RESEARCH

Preliminary findings with Cambodian adolescent refugees suggest future research directions in art psychotherapy. Comparative studies of phenomenology would provide information about recurring stylistic features in art across traumas. Hypotheses then could be made concerning whether psychological conditions associated with trauma in general produce certain expressive responses or whether artistic responses relate to specific stressors.

It would be interesting to investigate the effects of different traumatic stressors on creativity as well as to compare survivors of the same event who have and have not been diagnosed with post-traumatic stress disorder. One could explore whether correlations exist between aspects of imagery and different variables such as the nature of the stressor (e.g., natural or human induced), demographic data (e.g., age at the time of the trauma, psychological treatment since the catastrophe), and symptomatology (e.g., sleep disturbance, somatization). Longitudinal studies might examine the effects on imagery of different stages of flight and resettlement as well as phases in artwork and art therapy relative to mastery of trauma.

The profession would benefit from the development of new theories and methods of art therapy as they relate both to trauma and to cultural diversity in the therapeutic relationship. More concentrated effort needs to be made at discovering why our field remains rather homogeneous. Practitioners must engage more seriously in our own values clarification and must respond such that art therapy curricula better address issues and needs of a broader range of students and clients.

Appendix: Background Information for Cross-Cultural Art Psychotherapy[1]

THE TRAUMA

Pre-Trauma

What was the nature of any previous life stressors and the client's coping styles in response?

Trauma

Did the catastrophe occur precipitously? Was it human induced and if so by whom? A one-time event or sustained?

What happened and how did the client cope?

Was the client a victim, witness, and/or agent of traumatic events?

What were living conditions?

How often did the client feel that his or her life was in danger? Who taught him or her how to survive?

Did the client have social supports during the trauma?

Was the client separated from significant others and did he or she have a chance to say good-bye? Was he or she able to carry out rituals of burial and grieving?

Was the client allowed to express emotion without endangering his or her life?

Did the client receive any medical or psychological help during the trauma?

Post-Trauma

How did the client cope following the trauma?

Did the client have a support network or receive treatment after the traumatic events ceased?

What were the client's first contacts with rescue workers, immigration officers, border soldiers? Were there new traumas?

Did the client stay in a transit camp awaiting resettlement? For how long? What were the living conditions? Were there new traumas?

What were the circumstances of resettlement and the nature of first contacts with the host community? Were there new traumas?

Was there a reunion with or new information about family or friends after the last significant contact?

How does the client remember the trauma and relate to those memories?

Does the client have hopes of returning to the home country?

[1]Brownlee (1978) and Torrey (1973) are excellent resources for similar questions about cross-cultural dimensions of healing. Similarly, the reader may find useful those intake evaluations regarding traumatic history of Southeast Asian refugees (Kinzie, 1981; Rahe et al., 1978) and Vietnam veterans (Scurfield & Blank, 1985; Wilson & Krauss, 1980).

THE DIAGNOSIS

How do the client and his or her community name the problem?

What does the client state to be the presenting problem?

How are symptoms categorized?

Is there a physical locus of affect?

How are diagnoses made and by whom?

To what extent is the disorder culture bound?

THE ETIOLOGY

What do client and community consider to be the source of the illness? (Natural or supernatural? Biological, environmental, or metaphysical? Spirit possession? Loss of soul? Bad thoughts or acts? A block, loss, or imbalance of body energies? Microbes?)

THE GOAL

What should be the final outcome of treatment according to the client? (Reintegration into the community? Personal insight? Restoration of natural and social harmony? Symptom removal? Improved daily functioning? Relief of psychic tension? Change of attitude?)

How does visiting a western therapist contribute to or impede this desired outcome?

THE TREATMENT

What is the appropriate form of treatment given the cause of illness? (Exorcism? Divination? Isolation? Purification? Confession? Abreaction? Physical methods such as drugs, baths, or shock? Reeducation? Individual therapy?)

What are the appropriate means of taking the client's history?

What are the client's expectations of treatment?

Does the client understand the procedures and believe that they will help?

What are the client's styles of problem solving?

How active is the client in his or her own treatment?

Is the client's basic referent the self, family, or community? What implications does this have regarding treatment approach?

Is it appropriate for the client's social network to be involved in the treatment? In what roles?

What is the nature of follow-up treatment?

THE HEALER

Who is (are) the appropriate healer(s) given the client's concept of illness and its cause? (Shaman, sorcerer, singer, medicine man, herbalist, masseur, religious leader, relative, community members, western medical doctor, psychologist, art therapist? Male or female?)

Does the healer have the knowledge of physical methods of treatment that are publicly endorsed? Can he or she manipulate the spirits?

How did the healer receive this knowledge?

What prerequisite experience must the healer have had?

How active is the healer in the treatment compared to the patient?

Does the healer have extensive knowledge of the individual and the community, and the power and authority to mobilize group support?

THE RELATIONSHIP

What is the relationship between healer, client, and community?

Is community involvement necessary for successful healing?

What happens when cultures intersect in the therapeutic relationship?

What is the western healer's attitude toward the client's culture and concept of illness?

How does class difference between healer and client affect interaction?

How is the traditional healer regarded by the majority culture?

How will the client be regarded by the home community if he or she receives care from an "outsider"?

Does the client go to traditional healers for some aspects of care and to the majority health care system for others?

Has the client tried traditional methods first and come to the western healer only when the symptoms are acute?

Does the client want the western healer to work in conjunction with traditional healers or does he or she prefer to keep the two worlds separate?

What information does the western clinician feel would assist treatment? What are the culturally appropriate times and modes of obtaining this information?

Does it serve the community to maintain certain individuals in marginal roles?

THE ART

What is the relationship between art and life within the client's culture?

What is considered to be the source of creative powers?

What is the purpose of making art? Is art making designated as a specialization to be performed by certain people?

What is the role of the arts in healing?

Are specific uses of symbols in healing understood and endorsed by the client's community?

To what extent are elements of art products and process idiosyncratic, culture specific, and universal?

Is human figure representation acceptable?

Should certain images not be given form?

Are there toxic historical associations with particular shapes, colors, or symbols?

Are there traditionally correct ways to produce a work of art?

What roles do individuality and spontaneity play in artistic production?

How do cultural values about competition and the relationship between individual and community affect the nature of art?

REFERENCES

Abbenante, J. (1982, October). *Art therapy with victims of rape*. Paper presented at the Thirteenth Annual Conference of the American Art Therapy Association, Philadelphia.

Benedek, E. (1984). The silent scream: Countertransference reactions to victims. *American Journal of Social Psychiatry, 4*, 49–52.

Billig, O., & Burton-Bradley, B. (1978). *The painted message*. New York: Halsted.

Bloch, I., & Møller, G. (1986). *Rehabilitation of torture victims: Physiotherapy as a part of the treatment*. Unpublished manuscript.

Boas, F. (1972). *Function of dance in human society*. Brooklyn: Dance Horizons.

Boothby, N. (1983, January). The horror, the hope. *Natural History*, pp. 64–71.

Branfman, F. (1972). *Voices from the Plain of Jars: Life under an air war*. New York: Harper Colophon.

Brett, E., & Mangine, W. (1985). Imagery and combat stress in Vietnam veterans. *Journal of Nervous & Mental Disorders, 173*, 309–311.

Brett, E., & Ostroff, R. (1985). Imagery and posttraumatic stress disorder: An overview. *American Journal of Psychiatry, 142*, 417–424.

Brownlee, A. (1978). *Community, culture and care: A cross-cultural guide for health workers*. St. Louis: Mosby.

Burch, E., & Powell, C. (1980). The psychiatric assessment of a Vietnamese refugee through art. *American Journal of Psychiatry, 137*, 236–237.

Campbell, J. (1973). *Myths to live by*. New York: Bantam.

Carlin, J. (1979). The catastrophically uprooted child: Southeast Asian refugee children. In J.D. Call, J.D. Noshpitz, R.L. Cohen, & I.N. Berlin (Eds.), *Basic handbook for childhood psychiatry* (Vol. 1, pp. 290–300). New York: Basic.

Cohen, F., & Phelps, R. (1985). Incest markers in children's artwork. *Arts in Psychotherapy, 12*, 265–283.

Corbit, I. (1985). *Veteran's nightmares: Trauma, treatment, truce*. Unpublished doctoral dissertation, Union Graduate School.

Costanza, M. (1982). *Living witness: Art in concentration camps and ghettos*. New York: Free Press.

Di Maria, A. (1986, November). *Death in the media age: Children picture the shuttle explosion*. Paper presented at the Seventeenth Annual Conference of the American Art Therapy Association, Los Angeles.

Eliade, M. (1961). *The sacred and the profane*. New York: Harper & Row.

Eliade, M. (1964). *Shamanism: Archaic techniques of ecstasy*. New York: Pantheon.

Fong, K. (1983). *Developmental stages of cultural adjustment: From the perspective of cross-cultural foster parenting of Indochinese refugee unaccompanied minors*. Unpublished manuscript.

Garcia, V. (1975). Case study: Family art evaluation in a Brazilian guidance clinic. *American Journal of Art Therapy, 14*, 132–139.

Gardano, A. (1986). Cultural influence on emotional response to color. *American Journal of Art Therapy, 24*, 119–124.

Garrett, C., & Ireland, M. (1979). A therapeutic art session with rape victims. *American Journal of Art Therapy, 18*, 104–106.

Golub, D. (1984, February). *Portraits of survival*. Paper presented at the New England Regional Arts Training Symposium, Boston.

Golub, D. (1985). Symbolic expression in post-traumatic stress disorder: Vietnam combat veterans in art therapy. *Arts in Psychotherapy, 12*, 285–296.

Grossman, F. (1981). Creativity as a means of coping with anxiety. *The Arts in Psychotherapy, 8*, 185–191.

Harding, R., & Looney, J. (1977). Problems of Southeast Asian children in a refugee camp. *American Journal of Psychiatry, 134*, 407–411.

Hilsum, L. (1986, May). Children of war. *New African*, pp. 18–20.

International Rescue Committee. (1982). *Children of Kampuchea: Their nightmares and dreams*. Thailand: Author.

Japan Broadcasting Corporation (Ed.). (1977). *Unforgettable fire: Pictures drawn by atomic bomb survivors*. New York: Pantheon.

Jung, C. G., von Franz, M. -L., Henderson, J., Jacobi, J., & Jaffé, A. (1964). *Man and his symbols*. Garden City: Doubleday.

Kiev, A. (1972). *Transcultural psychiatry*. New York: Free Press.

Kiev, A. (Ed.). (1974). *Magic, faith and healing*. New York: Free Press.

Kinzie, J. D. (1981). Evaluation and psychotherapy of Indochinese refugee patients. *American Journal of Psychotherapy, 35*, 251–261.

Kinzie, J. D., Fredrickson, R. H., Ben, R., Fleck, J., & Karls, W. (1984). Post-traumatic stress disorder among survivors of Cambodian concentration camps. *American Journal of Psychiatry, 141*, 645–650.

Kinzie, J. D., Tran, K. A., Breckenridge, A., & Bloom, J. (1980). An Indochinese refugee psychiatric clinic: Culturally accepted treatment approaches. *American Journal of Psychiatry, 134*, 407–411.

Kovner, A. (Ed.). (1971). *Childhood under fire: Stories, poems and drawings by children during the Six Days War*. Tel Aviv: Sifriat Poalim.

Landgarten, H. (1981). *Clinical art therapy: A comprehensive guide*. New York: Brunner/Mazel.

Langford, A. (1980). Working with Cambodian refugees: Observations on a family practice ward at Khao I Dang. *Journal of Transpersonal Psychology, 12,* 117–126.

Levinson, P. (1986). Identification of child abuse in the art and play products of the pediatric burn patients. *Art Therapy, 3,* 61–66.

Lieblich, A. (1978). *Tin soldiers on Jerusalem Beach.* New York: Pantheon.

Lifton, R. J. (1969). *Death in life: Survivors of Hiroshima.* New York: Vintage.

Lofgren, D. (1981). Art therapy and cultural difference. *American Journal of Art Therapy, 21,* 25–26.

Malchiodi, C. (1986, March). *Child abuse.* Paper presented at the Joint Conference on the Creative Arts Therapies, Boston.

McConeghey, H. (1986). Archetypal art therapy is cross-cultural art therapy. *Art Therapy, 3,* 111–114.

McHammond, R. (1985, October). *Children of war: The use of art therapy in working with Southeast Asian refugee children.* Paper presented at the Sixteenth Annual Conference of the American Art Therapy Association, New Orleans.

McNiff, S. (1979). From shamanism to art therapy. *Art Psychotherapy, 6,* 155–161.

McNiff, S. (1981). *The arts and psychotherapy.* Springfield, IL: Charles C. Thomas.

McNiff, S. (1984). Cross-cultural psychotherapy and art. *Art Therapy, 1,* 125–131.

McNiff, S. (1986). *Educating the creative arts therapist.* Springfield, IL: Charles C. Thomas.

Moreno, G., & Wadeson, H. (1986). Art therapy for acculturation problems of Hispanic clients. *Art Therapy, 3,* 122–130.

Newman, C. J. (1976). Children of disaster: Clinical observations at Buffalo Creek. *American Journal of Psychiatry, 133,* 306–312.

The Open School. (1986). *Two dogs and freedom: Children of the townships speak out.* Braamfontein, South Africa: Author.

Rahe, R., Looney, J., Ward, H., Tung, T., & Liu, W. (1978). Psychiatric consultation in a Vietnamese refugee camp. *merican Journal of Psychiatry, 135,* 185–190.

Róheim, G. (1970). *Magic and schizophrenia.* Bloomington: Indiana University Press.

Sabatier, P. (1984). Thailand: In defence of traditional healers. *Refugees, 7,* 39.

Salant, E. (1976). Art and play therapy with a Vietnamese child. In R. Shoemaker (Ed.), *Proceedings of the Seventh Annual Conference of the American Art Therapy Association* (pp. 82–85). Baltimore: AATA.

Schwarcz, J. (1982). Guiding children's creative expression in the stress of war. *Stress & Anxiety, 8,* 351–354.

Scurfield, R., & Blank, A. (1985). A guide to obtaining a military history from Viet Nam veterans. In S. Sonnenberg, A. Blank, & J. Talbot (Eds.), *The trauma of war: Stress and recovery in Viet Nam veterans* (pp. 265–291). Washington: American Psychiatric Press.

Silverstein, S. (1984, October). *Intervention following a sniper's attack which traumatized an elementary school.* Paper presented at the Fifteenth Annual Conference of the American Art Therapy Association, Washington, DC.

Silverstein, S., Eth, S., & Arroyo, W. (1986, November). *Effects of psychological trauma on children.* Paper presented at the Seventeenth Annual Conference of the American Art Therapy Association, Los Angeles.

Spring, D. (1980). "Jane": Case study of a rape victim rehabilitated by art therapy. In J. Shorr, G. Sobel, P. Robin, & J. Connella (Eds.), *Imagery: Its many dimensions and applications*. New York: Plenum.

Steinhardt, L. (1986). Art therapy in Israel. *Art Therapy, 3*, 115–121.

Stember, C. (1977). Printmaking with abused children: A first step in art therapy. *American Journal of Art Therapy, 16*, 104–109.

Stember, C. (1980). Art therapy: A new use in the diagnosis and treatment of sexually abused children. In *Sexual abuse of children: Selected readings* (DHHS Publication No. 78-30161, pp. 59–71). Washington, DC: USDHHS.

Terr, L. (1981). "Forbidden games": Post-traumatic child's play. *Journal of the American Academy of Child Psychiatry, 20*, 741–760.

Terr, L. (1983). Play therapy and psychic trauma: A preliminary report. In C. Schaefer & K. O'Connor (Eds.), *Handbook of play therapy* (pp. 308–319). New York: Wiley.

Tobin, J., & Friedman, J. (1983). Spirits, shamans and nightmare death: Survivor stress in a Hmong refugee. *American Journal of Orthopsychiatry, 53*, 439–448.

Torrey, E. F. (1973). *The mind game: Witchdoctors and psychiatrists*. New York: Bantam.

Volavková, H. (Ed.). (1964). *I never saw another butterfly: Children's drawings and poems from Theresienstadt concentration camp, 1942–1944*. New York: McGraw-Hill.

Vornberger, W. (Ed.). (1986). *Fire from the sky: Salvadoran children's drawings*. New York: Writers & Readers.

Williams, C., & Westermeyer, J. (1983). Psychiatric problems among adolescent Southeast Asian refugees. *Journal of Nervous & Mental Disease, 171*, 79–85.

Wilson, J., & Krauss, G. (1980). *Vietnam era stress inventory*. Unpublished manuscript.

Wohl, A., & Kaufman, B. (1985). *Silent screams, hidden cries*. New York: Brunner/Mazel.

Wong-Valle, E. (1981). Art therapy as a tool in the acculturation of the immigrant mental patient. *Pratt Institute Creative Arts Therapy Review, 2*, 46–51.

CHAPTER 2

West Indian Children and Their Families

Art Therapy with New Immigrants

SHIRLEY THRASHER, EVELYN YEE, AND SARAH ZAHNSTECHER

The relatively recent and continuing immigration of hundreds of thousands of West Indians to the United States poses a significant clinical and service delivery challenge to the helping professions. This chapter presents a social service agency's work among West Indian families to prevent child abuse and neglect and placement of children in foster care through integration of art therapy and clinical social work.

West Indian immigrants are those natives from the English-speaking Caribbean, including Jamaica, Barbados, Trinidad, Tobago, Antigua, St. Croix, and other islands extending from the coast of Florida in the north to Venezuela in the south (Brice, 1982). The selection of this population came about because the Catholic Guardian Society's East Brooklyn Prevention Program was mandated to design a program to address the high number of reported incidences of suspected child abuse and neglect and the high number of children entering foster care in a geographical area populated by West Indians in the northeastern United States. The purpose of the program was to enhance family functioning in order to maintain children in the household.

As our program developed, it became clear that this population was not readily responsive to the traditional clinical intervention of talking and that the family unit did not fit the traditional nuclear typology: biological parents with their natural children exclusively. Although in recent professional literature there has been attention to ethnic minorities, a serious gap remains in systematic knowledge of the immigration patterns, characteristic immigrant experiences, and the treatment of West Indians in U.S. institutions. A number of authors, however, have underscored the lack of empirical research on the West Indian immigrant population and the magnitude of unanswered questions regarding the Caribbean populations (Bryce-LaPorte, 1979; Couch, 1979).

The task the agency faced was to develop guidelines even with gaps in knowledge of this target group. A research project of an exploratory descriptive nature followed 30 West Indian families who were in receipt of professional social services at the agency. The data were collected by interviews and a survey questionnaire from the case records. The findings of that study provided the guideposts for the development of the clinical interventions using art therapy discussed in this chapter.

EMERGING FAMILY PROFILE

The West Indian adult usually comes unaccompanied to the United States seeking employment and educational opportunities to make a better life for the family, often leaving children in the homeland to be cared for by grandparents and other relatives. This migration process is an uneven one; it is often the case that many years separate biological parents, spouses, and children. This prolonged separation means that primary caretakers have been other than biological parents, and biological parents have missed significant stages of their children's growth and development. The West Indian family household in the United States tends to be multigenerational and includes extended kin due to this population's commitment to sponsoring other relatives' immigration to the United States.

When the parents and children actually reconstitute in the United States, there seems to be a considerable amount of parent–child conflict in the family interactions. In addition to the adjustment from an agricultural and rural environment to an inner urban city, children and parents must reestablish their own relationships. The parents often respond by using physical punishment. Physical punishment is viewed by West Indians as an appropriate and desirable disciplinary technique. This pattern, however, has caused them to be in conflict with the dominant culture where it may be perceived as too severe, labeled *child abuse,* and brought to the attention of child protective services.

West Indians value self-help and believe in keeping problems within the family with the exception of looking to a religious leader for guidance. Professional counseling for problem resolution is generally not an option to them. This population displays stoicism, formality, and aloofness when relating to professionals and those in authority. This distancing is antithetical to the traditional clinical environment, which values open communication and verbal expression.

West Indians seek help outside of the family, however, if the children are experiencing school problems. This strong interest in education is reflected in the adults' pursuit of educational training in addition to full-time employment; coupled with their interest in education is an attention to upward mobility and property ownership. Owning one's own home confers status to an Islander's identity when he or she is transplanted in the new country. Working two and three jobs, scrimping and saving, borrowing from loan sharks when the banks refuse credit, and economizing are often seen in the pursuit of purchasing a house. Dual jobs may create problems for West

Indian parents, however, if their attendance is required at schools or social service agencies.

PRESENTING PROBLEMS OF TARGET POPULATION

Schools are the major source of family referral to the agency. The main problem areas identified by the family are conflicts in the parent–child relationship in the home and in the school. More specifically, the problems articulated by the parents about their children in the home are failure to obey curfew, disrespectful and rebellious attitudes in communication patterns with parents, fighting, stealing, and failure to perform household chores. In the educational setting the problems identified by the parents about their children are truancy, suspensions, poor educational achievement, inappropriate class placement, fighting with peers, and verbal abuse of school personnel. The children have identified sources of conflict in the home and school setting through complaints of being physically punished by their parents, rigidity of curfew and other rules of the household, lack of communication, failing grades, negative labeling because of special education placement, and feelings of discrimination due to Caribbean accent.

AGENCY FUNCTION

The agency is voluntary, and its purpose is to prevent child abuse and neglect through professional services that enhance family functioning. The families are not charged with abuse and neglect so the issue is not one of child protection, but there are underlying assumptions that the family dynamics and parent child interactions provide the potential for abuse and neglect in the absence of services.

To be eligible for agency services there must be present in the household at least one child who is 18 or under at risk of removal because of deterioration of parental or child functioning. The goal is to provide those services that will strengthen the family unit and maintain children in the household.

The model used by this agency was one in which the art therapist provided the art interventions and the clinical social work in the delivery of services to its West Indian clients using the cultural characteristics derived from a research study of the population.

CASE EXAMPLES

The following examples illustrate the way in which art therapy addresses the unique problems of the relocated and often separated West Indian families. To our knowledge, the only other report of art therapy with this population is the work of Moreno and Wadeson (1986), focusing on acculturation problems of female Hispanic immigrants with chronic emotional difficulties.

LOST HOMELAND

Mr. and Mrs. Ross came to the United States from one of the Caribbean islands 3 years ago with their three children, Chris, Monica, and Lisa, ages 8, 13, and 14, respectively. Two other children were left in the homeland to join the family at a later date.

Mrs. Ross brought Chris, now 11, into the agency at the suggestion of the school because of his disruptive behavior in the school environment including fighting with peers and verbally abusing school personnel. She also stated he was disrespectful at home, failing to follow the household rules and talking back to his parents. Mrs. Ross expressed a concern that her involvement with a social agency would jeopardize the immigration of her other children. She acknowledged that she was totally unfamiliar with the counseling process but had tried to alleviate the problem through talking, restrictive curfew, and physical punishment but to no avail and therefore was willing to consider other alternatives. She said she was also feeling unable to manage many of her daily responsibilities including full-time work and the care of her 2-year-old.

During Chris's first session the art therapist introduced drawing. Chris said that he hated art. Nevertheless, he did become intrigued with the therapist's use of Winnicott's Squiggle Game in which the therapist and the client take turns in making a squiggle or line on the paper and then develop it further (Winnicott, 1971).

In the next session Chris indicated that he did not feel his parents cared about him and he wanted to be placed in foster care. The therapist observed Chris's upset emotional state as he was talking, and she gave him a piece of clay and suggested that he manipulate it with his hands for relaxation as he talked. When the therapist said she would like to call Mrs. Ross in to discuss the situation, Chris said that his mother was working and would not have the time to come because she was more concerned with working. As he talked the clay began to take shape, and the therapist directed his attention to it by asking about its formation. Chris said it was a volcano that was ready to explode. The therapist empathized with the strong emotions evoked through the clay work and made a contract with Chris for him to try to negotiate regular appointments at the agency for his mother before taking any action on his request for placement.

When the therapist called Mrs. Ross, she said that Chris had come home and told her of his request for placement. She was upset and said she had not realized how lonely and neglected Chris felt, and she was eager to have the therapist intervene in whatever way necessary to help the family and Chris. Special arrangements were made so that Mrs. Ross could have regular appointments at the agency without jeopardizing her employment.

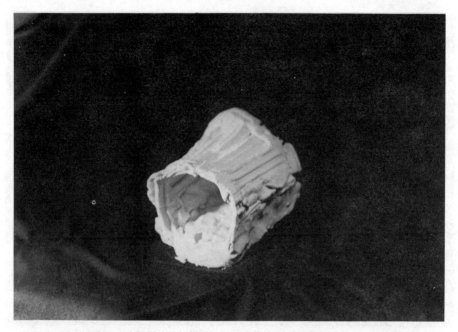

Figure 2.1. "Covered Bridge," bridging homeland and the United States, by Chris.

On Chris's arrival at the next session the therapist gave him the volcano, saying he might want to continue working on it as they talked about his home and school situation. Chris took the volcano and mashed it flat. The therapist began to explore with him his process of immigration and the differences between his homeland and his new environment. From each side of the flat clay emerged two arcs at each end. He began putting strips of clay across each end that were very sturdy and tight. On inquiry he said it was a covered bridge (Fig. 2.1). In this session Chris was able to say that he missed his homeland and his many friends there. He said he missed the wide-open spaces, the trees, greenery, and waterfalls. At the end of the session he said he was glad that his mother was coming to the agency. The covered bridge and arcs seemed to be the beginning of engagement and trust between Chris and the therapist.

In the next session, although the therapist produced Chris's covered bridge thinking he might want to work on it, Chris only looked at it and asked the therapist for additional clay. He began making triangles. The therapist inquired whether he had worked with clay before. Chris said that in his homeland at the bottom of the waterfalls was clay he had played and worked with over and over again, creating objects and figures. He put strips of clay over the triangles and said the finished product was tracks. He then selected gray clay and constructed two figures walking across the tracks. The sides of the tracks were completed to resemble a bridge (Fig. 2.2). Chris said he and his

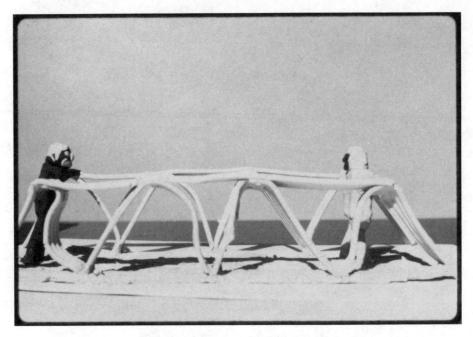

Figure 2.2. "Friends on a Bridge," by Chris.

friend were walking across the bridge. This symbolic representation of his feelings and thoughts was used to continue exploration of his lost homeland and his attempt to bridge the gap between the old and the new, the separation from friends and family, and his attempts to adjust to a new and strange city.

Chris has become more task oriented in his sessions, and his aggressive behavior has abated in school. His anger and impulsive behavior have continued to be worked through in his working with clay as he tries to bridge his two worlds. He is still mourning the loss of his friends. Structured recreation for him in his new environment has been proposed.

SEPARATION OF FAMILY

Mrs. Frank, a 41-year-old woman from one of the Caribbean islands, came alone to New York 4 years ago. She secured housing and employment and sent for her five children, ranging in ages from 8 to 21 after a 2½-year separation. Mr. Frank was still living in the Islands and employed there. Leon, their 13-year-old, was referred by the school because of his excessive truancy and lack of communication in the school setting. Mrs. Frank reported that she escorted him to the classroom every day but at some point during the day he would leave. Most recently he was found by the police during school hours on the subway tracks. She felt she had tried everything, in-

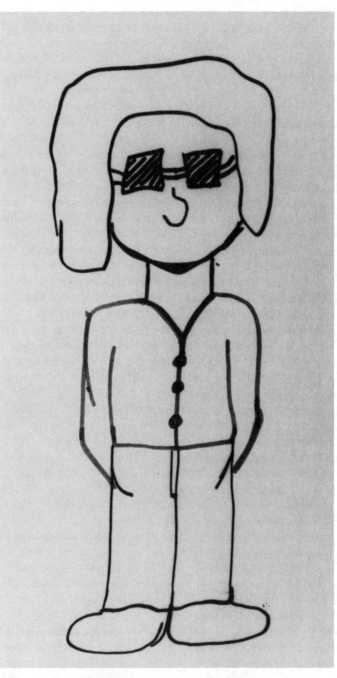

Figure 2.3. ''A Portrait,'' by Leon.

cluding physical punishment, but with no success. Leon was in the process of being evaluated for a special education placement by the committee on the handicapped.

The school reported that Leon was virtually nonverbal in the classroom, answering with a yes or no to questions and only after long delays. He was small for his age in the junior high school setting and had no friends.

To begin work with Leon, the therapist provided him with drawing material and suggested that he might want to draw himself so that she could get to know him and understand him. In his first picture Leon used colored markers to draw a boy with dark sunglasses, hair, a nose, but no mouth (Fig. 2.3). The boy's hands are either in back of him or in his pockets. The therapist used this drawing to begin to establish a relationship with Leon by focusing on the elements of the drawing and their reflection of Leon and his situation, a young boy who was having a difficult time attending school regularly and verbalizing those issues. The therapist told Leon that they would find a means of communicating with each other through the art materials. Leon smiled during these first mostly nonverbal sessions; if the therapist asked him a direct question, he would answer in one word or shake his head. He was successful in his exploration of the art materials and in his willingness to draw several pictures during each session.

In the beginning sessions Leon was still not attending school regularly, and the therapist proposed to Mrs. Frank that she abandon the practice of accompanying him to his classroom since she had indication from Leon that he was not happy with that arrangement. Although Mrs. Frank was reluctant to agree she was able to face the reality that it had proved ineffective. This action appeared to create a bond of trust between Leon and the therapist.

Leon was asked to draw his school (Fig. 2.4). The drawing was faint and bleak. The building has a lot of windows with one large door and one small door. Leon talked a little about a boy who attended the school. He said that the boy liked school and had two friends in school with whom he played. Since this was different from Leon's actual situation, the therapist empathized with Leon's wishes to be this boy. Leon was able to say that there was no play area in the school and there were too many people.

Leon missed his father a great deal. Mrs. Frank discussed the possibility with the therapist of sending him back to his father if his situation in school did not improve. She acknowledged her awareness of how much he missed his father and their farm, which had lots of space and animals. His longing for his father was expressed in his drawings. In one drawing Leon portrayed his father mowing a lawn, fixing flowers, and painting a wall.

Leon was still attending school only about once a week. Mrs. Frank was still concerned but manifested less anxiety about his lack of attendance at school. Arrangements were made for the therapist to make home visits on a regular basis in addition to the office sessions. On the first home visit the therapist discovered that Leon had constructed a model from index cards. It was truly a creative piece of art, and Leon was given support and rec-

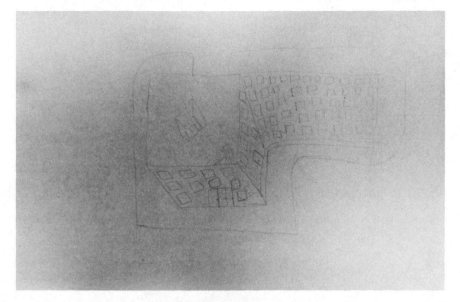

Figure 2.4. "The School," by Leon.

ognition for his project. It became evident that Leon was developing his creative talents when he was home, and he was encouraged to continue this endeavor by the therapist. The evaluation by the committee on the handicapped indicated that Leon was below his reading level but above average in abstract and reasoning skill. A small special education class was recommended because of his lack of socialization and verbal skills. Mrs. Frank began slowly to be able to appreciate Leon and give him support for his creative artwork at home and at the agency.

Leon appeared to enjoy expressing his feelings and thoughts in his artwork and having the therapist confirm and validate them. He began smiling and talking more as well. The therapist began making portraits of Leon as he worked, which was the beginning of their work together on his self-image and self-concept. They would discuss what he saw in what the therapist was able to capture. His feeling of importance soared as the therapist talked to him about her attempts to reflect his subtle moods and expressions as he worked in the sessions with the art materials. Time was devoted in talking about the changes in the portraits over the course of the treatment.

Leon was moved to a smaller class in a different school, and his attendance began to improve. Nevertheless, his longing for his homeland continued to be a pervasive theme in his artwork. After a year of treatment Leon did a drawing of the Islands that was full of greenery, birds, trees, and fruit with himself in the picture. The details were much richer than some of his earlier work of his homeland.

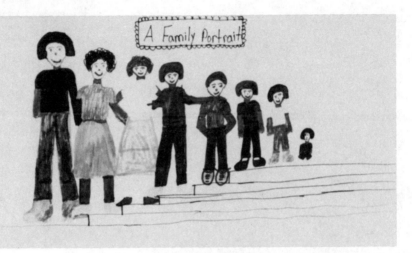

Figure 2.5. Leon's Family Portrait.

During the 1½ years of treatment Leon went to visit his father once and Mr. Frank came to visit the family once. Over this period the family talked about relocating and began to explore that possibility. Leon was asked to draw a picture of his family (Fig. 2.5). The colors he chose were bright. The older members of the family are joined in hands but separated from the younger members of the family. The drawing is a full view of the family with all the features intact. Leon included both parents, which was a reflection of his desire to have both parents together as a complete family unit. His earlier drawings of the family had excluded his father. Mr. and Mrs. Frank secured employment in a small community in a suburb of a city on the northeast coast of the United States and the family moved. Leon could now have his family together again. Before the move, the therapist arranged a trip in which she took the entire family for a last view of the city. Termination sessions focused on Leon's progress and development from an isolated and nonverbal hidden young man to a creative and emerging person, with strong feelings about his family and his inner life, as exemplified in his artwork and creative projects.

AFTER THE FAMILY IS RECONCILED

Mrs. Bell, a 38-year-old female, came alone to the United States leaving four children in the Caribbean. It took 9 years for her to reconstitute the family, bringing one child at a time during that period. The household consists of six children, ages 4 to 20. The last two children, ages 4 and 6, were born in the United States. Mr. Bell is the father of the last two children. The identified client is Lee, a 14-year-old, who was the last of the four children to arrive in this country and the fourth child of Mrs. Bell. Lee had lived with his maternal grandmother in the Caribbean from 3 to 12, until his arrival in the United States. Lee was referred to the agency by the local school because of his third suspension for fighting. Both Mr. and Mrs. Bell were employed because they were eager to buy a house to improve the family's crowded living quarters.

Mrs. Bell was feeling overwhelmed and distressed on arrival at the agency because of the time that had been required for recent school visits, which was jeopardizing her job as a hotel housekeeper. She requested the intervention of the therapist in the school situation. Lee had been in special education for a year but there had been little improvement in his academic performance. His mother said she felt puzzled by Lee's aggressive behavior because he really did not know how to defend himself. Because he would be taken advantage of, she did not trust him to go out with friends. She had become more strict and rigid and kept him close to home because of his school problems. She said the long separation of 9 years had made them strangers.

In the initial session Lee said that he missed his grandparents very much after living with them for so many years. He said that he did fight but only to impress girls and make friends.

Treatment began by asking Lee to draw a picture of home every week and construct a book of his past environment in the Caribbean, which he missed. He drew rural scenes of his grandparents' farm where he cooked and slept outdoors a great deal. He expressed vividly his love of nature in these illustrations. His book of the Caribbean and subsequent discussions of his homeland provided an entry into his present family life. He spoke of how hard it was for him to adjust to New York even though he loved being with his mother. He began to express animosity toward his younger siblings, whom he did not know since they had been born in this country and did not share his father. He also resented the attention the younger siblings received from his mother. When asked to draw his present family, Lee depicted his mother, father, and himself on a picnic together, revealing his desire for an intact family in which he is the only child (Fig. 2.6). This is not an intimate joyous scene but a rather isolated one in which Lee is jumping off a diving board into the proverbial waters of the unconscious, as his subsequent behavior seems to reveal.

Lee was suspended from school a fourth time for carrying a butcher knife to school. Mrs. Bell was distraught. Intensive and active counseling was necessary to prevent Mrs. Bell from using physical punishment as discipline. The therapist attended the suspension hearing with Mrs. Bell and obtained agreement that the school reconsider educational placement for him after psychological testing by the agency. The testing revealed a tremendous sense of isolation, depression, and repressed rage at the mother. The psychologist hypothesized that because of Lee's dependency on his mother, he was afraid that the expression of his anger would destroy her. Some of the hostility was manifested in school fighting, which resulted in negative reactions to

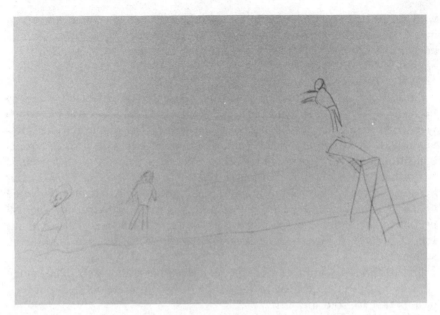

Figure 2.6. Lee's "Family Picnic," lacking his siblings.

Lee, adding to his isolation and depression. Lee said he brought the knife to school in order to be sent back to his grandmother's in the Islands.

During this difficult time the therapist asked Lee to draw the animal he would most like to be. He drew a white dove looking down on the city from a high safe tree. He then drew a frog in a swamp on the other side of the page and described it as a "filthy disgusting thing." He said this is the way people really see him. He said that the frog could stop wallowing in the mud and become the dove if it really tried. As Lee continued the artwork he gained some mastery over using it to help him accept some of his deep feelings. He eventually expressed a desire to become task oriented, and the therapist helped secure a tutoring program that facilitated Lee's placement in the vocational school he wanted. His behavior and performance improved in the new school setting.

Lee was never able to become directly angry with his mother. Nevertheless, Mrs. Bell gained some insight into Lee's longing for his homeland and grandmother who had been his primary caretaker during his early childhood. The therapist helped Lee to secure a summer job, and he sent the first five dollars of his earnings to his grandmother and told her proudly to have a good meal. The family was finally able to move into their own home. Ongoing home visits with the mother, who was too frightened to come to the office, focused around the quality of her interactions with Lee. This eventually led to a revelation of her difficult and abused childhood. This process resulted in a new openness between mother and son.

SEXUAL ABUSE IN THE FAMILY

Mrs. Hall, a 33-year-old divorcee of Caribbean descent, was referred to the agency by the guidance counselor of the local school for professional counseling for 10-year-old Linda. Linda was disruptive in class, provoked the other children, and talked inappropriately in the classroom. Linda had also reported during a group discussion in school that she had been fondled in her genital area by her 76-year-old grandfather. The school had confronted Mrs. Hall, who had denied the incident but followed the directions of the school officials to bring Linda to the agency.

On arrival, Mrs. Hall reported that she was reluctant to believe the daughter's story of sexual molestation by her grandfather. Nevertheless, her respect for the authority of the school was the impetus for her coming to the agency. She said her father had come from the Caribbean alone to seek employment for a better life for the family leaving the children and spouse in the homeland 15 years earlier. She is the seventh child of nine siblings who were brought to the United States two at a time until the entire family arrived. She was 13 years old when she arrived in this country. Her biological mother died when she was 1 year old and her father married her aunt (the mother's sister) immediately.

The family all lived in one household until Mrs. Hall married Mr. Hall, whom she knew from the Islands. They had two children by this union, 10-year-old Linda, the identified client, and 8-year-old Peter. Mr. and Mrs. Hall had been separated and divorced for 3 years and he lived in another country.

Mrs. Hall lived apart from her parents with the two children and two of her brothers in one household. She was employed full-time as a housekeeper in a hospital and worked evenings. The children went to the home of her sisters after school every day. Living in the home of the grandparents were four other siblings of Mrs. Hall, two brothers and two sisters, and their children. Mrs. Hall described having a close relationship with her family and siblings. She visited her parents twice a month.

Mrs. Hall expressed annoyance that Linda had told the school about family matters. It is a characteristic of this population that intimate matters be kept within the family. She said her mother and siblings would be watching the grandfather to see whether there were any further incidents, although she still doubted the validity of the story. She said Linda was old enough to say "no" if she was approached and it was time now to put the incident in the past and forget it.

Mrs. Hall was asked to draw her family during this initial session of background and history taking. She chose to draw a house, a tree, and a person (Fig. 2.7).

Although Mrs. Hall described a large, close-knit family, her symbols portrayed a separateness and aloneness possibly even to the exclusion of her own two children. Keeping conflict within the home and maintaining privacy is a cultural phenomenon. Her manner was distancing toward the

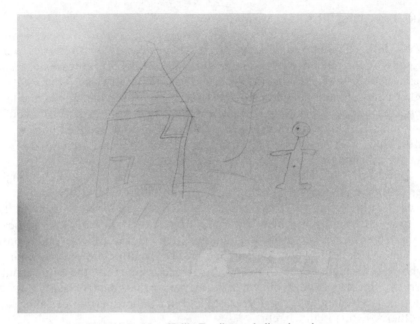

Figure 2.7. Mrs. Hall's Family, excluding the others.

therapist, and the nonverbal communication depicted by her drawing illustrated loneliness and an emotionally impoverished woman.

Linda, on the other hand, was more open to verbal expression and art therapy. In the initial session, when she was asked to draw her family, she chose to draw her extended family, which included three aunts and two uncles and a cousin. She spent a lot of time with extended family so perhaps she felt safer in depicting all of them. During the first session she was able to talk tentatively about the sexual incident with the grandfather and said it had occurred on many occasions in the past although it had stopped.

During the second session Linda was in the waiting room with stuffed animals all around her that she had gathered from the shelves and floor of the playroom. During this visit she inquired about the family drawing of the previous session. The therapist suggested a theme in which she would draw her most favorite and least favorite person. She drew one of her aunts as her most favorite person and her grandfather as her least favorite person. She drew two other people and said an uncle was a favorite because he paid her $1 for giving him a back massage. She then reversed roles with the therapist and instructed the therapist to draw and asked if the therapist had had an experience like Linda's with her grandfather. This identification with the therapist was the beginning of their working alliance together.

After several sessions Linda was asked to draw people that she wanted to say no to (Fig. 2.8). She had said during previous sessions that it was difficult for her to say no because she wanted to have friends and be liked. The first is labeled *brother* though it looks more like her mother. The second

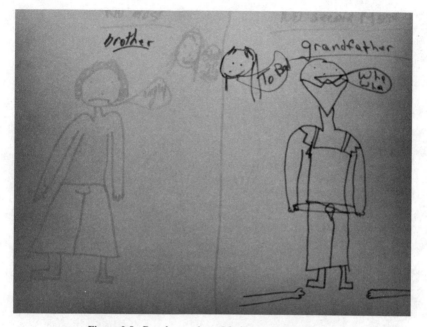

Figure 2.8. People to whom Linda wanted to say no.

is her grandfather. She cut his arms off at the shoulders and they fell to the ground. In this way she was able to protect herself from his touch. At first she cut only one arm off and gave a support to the other arm that crossed out the genital area. She said that she used to love her grandfather.

Play, art therapy, and verbal expression were combined, each facilitating the other, in the process of meeting the needs of this client. Anger was the most forbidden feeling. Linda was able to use the punching bag gingerly only after the therapist, understanding her need to express anger, facilitated this process by demonstration. In one session she played a game in which she killed her brother and then immediately changed it to her mother, killing her by mistake.

In an interactive drawing of pictures and storytelling between the therapist and Linda, much of Linda's external and internal world emerged (Fig. 2.9). The therapist began by drawing a spiral with a red knot in the middle to depict Linda's internal state on entering this session. As the story and pictures progressed, Linda related a story of a car crashing and catching fire in which the mother, father, and baby were able to escape. According to Linda, the mother and father blamed each other for the crash. Linda said they needed a new car. The therapist drew the family a new car but Linda crashed the new car and drew money to save the family by using it to buy a new house. She said both parents and baby were in the house, perhaps expressing a desire once again to live with father, perhaps communicating her abandonment issues once more.

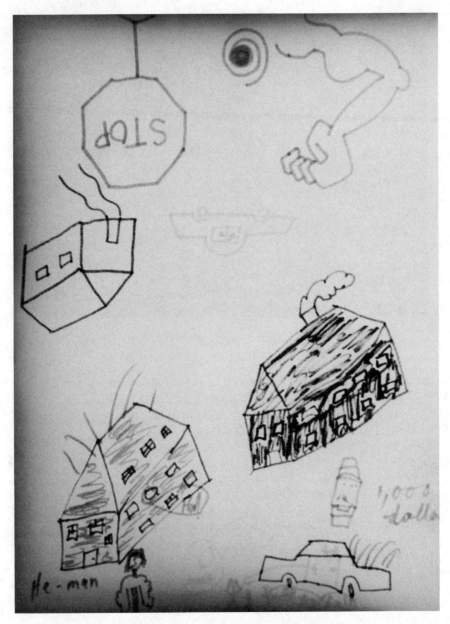

Figure 2.9. "Repairing the Family," by Linda and the therapist.

In this culture adults must be treated with great respect, although it is permissible to express anger toward siblings. Linda may never be able to verbalize her angry feelings toward her mother but she began to work them through in her drawings. Linda's behavior improved dramatically in school, and she became more task oriented in her work. Mrs. Hall took responsibility for supervising Linda differently and reduced visits to the grandfather's home.

CONCLUSION

Art therapy has proved to be a useful intervention in the social services provided for West Indian immigrant families. The unique problems of separation from homeland, culture, friends, and often close family members are readily addressed through the more imagistic and less verbal activity of art therapy.

The practice of integrating art therapy and clinical social work in a functional social service agency has proven effective in working with these families to prevent child abuse and neglect and placement of children in foster care. This model illuminates the need for attention to the cultural specificities of ethnic minorities if they are to become full participants in this society. Integrating art therapy with social work is likely to be applicable to other ethnic minorities who face problems similar to the West Indian families in this program.

REFERENCES

Brice, J. (1982). West Indian families. In M. McGoldrick, J.K. Pearce, & J. Giordano (Eds.), *Ethnicity and family therapy*. New York: Guilford.

Bryce-LaPorte, R.S. (1979). A challenge to immigration: Implications for the United States and the international community. In R.S. Bryce-LaPorte, D. Mortimer, & S. Couch (Eds.), *Sourcebook on the new immigration*. Washington, DC: Research Institute on Immigration and Ethnic Studies, Smithsonian Institute.

Couch, S. (1979). Where do we go from here? In R.S. Bryce-LaPorte, D. Mortimer, & S. Couch (Eds.), *Sourcebook on the new immigration*. Washington, DC: Research Institute on Immigration and Ethnic Studies, Smithsonian Institute.

Moreno, G., & Wadeson, H. (1986). Art therapy for acculturation problems of Hispanic clients. *Art Therapy, 3,* 122–130.

Winnicott, D.W. (1971). *Therapeutic consultation in child psychiatry*. New York: Basic.

CHAPTER 3

Art Therapy for Bereaved Children

GRACE C. ZAMBELLI, ELIZABETH JOHNS CLARK, AND MARGE HEEGAARD

Experiencing a significant loss at an early age creates intense confusion and pain; intervention is required to prevent long-term psychological problems. Art therapy is an effective means of identifying misconceptions and issues of conflict, thereby promoting fuller expression for feelings of grief. Art therapy is therefore emerging as a viable new intervention for working with bereaved children.

Few reports of programs established for this purpose have appeared in the literature, despite the recognition of the need for such services to be made widely available. This chapter presents child bereavement programs developed at a hospice and an elementary school. Prior to describing the actual work of these programs, a discussion of bereavement and the special problems and needs of bereaved children is presented to place the goals of art therapy intervention in the larger context of the child's grieving process and maturational development.

ART THERAPY AND GRIEF

The tenets of art therapy involve humanism, creativity, reconciling emotional conflicts, fostering self-awareness, and personal growth (American Art Therapy Association, 1977). These beliefs and goals are consistent with bereavement counseling in general and with the hospice philosophy specifically, which is essentially humanistic. Hospice care includes medical and psychosocial intervention, which helps terminally ill patients and their families live their lives to the fullest. Art therapy and other creative, humanistic intervention strategies are becoming popular methods for working with the life-threatened patient and for working with the family members of patients who die—particularly bereaved children.

Editor's Note: The authors of this chapter initially wrote two separate chapters. The editors have combined them, so the work reported is a composite of bereavement art therapy programs at The Hospice, Inc., in Montclair, New Jersey (Zambelli & Clark), and a Minneapolis, Minnesota, elementary school (Heegaard).

Professionals such as Kübler-Ross (1983) and the Simontons and Creighton (1978) have done much to popularize nonverbal communication techniques, such as drawing and visualization, to deal with the emotional stress arising from catastrophic illness and grief. In fact, the number of workshops and articles about creative, nontraditional psychosocial intervention strategies has steadily risen at hospice conferences and in the hospice literature since the early 1970s. Professionals outside the field of art therapy are recognizing the value of using nonverbal forms of therapy in their work with the dying and bereaved.

The art therapy literature also shows an increasing number of articles about hospice and bereavement counseling within the past 8 years. The use of a short-term art therapy group for children was first described in the literature by Cocuzza-Zambelli in 1981. Simon (1981) reports how art therapy stimulates the conscious and unconscious expression of the mourning·process in adult and child patients. Plank and Plank (1978) trace children's reactions to death in art and autobiographies. Miller (1984) describes how art therapy enables the elderly and terminally ill to face their feelings about death. Segal (1984) finds creative arts therapy to be an effective method for cutting through communication barriers erected by grieving children. Junge (1985) discusses the use of art therapy in helping a family cope with the death of one of its members.

It is vital for an art therapist to gain a strong foundation in death education and an understanding of the grief process to work effectively with a grieving child. Children want answers to their questions about loss and grief. Further, it is often difficult to distinguish normal grief from pathology.

The Grief Process

The grief process is sometimes confused with the stages of dying that have been defined by Elizabeth Kübler-Ross (1969) as: (1) denial, (2) rage and anger, (3) bargaining, (4) despair and depression, and (5) acceptance. Bereaved persons whose loved ones' deaths were anticipated may have worked through some of these stages prior to the death. They will still need to work through the grief process, but it may begin later and have some additional differences.

The grief process begins with *protest* and moves into the second phase, which can be described as *despair*. The last phase is a time of *reorganization* (Bowlby, 1980), but the entire process is a normal movement back and forth from one phase to another and lasts for an indefinite length of time. Grief creates tasks of mourning, and for many this may take 2 years to complete (Worden, 1982). Some complete their grief much sooner, some never. It is a confusing time for both adults and children.

Childhood Bereavement

Five percent of children in the United States (about 1.5 million) lose one or both parents by age 15, and this proportion is substantially higher in lower socioeconomic groups (Krupnick, 1984). It is unclear how the death of a parent impacts on the subsequent emotional, cognitive, and physical development of a child. However, the literature clearly suggests that children who have experienced the death of a parent are more at risk for psychiatric, medical, and behavioral consequences than children who have not experienced such a loss (Arthur & Kemme, 1964; Black, 1974; Kaffman & Elizur, 1983; Kliman, 1980; Rutter, 1966).

Despite the prevalence and significant implications of childhood bereavement, little has been written about preventive strategies that may positively facilitate adaptation to parental loss. Krupnick (1984) notes that there is a paucity of scientific evidence regarding the effectiveness of intervention prior to, or subsequent to, bereavement during childhood. There seems to be a general consensus in the literature that both long-term and short-term stress are common, and that professional mental health intervention may be useful, especially when troublesome behavior appears (Berlinski & Biller, 1982; Kliman, 1980; Krupnick, 1984).

The signs and symptoms of childhood grief are less obvious and of shorter duration than those of adult grief. This is due to the child's incomplete emotional and cognitive development (Furman, 1974; Nagara, 1981; Schowalter, 1975). There is a tendency to use the most typical adult model of bereavement, the stage theory model of adult bereavement, to explain childhood grief reactions. This consists of testing and accepting the reality of the loss; remembering and decathecting memories of the lost object; and cultivating substitute object relationships (Kliman, 1968). This can lead to much confusion and misunderstanding about the grieving process of children (Krupnick, 1984). While sharing some similarities with adult grief, children's reactions to death differ both in their specific manifestations and in their duration. Because the continuing maturation of cognitive and emotional processes interferes with the child's ability to resolve loss at certain ages, the concept of "stages" does not adequately describe the bereavement process in children.

Johnson and Rosenblatt (1981) distinguish between grief that is due to maturation and incomplete grief. When either is present in a child who has lost a parent, there are important implications for the duration of the grief and for the type of psychotherapeutic intervention required. Maturational grief typically requires supportive counseling and is expected for those who have lost a significant other, especially when the death occurred in the early part of an older child's life. Incomplete grief, on the other hand, usually necessitates in-depth therapeutic intervention, and is associated with long-standing pathological problems that have resulted in response to the death.

Because of the powerful influences of maturation, there is controversy in the literature about whether children have the developmental prerequisites for complete mourning and about the likelihood of achieving a healthy outcome if bereavement occurs before that time (Krupnick, 1984; Palumbo, 1981). It is agreed that children prior to the age of 3 or 4 are unable to achieve complete mourning, and that by adolescence, most children can mourn. Despite the controversy, there is no doubt that children can, and do, react to loss at any age.

The most common initial reactions to parental death include sadness, anger, fear, appetite and sleep disturbances, withdrawal, concentration difficulties, dependency, regression, restlessness, and learning difficulties (Worden, 1982). These symptoms vary according to the age at which the child is bereaved. Thus when assessing children's grief, it is important to have a working knowledge of specific age group reactions.

The major differences between adult and childhood grief are the time frame and overt processes of grieving (Johnson & Rosenblatt, 1981). In general, due to the developmental differences in cognitive abilities and personality structures, children are more likely to use primitive defenses (i.e., denial and regression) than adults when coping with death. The use of denial may make it appear that the child actually has resolved the death since no obvious signs of grief will be present. Children's regressive behavior also may be associated with other causes. Consequently, children are at greater psychological risk than adults because their grief is less overt and can occur months or even years after the death (Krupnick, 1984).

Due to these difficulties, there is a need for more death education at all levels for children and adolescents. Understanding the concepts of loss and feelings could be a natural part of mental and physical hygiene taught at the appropriate cognitive level. Learning to cope with home/school separation or early pet loss would be the natural foundation for developing patterns to cope with future significant losses. Since it is not being taught to most children, art therapists need to be able to include death education as part of grief intervention.

Death Education for Children

Children want to know about death. They want to know why someone dies, what happens after someone dies, where the dead go, and whether the spirit continues to exist after the body dies. The child's personality, life experience, and family and social resources available for learning about death all influence a child's understanding. Self-concept influences a child's ability to cope with death.

Children need to know that death is permanent and not reversible and that physical function stops with death. They need to know that death is universal and inevitable. Persons working with grieving children must be aware of the effect of assigning their own attitude to children in the areas of death and grieving. Healthy death education needs to come from someone open and honest, with good communication skills at the child's level, and at an appropriate time, preferably before the crisis. Children want and *need* to know physical circumstances concerning death. They want to know about caskets, funerals, and cemeteries. Terms like *die* and *dead* need to be used instead of vague terms like *pass away* and *expire*, which just create confusion and anxiety. Children do not need to equate death with sleep, aging, or hospitals. They need to know the difference between common minor illnesses and the more serious ones, so they will not fear physical symptoms. Religious beliefs can be shared if they are presented as personal beliefs and care is taken not to confuse the child. An adult's concept of afterlife may be quite different from what a child envisions. Telling a child that God has taken a person can cause resentment against God or a conflict in a child's mind about being loved by God.

Children's Emotional Needs

The death of a young child's parent is always untimely, whether violent or due to disease. The death of a parent usually means overwhelming changes creating excessive upheaval and anxiety. At all ages, a person's ability to mourn generally depends on the assurance that needs will be met and other relationships will continue. The younger the child, the more he or she will rely on someone else to fulfill needs. Wolfenstein (1966) points out that the parent withdrawn in grief is able to provide little support so the child often feels and acts as though both parents are lost. A child's ability to mourn is helped when the surviving adult has the ability to mourn and accepts and supports the child's reaction. Prelatency children especially have difficulty in this area. Too often, the family tries to hide true feelings from a younger child.

Bowlby (1960) points out that the stages of separation for children are similar to the process for adults with the exception that a successful completion of the process of mourning for the child entails a new attachment to a new adult parental figure. It is important for a child younger than adolescence to find a new parental figure to invest with love for healthy development, whether this be a relative or a stepparent. Yet stepparent relationships may interfere with the unresolved aspects of mourning, and loyalty conflicts may create further emotional difficulties.

It is likely that bright, emotionally mature, healthy adolescents can deal with thoughts of death better than poor achievers. For adolescents, death fears are closely related to other conflicts, and they may not admit to themselves the anger and violent feeling they have toward parents, schools, or authority so they may externalize their feelings. The death of a parent may be seen as abandonment and cause feelings of self-blame and poor self-esteem.

The Committee on Healthy Consequences of the Stress of Bereaved for the Institute of Medicine (Osterweis, Solomon, & Green, 1984) reports that controversies still surround the question of whether children and adolescents are capable of mourning the loss of a parent until they have worked through the natural adolescent parental separation process. Until adolescence, children have not developed formal operational thinking, physiological maturation, and the ability to separate from their parents into their own identity (Wolfenstein 1966). The separation process that occurs with adolescence may serve as the pattern for future separation. Children often seem to understand what death is, but have difficulty mourning.

Bereaved children need to discuss their uncertainties with an understanding adult, but family members are often unable to be supportive because of their own grief. Bereaved children need to feel secure, loved, and understood. They need to be reassured with calmness and confidence in order to grow through the painful experience and become adults strong enough to meet future life crises. They will then be less likely to develop unhealthy defenses to avoid difficult feelings.

Children's Response to a Significant Death

Silence or evasion teaches children that death is a taboo subject. Children are capable of talking about death, and seem to want to. They need to talk and are pleased by the attention of an understanding adult.

Children show their feelings and grief more in behavior than in words. There may be anger manifested by breaking things. The acting-out child may be feeling a great fear of abandonment, especially if he or she comes home to an empty house. Silly, noisy, boisterous behavior may be an attempt at reassurance regarding fears about the remaining adult.

When a child's parent dies, the child's most immediate concern is of how his or her needs will be met. It is common to see a child survivor of a parent's death become compulsively self-reliant or very narcissistic. This can lead to relationship problems as an adult. There may be anxiety relating to the cause of death. Bowlby (1960) says children often mistakenly blame themselves or the surviving parent for having caused or contributed to a parent's death because seldom are they given a clear explanation of the cause. The younger the child, the greater the difficulty in appropriate differentiation from the dead parent. Circumstances of death, effect of developmental concerns, and support received influence this differentiation.

The death of a sibling is another traumatic experience, and can promote guilt in the surviving children because of sibling rivalry and death wishes, or survival guilt (Klein, 1982). They may "feel helpless, or a burden for the sad parents, and perhaps harbor resentment over the attention received by the dying sibling. They may feel guilty about benefits gained from the death (such as room or toys) and worry about inadequate feelings of grief. They may feel the need to be a substitute for the child who died. To preserve their own identity, some rebel to become as different as possible from the dead child.

Factors such as intensity and duration are usually used to differentiate normal from pathological response. Signals of a need for help include: persistent anxieties of further loss; fear of or desire to die; persistent blame and guilt; pattern of overactivity with aggressive and destructive outbursts; compulsive caregiving and self-reliance; euphoria with depersonalization and identification symptoms; and accident proneness (Bowlby 1980).

Raphael (1983) categorizes destructive behavior as: suppressed or inhibited bereavement responses; distorted grief or mourning; and chronic grief, possibly manifested by acting out.

Kliman (1968) adds to this list: inability to speak of the deceased; exaggerated clinging; expressions of only positive or negative feelings about the deceased; strong resistance to forming new attachments; prolonged dysfunction at school; and illegal acts.

Kliman believes all children who lose a parent through death are "at risk" and recommends at least some time-limited interventions in all cases.

Furman (1974) suggests the validity of making professional guidance and support available to the parents of small children. It is difficult for a nonprofessional to evaluate a child's grief. Teachers and parents often do not recognize grief behavior for what it is.

Rationale for Group Therapy for Bereaved Children

Since many bereaved children are at risk for psychological problems, preventive intervention strategies are warranted (Berlinski & Biller, 1982; Krupnick, 1984). The fact that children's grief is intermittent and is influenced by changes in their cognitive and emotional development suggests that a time-limited, content-oriented supportive approach may be the most efficacious when dealing with the newly bereaved child who has lost a loved one and/or is experiencing maturational grief.

The goal of a group therapy program for bereaved children is twofold: (1) to provide social sanction for the expression of grief; and (2) to promote adaptive mourning responses. The activities should be designed in accordance with the children's level of emotional and intellectual development and address specific conflicts that result when a significant family member dies.

Involvement in a short-term bereavement counseling group provides children with the necessary social sanction and permission to express their feelings. Research in the area of death education has shown group counseling to be an effective intervention with children (Berg, 1978). The group allows for the formation of therapeutic alliances among the members. This therapeutic bond helps to alleviate the anxiety associated with the discussion of death. Thus children find comfort and relief in knowing that others feel the way they do. This, in turn, allows them to feel less threatened, and fosters the open discussion of their feelings surrounding the loss.

Slavson (1986) notes that substantial changes can occur in the child's psychic structure through the group process. If a child can be assured of self-worth, he or she can overcome blocks in self-expression caused by frustration and repressive and fear-producing experiences. Group therapy can provide an adaptive and corrective mourning experience for those children who feel rejected and worthless as a result of their parents' deaths.

Applicability of Art Therapy Techniques to Childhood Bereavement

Several factors contribute to the usefulness of group art therapy as a tool for ameliorating childhood grief. The clinical process of art therapy can be differentiated from other forms of intervention such as play therapy and individual counseling and from traditional psychotherapy by its unique use of nonverbal activities. Nonverbal activities allow children to act out conflicts that they might be unable or afraid to express with traditional insight-oriented talk therapies. This is particularly important during bereavement because of the societal taboos concerning the discussion of death. Both Segal (1984) and Simon (1981) discuss the natural tendency for children to repress painful mourning feelings and how these feelings find covert expression in bereavement art. In an art therapy program, these feelings are initially addressed through the safety of drawing or painting, and later through the child's direct verbalizations about his or her artwork. These combined nonverbal and verbal methods allow the child to become effectively involved in the mourning process, and help to promote open communication about the grief, which is necessary if the death is to be resolved (Bowen, 1976; McGoldrick & Walsh, 1983).

Art therapy enables bereaved children to transcend the intellectual and emotional limitations associated with understanding and conveying feelings about death. An art therapy program places an emphasis on enhancing creative capacities. Pollock (1978) describes creativity as an essential factor in the grief process. He conceptualizes creativity in mourning as restitution and discharge. These reparative drives restore the loved internal and external objects and are the basis of creativity and sublimation. The restoration preserves the lost object and gives it eternal life. Since creativity seems to play a central role in the mourning process, the art therapy program for bereaved children has specific art activities that promote the creative and adaptive expression of feelings.

Creativity also is encouraged through problem solving. Children play games that promote the discussion of feelings and generate solutions to problem situations. Segal (1984) notes that games are a familiar, nonthreatening activity associated with fun. They are traditionally used in therapeutic work with young children because they provide a natural and preferred mode of expression. The playing of a game allows the child to try out and practice new ways of coping and relating (Nickerson & O'Laughlin, 1983). Creative and fun activities used in conjunction with each other allow children to learn corrective coping strategies in a relaxed manner and result in productive mourning and eventual resolution of the grief.

THE HOSPICE, INC.

A Creative Arts Therapy Bereavement Intervention Program has been in existence at The Hospice, Inc., of Montclair, New Jersey, since 1984. Since that time more than 67 children from 45 families have been enrolled in the program. The ages of the children range from 4 to 16. A small-group format is used. Groups are composed of children who are similar in age. Most of the children have experienced the death of a parent within a year of enrolling in the group.

The program for the children is offered in conjunction with a parent support group. While the structure and content of the parent group are not the subject of this chapter, it is important to note that the child's overall adaptation to death is highly influenced by the surviving parent's response to the loss. When family variables are analyzed in conjunction with child behavioral outcome data, the functioning of the family system as a whole often is found to be of primary importance, perhaps even more important than the actual absence of the deceased parent (Berlinski & Biller, 1982). Thus working with the parent is essential when intervening with the child. Goals for the children's group are: developing rapport among group members; providing grief education; memorialization of the deceased; examination of personal support systems; the development of coping strategies; and a discussion of future expectations. These goals remain consistent from group to group.

The groups are designed to meet weekly for an hour for a period of 8 weeks. Most children who have been involved in the program end up contracting for two 8-week sessions. However, some children have found the 8-week format sufficient. Additionally, signing up for an 8-week series (rather than a 16-week stint) seems to be an easier commitment for most families. The break at the end of the first 8 weeks and the alternative schedule of activities for the subsequent 8 weeks allow new children to enter the group without having to wait more than 2 months and earlier members to continue in the program without experiencing a duplication in activities. Children who need to continue in the program for longer than 16 weeks are usually referred for more open-ended counseling.

A family intake interview and ending evaluation are required for the Creative Arts Group. Additional family consultation meetings are held as needed during the 8-week period. New members can join the group up to the third meeting.

Evaluations of the program have been very positive. In general, parents have described their children as being better able to discuss their feelings about the death. They cited improvement in family communication. The children reported that they felt better knowing others in the same position. They enjoyed the variety of the activities offered through the program. All the families who participated in the program evaluation felt that the group helped to promote acceptance of the death as well as the facilitation of their grieving process.

CASE EXAMPLE: DANIEL

The father of a 5-year-old boy, Daniel, died within a year after being diagnosed with cancer. Daniel was close to his father and was quite affected by his death. This physically healthy child who had no previous history of emotional illness began to show dramatic behavior changes in school and at home. His usual friendly disposition changed to one of stormy aggression. He began biting and kicking other children. He refused to write previously learned words and letters. He repeatedly used black in his paintings in kindergarten. At home, he was provocative and mischievous. He bullied his 2-year-old brother. His mother eventually brought Daniel for art therapy because his behavior was becoming increasingly problematic both at home and in school.

Daniel was a shy child who initially had difficulty relating to the other children in the group or even speaking to the group leaders. While he participated in the various group activities, he made repetitive drawings and paintings of a tornado (Fig. 3.1). It is possible that this image depicts a regression to an earlier level of graphic development in which sensorimotor scribbling is the prime method of expression. Daniel displayed his anger through his chaotic brush strokes. The title "Black Tornado" aptly describes his sense of confusion and vehement protest against his separation from his father.

Figure 3.2, an untitled finger painting, was made after several group sessions when he was asked to draw a picture about his grief. Although color has returned to his painting, this production imparts a more direct expression of rage. The black spots in the center of the painting are actual holes that Daniel made in the paper as he angrily applied the paint. This picture was a departure from his stereotypic reproductions and might suggest that Daniel was feeling less depressed and was attempting to develop control over his angry feelings.

Figure 3.3 is an example of a kinetic family drawing. This picture illustrates the family disequilibrium. The images show the home as an active battleground. The rectangular figure in the center of the picture is Daniel's father. While he knows his father is dead, Daniel wishes him back. This is typical preoperational thinking, since children of this age cannot view death as permanent. It also depicts Daniel's ambivalence about accepting his father's death. Since human figures have returned in this drawing Daniel also shows that he is beginning to use more age-appropriate coping mechanisms in attempting to deal with his anxiety over his father's death. It should also be noted that his mother was involved in the program's parent counseling component at this time and was learning to cope with the changes occurring in the family system.

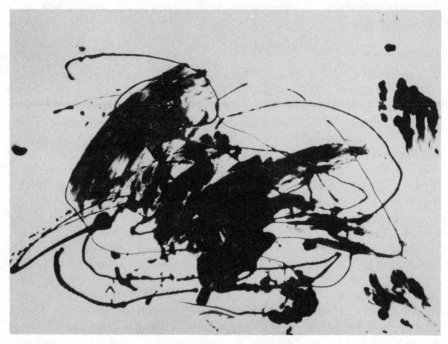

Figure 3.1. "Black Tornado."

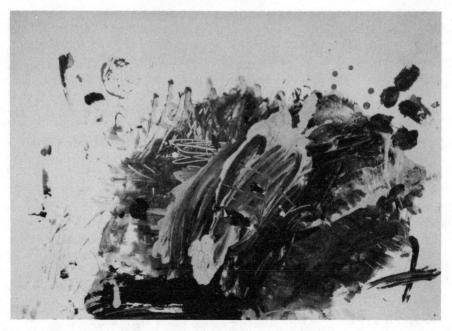

Figure 3.2. Finger painting.

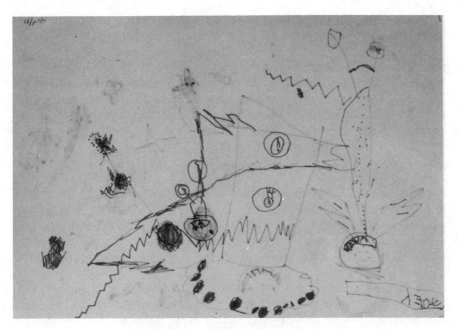

Figure 3.3. Kinetic family drawing.

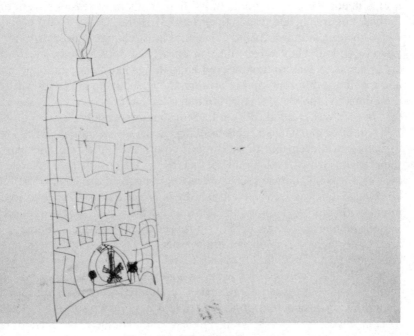

Figure 3.4. ''Good-bye.''

The last drawing (Fig. 3.4) was made on Daniel's final day in the group (approximately his sixteenth session). His behavior had improved tremendously at home and in school. The family was in a much better state of mental health. Daniel drew a building with a door and an exit sign. This was his way of saying good-bye to the program where he had received much help and support over the past 4 months. Figure 3.4 varies markedly from Figure 3.1. Daniel made a dramatic progression in representing his ideas and coping with the anxiety created by his father's death.

AN ELEMENTARY SCHOOL PROGRAM

Art therapy as bereavement intervention was offered in an elementary school in Minneapolis in 1984 (Heegaard). The school social worker notified the staff that an art therapist would be available to work with children who had experienced the death of someone special. Some children were referred by their teachers, and some teachers made a class announcement, and interested children signed up.

Three groups were formed. One was for children ages 5 to 7; it was discontinued in favor of individual art therapy because it was more appropriate for their needs and developmental level. The other two groups, for ages 8 to 9 and 10 to 12, met weekly for 8 weeks in the spring, and the sessions were offered again the next year. Most of the significant adults were not receiving their own grief support and education, and some of the children's needs were very great. Individual art therapy sessions were offered to these children in addition to the groups. The staff became very supportive.

Death education was included because most young children do not receive any elsewhere. They were told that an art therapist is someone who uses art as a special way to look at confusing things like family loss and change, and that it is a different kind of art than they usually do in school, with fewer directions to follow and no need to make the pictures pretty. They were told that the art would be used to tell a story and express feelings.

Therapy began with scribble drawings and a discussion of feelings related to colors. Children like to talk about colors they like best and least, and their reasons why they do or do not like them. One boy disliked green because his uncle was killed in a green car, and a girl disliked the same color because her God-sister was wearing a green dress in her coffin. They like to experiment with different colors to determine which colors best express their various feelings. They generally choose red to express anger. Some children are comfortable scribbling an entire sheet solid red, and others need encouragement to scribble a few pale marks.

The children were given a predrawn gingerbread man shape and told that feelings are what make people real. The children were asked to identify on their drawing designated colors, where they experience specific feelings such as fear, anger, guilt, depression, sadness, and happiness. Confusion, repression, and comfort with feelings can be recognized in even the youngest children.

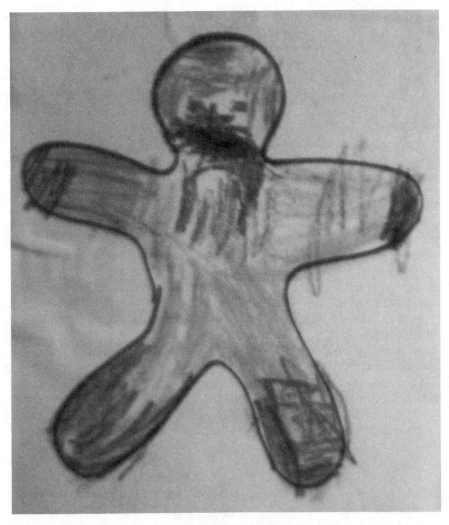

Figure 3.5. "Feeling Person."

CASE EXAMPLE: ROBERT, CHARLES, AND RONNIE

Robert, Charles, and Ronnie are three boys whose father died of a heart attack after being disabled and unable to work for several years. The boys, 6, 7, and 9½, reacted to their loss in different ways, as revealed in their artwork.

Robert (6), the youngest brother, seemed to be the least affected by his father's death, but was able to recognize and express feelings within a pre-drawn gingerbread man shape (Fig. 3.5). He said he felt his anger all over and liked to punch and kick. He colored the hands and feet red. He was also comfortable crying. He said it was okay for kids to cry at school, home, shopping, funerals . . . anyplace. He said his father had died because he caught a little cold and got pneumonia. After this misconception was cleared up he later said that his father died because he was 199 or 96. It is necessary to teach children that aging alone does not cause death. The group drew "Causes of Death," and it was stressed that nothing they did or said caused the death. It is important to continue to explain the issues of the death to the children as they mature or they may remain confused.

Charles (7) was more uncomfortable with his feelings. He repressed most of them and pretended that nothing had changed in his life. His behavior at home and at school was problematic as he acted out his feelings. In responding to "draw something sad" he drew a man, crossed him out, turned the paper over and drew pac man eating circles. His preferred medium was clay, and he made many dinosaurs. He repressed his anger and was hyperactive and uncooperative in group situations, but he worked hard in individual sessions.

In a "sequence story" he began with a "Happy Halloween Party" with lots of fun and food (Fig. 3.6). It moved from trick-or-treating at a haunted house during a thunderstorm to a house where they "finally" got one treat, and then to a very lonely looking room at home.

A later picture suggested by a stimulus card continued this theme of loneliness (Fig. 3.7). Charles said the dinosaur felt very lonely so he added some food to eat (tree) and a lake to play in. He titled his next picture "The Lonely Worm."

Community intervention was requested through the social worker, but nothing seemed available. Charles retreated into a fantasy life and, after working with him for many months, the art therapist chose to confront his denial. His next picture was about a man who had been killed by being hit by a car in a heavy rainstorm (Fig. 3.8). Eventually, he was able to personalize his loss (Fig. 3.9).

As he became more comfortable talking about death and the changes in his life, his behavior at home and at school improved and he no longer had a frightened, wild-eyed look.

Ronnie (9½), the oldest, was repressing most of his feelings. He seemed most comfortable with sadness, which was the feeling he drew on the outside of a brown paper bag. Symbols were placed inside the bag to represent his difficult feelings. However, he was able to recognize his defenses. He knew he chose to fight with his brother to avoid feeling sad. Their apartment had been robbed twice and a person had been killed in the building. He was fearful, insecure, and resentful about being poor and different and didn't like his life very much (Fig. 3.10).

During one session the children were asked to draw the letters for the word *death* and add symbols associated with each letter. Ronnie made a ball out of his first picture and threw it in the wastebasket. The second picture also revealed a great deal of rage and destructive feelings (Fig. 3.11). After a discussion about Ronnie's art therapy, the social worker and school psy-

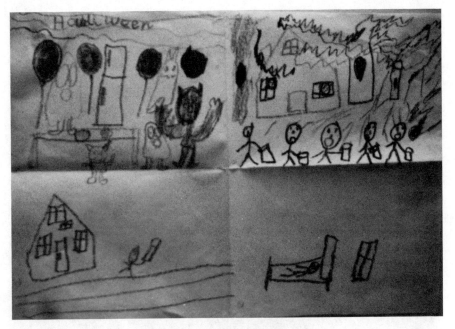

Figure 3.6. "A Halloween Story."

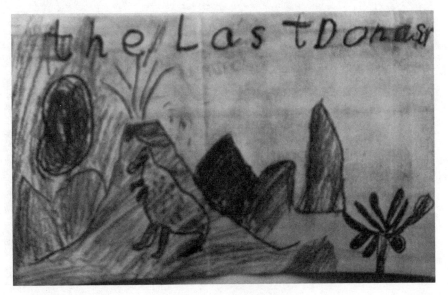

Figure 3.7. "The Last Dinosaur."

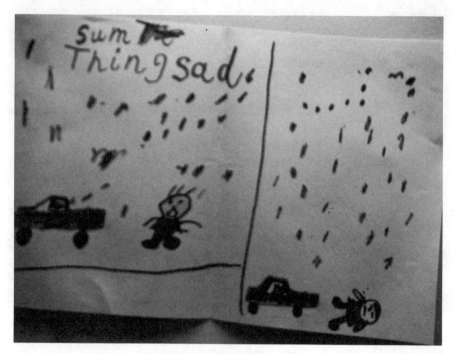

Figure 3.8. "Something Sad."

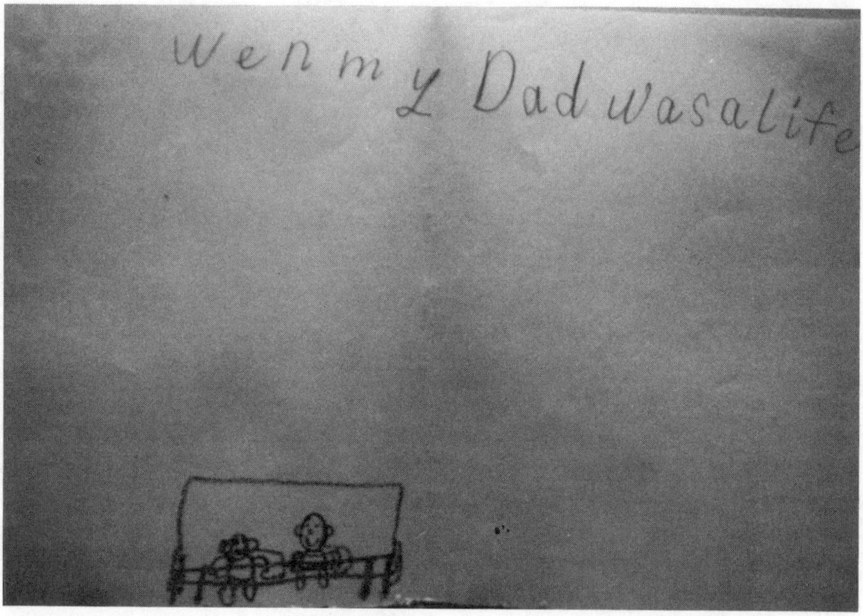

Figure 3.9. "Memories."

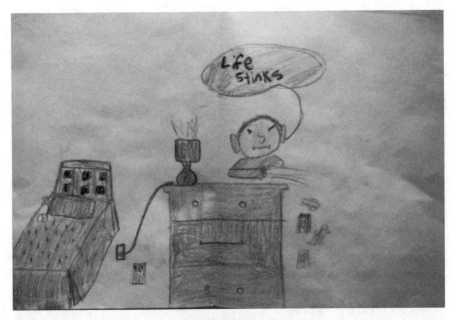

Figure 3.10. Free Choice Drawing.

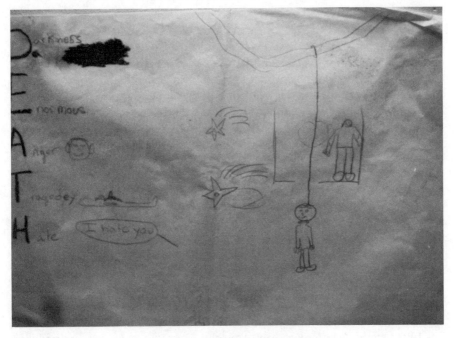

Figure 3.11. "Symbols of Death."

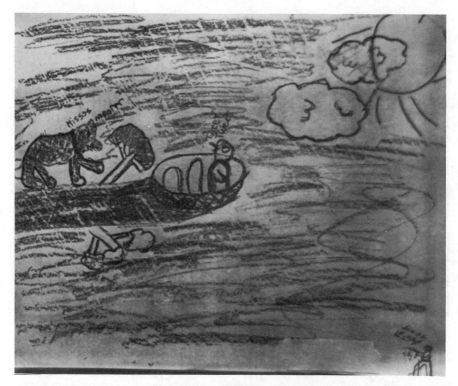

Figure 3.12. "The Life of a Bird."

chologist considered him a suicide risk and the family finally received additional intervention. Ronnie said he was often picked on by other kids and teased about being poor. In role playing he learned remarkably quickly to act with more confidence. He became more accepted by his peers, and his last pictures included some intervention in life's dangers. He drew a dog attacking a person who was going to shoot a bird, and in Figure 3.12 a tiny figure (lower right) shoots the cat before it can eat the bird. His pictures became less violent and more hopeful from then on.

At the end of the school year, the boys were expressing their feelings appropriately verbally as well as nonverbally through artwork. A follow-up evaluation a year later showed no regression. They were doing well socially and academically according to reports from school and home. The school staff was enthusiastic about the progress they observed and credited it to the art therapy intervention.

CONCLUSION

Effectiveness of grief support groups and art therapy intervention may be difficult to evaluate completely until the child is grown and able to individuate and form significant relationships. However, awareness, understanding, and expressing feeling do help prevent inappropriate defenses. Art therapy can assist development of a sense of self-worth, communication skills, social cooperation, problem solving, and increased personal efficacy.

Children may need intervention follow-up as they mature, reach adolescence, and experience subsequent losses. Our society needs to find better ways of providing the needed education and support. Art therapy can provide an effective intervention for the bereaved child.

REFERENCES

American Art Therapy Association (1977). What is Art Therapy? In R. Shoemaker & S. Gonick-Barris (Eds.), *Creativity and the art therapist's identity. Proceedings of the Seventh Annual Conference of the American Art Therapy Association.* Baltimore: AATA.

Arther, B., & Kemme, M. (1964). Bereavement in childhood. *Journal of Child Psychology & Psychiatry 5,* 37–49.

Berg, C. (1978, September). Helping children accept death and dying through group counseling. *Personnel & Guidance Journal,* pp. 169–172.

Berlinski, E., & Biller, H. (1982). *Parental death and psychological development.* Lexington, MA: Lexington Books.

Black, D. (1974). What happens to bereaved children? *Proceedings of the Royal Society of Medicine, 69,* 842–844.

Bowen, M. (1976). Family Reaction to Death. In P. Guerin (Ed.), *Family Therapy.* New York: Gardner.

Bowlby, J. (1960). Grief and mourning in infancy and early childhood. *Psychoanalytic Study of the Child, 15,* 9–52.

Bowlby, J. (1980). *Loss: Sadness and depression.* New York: Basic.

Cocuzza-Zambelli, G. (1981). The use of art therapy with children in the bereavement process. In A. Evans, E. Kramer, & I. Rosner (Eds.), *Art Therapy: A Bridge Between Worlds.* Falls Church, VA: American Art Therapy Association.

Elizur, E., & Kaffman, M. (1983). Factors influencing the severity of childhood bereavement reactions. *American Journal of Orthopsychiatry, 53,* 668–676.

Furman, E. (1974). *A Child's Parent Dies.* New Haven: Yale University Press.

Johnson, P., & Rosenblatt, P. (1981). Grief following childhood loss of a parent. *American Journal of Psychotherapy, 25,* 419–425.

Junge, M. (1985). The book about Daddy dying. A preventive art therapy technique to help families deal with the death of a family member. *Art Therapy, 2,* 410.

Klein, K. M. (1982). *Topics in pediatrics/spring 1982.* Minneapolis: Children's Health Center Publications.

Kliman, G. (1968). In G. Kliman (Ed.), *Psychological emergencies in childhood.* New York: Grune & Stratton.

Kliman, G. (1980). Death: Some implications in child development and child analysis. *Advances in Thanatology, 4,* 43–50.

Krupnick, J. (1984). Childhood and adolescence. In M. Osterwies, F. Solomon, & M. Green (Eds.), *Bereavement: Reactions, consequences, and care*. Washington, DC: National Academy Press.

Kübler-Ross, E. (1969). *On death and dying*. New York: Macmillan.

Kübler-Ross, E. (1983). *On Children and Death*. New York: Macmillan.

McGoldrick, M., & Walsh, F. (1983). A systemic view of family history and loss. In L. Wolberg & M. Aronson (Eds.), *Group and family therapy*. New York: Brunner/Mazel.

Miller, B. (1984). Art therapy with the elderly and terminally ill. In T. Dalley (Ed.), *Art as therapy*. New York: Tavistock.

Nagara, H. (1970). *The developmental approach to childhood psychopathology*. New York: Jason Aronson.

Nickerson, E., & O'Laughlin, K. (1983). *Helping through action: Action-oriented therapies*. Amherst, MA: Human Resources Development Press.

Osterweis, I., Solomon, M., & Green, M. (Eds.), *Bereavement: Reactions, consequences, and care*. Washington, DC: National Academy Press.

Palumbo, J. (1981). Parent loss and childhood bereavement: Some theoretical considerations. *Clinical Social Work Journal, 9*(1), 3–33.

Plank, E., & Plank, R. (1978). Children and death. *Psychoanalytic Study of the Child, 33*, 593–620.

Pollock, G. (1978). Process and affect: Mourning and grief. *Journal of Psychoanalysis, 59*, 255–276.

Raphael, B. (1983). *The anatomy of bereavement*. New York: Basic.

Rutter, M. (1966). *Children of sick parents*. London: Oxford University Press.

Schowalter, J. (1975). Parent death and child bereavement. In R. Schoenberg, L. Schoenberg, A. Gerber, A. H. Wiener, A. Kutscher, & D. Peretz (Eds.), *Bereavement: Its psychosocial aspects*. New York and London: Columbia University Press.

Segal, R. (1984, December). Helping children express grief through symbolic communication. *Social Casework: The Journal of Contemporary Social Work, 65*, 590–599.

Simon, R. (1981). Bereavement art. *American Journal of Art Therapy, 20*, 135–143.

Simonton, O., Matthews-Simonton, S., & Creighton, J. (1978). *Getting well again*. New York: Bantam Books.

Slavson, S. (1986). Differential methods of group therapy in relation to age levels. In A. Riester, & I. Kraft (Eds.), *Child group psychotherapy: Future tense*. Connecticut: International Universities Press.

Wolfenstein, M. (1966). How is mourning possible? *Psychoanalytic Study of the Child, 21*, 93–123.

Worden, J. W. (1982). *Grief counseling and grief therapy*. New York: Springer.

CHAPTER 4

A Mothers' Art Therapy Group in a Short-Term Psychiatric Setting

MARY CAIRNS

In starting a mothers' art therapy group, I came to this new experience with a set of questions and expectations. Being the mother of a small child, I speculated about what would be important to a mentally ill hospitalized mother. Among the questions I formulated were: How did they cope with being separated from their children, and how did that impact on their mental illness? How did their mental illness and/or multiple hospitalizations affect their relationship with their children? How did they feel about the surrogate child-care arrangements during their absence? How did they perceive their roles, and what was important to them as mothers? I thought about how art therapy could serve as an added avenue for expression for these issues and the presumably painful feelings they evoked. I felt that this group of people had unique problems that were largely overlooked in their general treatment. As a result, I designed a mothers' art therapy group to provide a supportive atmosphere where their concerns could be explored, their anxiety could be relieved, and their self-awareness could be increased, all in the company of other mothers who had been through similar experiences.

The art therapy literature is lacking in works focusing on mentally ill mothers. Landgarten (1975) and Rubin (1978), however, both ran mother–daughter art therapy groups in which issues of hostility and expectations were addressed. Although some of these findings were relevant to this chapter, they worked only with healthy mothers and their young daughters who have no children.

The general literature, however, reveals that Grunebaum, Weiss, Cohler, Hartman, and Gallant (1975) developed a joint mother–child hospital admissions program. Their report outlined the dilemma experienced by most mothers suffering from postpartum depression upon being admitted to a mental hospital *without* their children: (1) separation, usually sudden; (2) feelings of ambivalence about the surrogate care; and (3) guilt and shame about what they perceive as abandonment of their children and having become failures as mothers. Stott et al. (1984) reported that supportive treatment is essential for disturbed mothers, while insight therapy is the least useful with this population until a mother can handle internal conflict. Both reports, however, focus primarily on working with mothers and children together as a means of addressing issues as they occur, which is a privilege not afforded to the mothers at the hospital where I work, or most hospitals, for that matter.

The Illinois State Psychiatric Institute (ISPI), is a short-term hospital that serves Chicago's socioeconomically depressed south and west sides. The average length of stay is 3 weeks. The patient population is primarily Black, with one-third Hispanic and White, covering a wide range of mental disorders, mostly psychoses. The mothers described in this chapter are Black and were diagnosed as schizophrenic, manic-depressive, or having a major depression. Most had experienced multiple hospitalizations. They were drawn from six different units in the hospital to ensure an adequate supply of mothers, and yet the group still remained small, between two and five patients. The age of the mothers and their children varied and was not a determinant in eligibility, as long as the mothers had dependent children. Higher-functioning mothers were invited after an initial interview to assess their interest in such a group and to see whether they were reasonably well organized to handle the inherent conflicts of group therapy. Blatantly delusional or psychotic patients were not invited until they became better organized.

The mothers met twice a week for an hour in the activity shop on my unit. Simple art materials were provided: pastels, markers, and occasionally clay. Tea, cocoa, and cookies were served. I explained the purpose of art therapy and the mothers' group at each session and invited the participants to bring up issues or problems to discuss and address in a drawing. Since the mothers were usually reluctant to do this, I assigned topics to draw and discuss, such as "How do you feel about being separated from your children?"; "What do you like most about motherhood? Least?"; "How do you and your children cope with your illness?"; and "Draw you and your mother." Each patient was invited to share her drawing with the group members, who then responded to them, noting similarities and differences of experiences. The mothers' art therapy group lasted for 5 months, although the average patient attended only 3 or 4 weeks, or six to eight sessions due to the high rate of turnover in a short-term setting.

RESULTS

The mothers in this study all differed in their experiences, attitudes, motivation for change, and level of pain or frustration. However, because they all had children, were primarily Black, mostly divorced or separated, mentally ill, and hospitalized, they were bound to have some commonalities in experience. One of these, contrary to my expectation, was that without exception, the mothers experienced relief from the burdens of child care while in the hospital, and were not intent upon rushing home to their children.

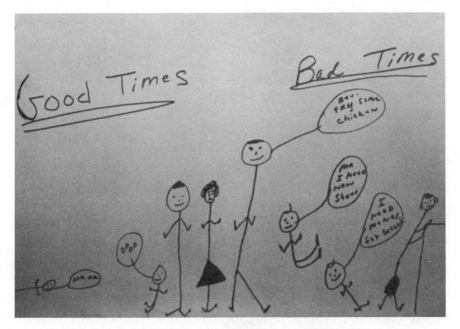

Figure 4.1. Beverly's picture of the best and worst times of motherhood.

They perceived the hospital as a haven and escape from the intolerable difficulty of trying to care for small children while feeling overwhelmed by a crippling mental disorder and often lack of family support. However, as their mental health improved, they began to speak of missing their children, and as their discharge dates approached, they became increasingly anxious about returning to them and their uncertain futures.

Beverly, for example, is a 40-year-old mother of two boys, 11 and 12, who were home with their father. She had had multiple hospitalizations since the age of 18 for schizophrenia, and blames her current mental illness on a "curse" someone put on her. When asked to draw the best and worst aspects of motherhood, Beverly made a drawing reflecting two very different periods in her life (Fig. 4.1).

On the left side of her drawing, she recalled the good times, when her boys were babies, and when she felt best as a mother, more than 10 years ago. The right side of her drawing, however, reflects her low level of functioning prior to her current hospitalization, as her two boys and husband are shown "demanding something from me." She appears to cower over the stove. Beverly acknowledged that she felt overwhelmed and used up upon admission to the hospital because she couldn't cope with the demands of an active family. She also expressed feelings of guilt over her failure to carry on her responsibilities as a housewife and the marital conflict it created. The other group members nodded in agreement that those were contributing factors in their breakdowns, too. They were very supportive of Beverly,

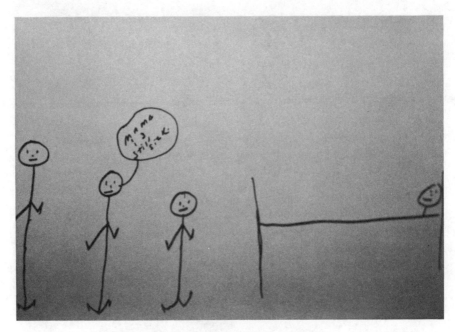

Figure 4.2. Beverly's home visit.

and offered religious advice, many feeling that religion was their only salvation.

Over the course of her hospitalization, Beverly improved dramatically, but as discharge approached, she drew a recent home visit (Fig. 4.2) in which she lies in bed, with only a head and no body shown, while her husband and children look on. Says one son, "Mama is still sick," suggesting that her family wonders whether she'll ever be a part of the family again. She expressed her fears of another collapse once home. Beverly's use of stick figures was probably a reflection of her feeling "used up," powerless, and depressed.

Claudette, an obese 33-year-old divorced mother of three children, ages 10, 6, and 16 months, was admitted after a suicide attempt and a history of major depression. This was her second hospitalization. She expressed her inability to cope with motherhood and unemployment in a drawing (Fig. 4.3) representing "being cut off from my children by my depression" (black area around her). Her three children were "happy because they are not with me" (yellow area around children). She said that she knew that it was very difficult for them during her long periods of depression when she was unavailable to them emotionally. She worried especially about the effect of her illness on her 10-year-old son. During those periods, he would take over some of her responsibilities, such as feeding and caring for the baby, his sister, and his mother. Her suicide attempt, she believes, was a way to help her children to be free of her and in the care of a foster home. Because Claudette was

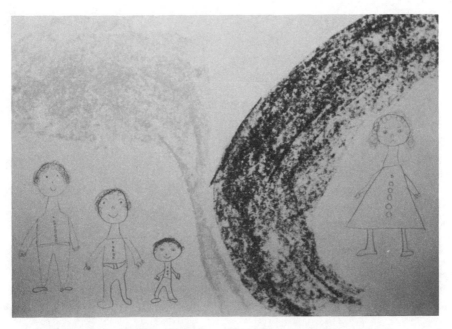

Figure 4.3. Claudette "being cut off from my children by depression."

aware of the potential damaging effects of this role reversal on her son, she wanted to follow up after hospitalization with therapy for herself and him.

Claudette was unusual in this respect, however. Most of the other mothers reported good relationships with their children, stating that they had no problems whatsoever. Their children were their "best friends" in whom they confided and who kept them from feeling lonely. They felt that their children were accustomed to having a mother who was sometimes "sick" and who had adapted "well" to the situation. What they meant by adapting "well" is unclear. It may be that these mothers are "enabling" (Stott et al., 1984); that is, that they have allowed their children to turn to significant others within their environment (in these cases, usually their grandmothers), enabling them to use positively what is offered to enhance their development. These children usually fare much better than those who do not have enabling mothers; this may explain in part why they reported that their children were conflict free regarding their repeated separations.

It is therefore not surprising that these mothers were for the most part uninterested in talking about their children. They felt confident that their children were well cared for and harbored no resentment toward them for loving grandma. However, while the children were free to form close attachments with their grandmothers, the mothers expressed tremendous hostility between themselves and their mothers. These conflictual relationships, they said, were of long standing, antedating their children's births and their mental illnesses.

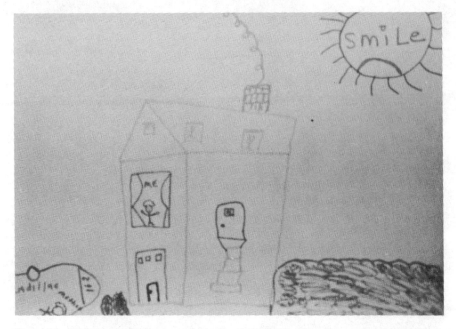

Figure 4.4. Shirley locked in the house by her mother, who is shown in an automobile accident.

Shirley, for example, is a 37-year-old manic-depressive mother of two boys, 11 and 15. She has had three hospitalizations. She described her mother as dominating and abusive and said that she married and had children to get out of her mother's house, but after divorce 8 years later found herself back there because "even my mother was better than my husband." When asked to draw herself and her mother, Shirley drew an episode where her mother locked Shirley and her two sons in her house before going out, apparently because she didn't want them to leave (Fig. 4.4). Shirley shows herself standing in the window while her mother is lying down in her overturned Cadillac after an accident in which she was "unfortunately" not hurt. Next to the house is a sun with the word "smile" inside of it and "an upside-down smile" representing "my stepfather because he is controlled by her, too." This drawing seems to be full of conflicting messages; I suspect it represents her ambivalent feelings toward her mother. Shirley says she is "controlled" by her mother and yet is shown standing up with her arms stretched out looking over her mother who is lying down in the car. She seems to bask in her role as the "helpless victim," perhaps because her dominating mother is her excuse for remaining dependent on her. Shirley acknowledged that she "should" be independent of her mother but states that she will probably be with her all her life because "there's nowhere else to go and besides, she needs me to be her slave."

In the following session, Shirley drew herself before and during a manic

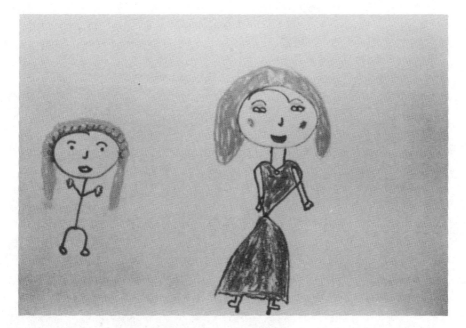

Figure 4.5. Shirley before and during a manic episode.

episode (Fig. 4.5). She said she is normally the one on the left, but when she is manic, she dyes her hair blonde and wears "jazzy" makeup and clothes as in the figure on the right, probably, she said, because she feels ugly inside. Shirley feels that she has had a manic-depressive episode every time she considers independence from her mother. This was the first time she had made a connection between her manic-depressive illness and her hostile–dependent relationship with her mother, although she did not understand why this happened. The small figure on the left may represent her depressed–dependent self. But the larger figure on the right represents her manic self, which motivates her toward independence but soon succumbs to internal pressures to conform and remain dependent (depression). This may be due to an unconscious fear of the loss of her mother's love and guilt over abandoning her mother, who struggles to keep her close.

Cheryl, a schizophrenic 29-year-old separated mother of three children, 10, 5, and 2½, also voiced discord between herself and her mother. She made a self-portrait (Fig. 4.6) relating to her relationship with her mother.

About her drawing, Cheryl said, "I'm incomplete, because no one ever filled me up," referring to the large empty head with one eye. She said she left out her hands because she didn't want to do any more work for her mother. The drawing looks like a large baby bird, unformed and unable to survive in the world.

The other group members empathized and related to Cheryl's powerful

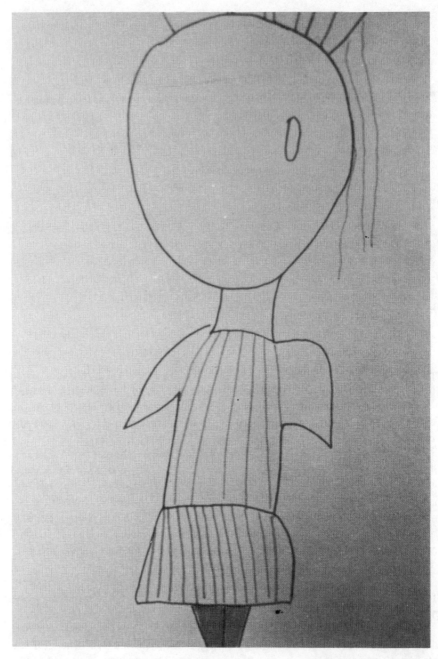

Figure 4.6. Cheryl's self-portrait, which she related to her mother.

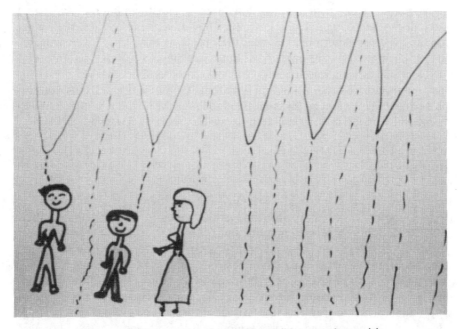

Figure 4.7. Shirley taking charge of her children on a home visit.

drawing. They felt that they did not receive the love and nurturance they needed from their mothers and doubted that they'd ever get it.

Power struggles between the mothers over the children also seemed to be an issue in the group. Shirley made a drawing of a recent home visit in which she went out to get her children out of the rain because she said, "When I'm home, they take orders from me!" (Fig. 4.7).

The jagged clouds give this drawing an ominous appearance, suggesting a threat to her role as mother and caretaker. In this sense, the mothers are in a terrible bind. On the one hand, they would like to be free of their mothers. On the other hand, however, they know that they need their mothers because they have nowhere else to go and because their mothers must care for their children during their hospitalizations. With their lack of financial resources to find adequate child care or housing for themselves, coupled with their mental illnesses and perhaps expectations for love and acceptance from their mothers, these women remain dependent on them. They resent their mothers' control over their lives and their children's lives and feel overwhelmed by their sense of powerlessness.

Adding to their frustration and helplessness is their shame about being in a mental hospital and being labeled "crazy" by their mothers, friends, and/or children. As their discharge dates approached, they worried that their children would forget or reject them. They experienced increased anxiety about going home, back to their uncertain futures, and their unpredictable and difficult mother–daughter relationships. Despite these fears, however, most mothers seemed determined to meet their mothers head on. Power struggles with their mothers were unpleasant but what they were used to, after all.

Receiving affirmation and support in the mothers' art therapy group for their pain and frustration lent each member a vitally needed sense of empowerment. This allowed these mothers to leave the hospital better equipped to meet the needs of their children as well as their own needs.

DISCUSSION

In consideration of the total context of these patients, it is not surprising that the mothers were more absorbed in their roles as daughters than in their roles as mothers. Still searching for their identities in the mother–daughter relationship, they seek love and nurturance from both their mothers and their children. Women often admit that one motive for becoming a mother is to gain a sense of being mothered themselves (Flax, 1981). The transgenerational patterns become visible then. The hostilities between the mother and daughter seem as yet to be absent in the mother–child relationship. However, the dependency issues are present in both and are passed on and on through the generations, unless interventions are made to help these very needy families.

The mothers' art therapy group was one such intervention. Not insight oriented, the group served more as an anxiety absorber. These mothers wanted to talk, for they had a lot to say. Thus the artwork helped to slow down the process so that each issue could be addressed more completely. They were able to compare and contrast their experiences of being a mentally ill mother through the artwork in a way they couldn't through discussions alone. Since these women felt so profoundly isolated, the group served to create a sense of community for them within their total hospital treatment milieu. They offered support and encouragement to each other while the art facilitated both self-exploration and group cohesiveness.

CONCLUSION

While these mothers gained strength and encouragement in the group, more is needed. For example, more mental health professionals working with mothers could be alerted to a possible mother–daughter conflict as a dynamic in their mental illness. "Do for the mother so she can do for her children" (Stott et al., 1984): This statement should reflect our approach in working with these mothers by offering support, affirmation, and guidance through their very difficult struggles, so that they can give back to their children more affirmation and positive regard.

I plan to include in my own future work an art therapy group with mothers and their mentally ill daughters who have children. Not only would art therapy facilitate the expression of dependency and autonomy conflicts but it would also provide the mothers and their daughters with a more positive experience together. Helping both mothers to explore and resolve their dependency issues with each other will enable them to be more free to attend to the needs of their children and their own personal growth.

REFERENCES

Flax, J. (1981). The conflict between nurturance and autonomy in mother–daughter relationships and within feminism. In E. Howell & M. Bayes (Eds.), *Women and mental health*. New York: Basic.

Grunebaum, H., Weiss, J. L., Cohler, B. J., Hartman, C. R., & Gallant, D. H. (1975). *Mentally ill mothers and their children*. Chicago: University of Chicago Press.

Landgarten, H. (1975). Group art therapy for mothers and daughters. *American Journal of Art Therapy, 14,* 31.

Rubin, J. (1978). *Child Art Therapy*. New York: Van Nostrand Reinhold.

Stott, F., Musick, J., Cohler, B., Spencer, K., Goldman, J., Clark, R., & Dincin, J., (1984). Intervention for the severely disturbed mother. In Cohler & Musick (Eds.), *Intervention with psychiatrically disabled parents and their young children: New directions for mental health services*. San Francisco: Jossey-Bass.

CHAPTER 5

Art Therapy for Battered Women

ROSEMARY LAGORIO

Growing societal recognition of the pervasiveness of the battered woman received its impetus in the United States from the women's movement and President Carter's establishment of an Office of Domestic Violence with the Department of Health and Human Services. Shelters specifically for battered women and children are a recent phenomenon, having been started in 1972 by Erin Pryzey in England.

As the awareness of the existence of domestic violence increases, so do the research and literature. My purpose in writing this chapter is to introduce the reader to the valuable impact art making can have in assisting the battered woman toward a more complete and realistic view of her situation, her self-worth, choices, problem solving, and personal empowerment. Those charged with developing programs and services for this population can be well served by the contribution art therapy can offer in identifying and confirming both personal and societal issues that allow domestic violence to be tolerated. Art therapy can also effect change in a period of crisis.

LITERATURE REVIEW

While there may, in fact, be a number of art therapists actively engaged in working with battered women in a shelter setting, there is, to my knowledge, no documentation or published work regarding art therapy and sheltered, battered women.

However, the reader will find reports of the art findings of Wohl and Kaufman (1985), Spring (1985), and Malchiodi and Peterson (1985) of general related interest. Wohl and Kaufman (1985) have made a significant contribution in their work in relating battering of children to symbols used in the children's artwork. However, these words do not include battered women or art itself as a treatment modality.

Spring (1985) wrote of her art experience in a shelter for sexually abused and/or chemically dependent clients. While it is possible that some may have also been battered, this was not addressed, nor was it necessarily a constant factor.

Malchiodi and Peterson (1985) have written a practical guide to applying the creative, expressive arts of art, music, movement, writing, and poetry to working with children who, along with their mothers, are living in shelters due to domestic violence.

Most of the general literature available to professionals covering the dynamics and case management of battered women has come into print in only the last 10 years. It is important to note that the Family Violence Research Program at the University of Texas at Tyler has set up a central clearinghouse regarding spouse abuse. Their data base is a source of printed, unprinted, and research studies in the United States and beyond. A quarterly updated bibliography is available for a modest fee.

Lenore Walker (1979, 1984), an authority in the area of battered women, offers comprehensive, insightful work that dispels the myth of why a woman often stays in or returns to a physically abusive situation. Walker's analysis of the cycle of violence, female personality characteristics, and an expanded definition of abuse serves as a firm basis for understanding this population.

While less academically oriented, of great value to the professional as well as the general public are the books by Norwood (1985), Shainess (1984), and Forward and Torres (1986). All of these popular books can serve as adjunctive therapy tools in providing the woman with a basic understanding of the violence in her life. Shainess emphasizes general family and societal conditioning of women as one of the most important aspects of the problem. Norwood contends that the battered woman exists in an addictive relationship and presents a valuable graph modeled after the Alcohol Addiction Recovery Model, which she titles the "Progression of 'Loving Too Much' and Recovery." In one of the most recent additions to the popular literature, Forward and Torres (1986) explore the traits of the abuser, whom they view as a mysogynist, as well as traits of the victim. They make a valuable contribution to the literature in offering how both personality types are formed, why the trapped relationship continues to exist, and what can be done to break the addictive part of the relationship.

The professional working with battered women also requires more specific knowledge and the specialized skills in the area of crisis intervention. Aguilera and Messick (1986) present theory, methodology, and case situations in working in crisis intervention. The work of Puryear (1979) presents a type of "how to" guide regarding intervention, assessment of problems and strengths, and assisting clients' action.

DESCRIPTION OF SETTING AND POPULATION

The Evanston Shelter for Battered Women and Children is a large, rambling, Victorian structure that presents somewhat of a paradox in that it resembles a typical warm home setting with separate sleeping space and common areas for activities, yet it is in fact an institution with specific circumscribed house rules that, if broken, could result in residents being asked to leave.

The shelter provides living space for 30 occupants. Women who do not have financial resources, family, or friends with whom they could be safe are eligible. Male children under age 12 can be housed at the shelter. Active drug or alcohol use is a disqualifying factor as there are no programs to meet these specific needs. Occupants are housed free of charge, from a brief overnight stay to a maximum of 3 months.

The primary function of the shelter is to provide a safe place away from the abuser. It is hoped that the women will benefit from assistance with advocacy, counseling, nurturing, and empowerment. Occupants also benefit from a sense of commonality with other women of similar experience, thus breaking their sense of isolation. Each woman is assigned a primary counselor. In addition, the shelter requires all residents to attend an evening support group once a week. This allows an opportunity for peer and staff support. While this is a mandatory meeting and sometimes an inconvenience to tight scheduling, most women find it comforting. This meeting provides support and counseling, the aim of which is to preclude a revolving-door syndrome.

The resident population varies in number at any given time. Typically, the residents are middle to lower middle class, with a mixture of White, Black, and Hispanic included. Most are women seeking a sanctuary from the abuser. They are generally in need of financial as well as job-seeking assistance. All women are 18 or over, and are victims of personal or physical abuse by a spouse or significant other, or family member.

In many instances, in addition to suffering environmental abuse, the children have been physically or verbally abused.

METHODOLOGY

Because of the fluctuating numbers of residents as well as the variance in their length of stay in the shelter, I decided my approach would need to offer both structure and flexibility.

Clients for whom I was to serve as primary counselor were required to meet with me individually once each week for an hour. Other residents were referred by the primary counselors for work on specific issues, or for regularly scheduled adjunctive art therapy.

Shortly after I arrived, the social worker who led one of the two evening group sessions each week left the shelter, giving me an opportunity to use art therapy on a weekly basis for 9 months.

I had particular interest in the repetition cycle evidenced by the battered women, remaining in the abusive situation or, after having left the situation, making the decision to return to it. What was the basis for the sense of entrapment or addiction to a situation that subjected them to great stress and sometimes put their lives in jeopardy?

   In exploring the repetition cycle, I would focus on what they viewed as positive and negative about the situation, where these attitudes might stem from in their early history, their own sense of self-esteem, and where they fit into the situation.

   My style was, I would say, a gentle rather than confrontational one. I recognized that among the primary needs of this group are safety, security, and trust. This supportive milieu offered opportunities for education regarding interpersonal dynamics and personal resources, and brought forth a sense of self-worth and empowerment.

   While I was free to work with both women and children at the shelter, I chose to devote a major portion of my time to working with the adult females. My rationale for this was twofold. First, art therapy has already made some significant inroads into helping the abused child and is just beginning to explore the abused woman. Secondly, the child is, in the final analysis, subject to the insightfulness and resolve of the adults who act as guardians. Therefore, I felt it imperative to assist the woman toward empowerment over her abusive situation, thereby allowing a greater possibility for effecting a more lasting change. I recognized that a family system can indeed change with intervention in any area, but I felt we could get closer to the crux of the problem by addressing adult needs as a major priority.

   While I enjoyed the welcome of the existing staff, I soon came to the stark realization that I was faced with an impoverished budget. This deficit was ameliorated as I made personal visits and phone calls to local art supply stores, manufacturers, and distributors to secure the necessary supplies. This situation drained much energy and time that were needed elsewhere to initiate the art therapy program. However, a major benefit of my ''campaign'' for supplies was that it stimulated interest in domestic violence as a social ill and allowed individuals and companies to make a contribution toward effecting change in this area.

   Art therapy availability was made known to residents by posting a visually attractive notice on the resident bulletin board announcing life mask making. I encouraged response by personally inviting residents to experience this fun-filled and relaxing adventure. I expected this to stimulate interest and bring forth volunteers. It did. Having a life mask made from plaster-gauze bandages allowed the women an excuse for taking time for themselves and escaping from their crisis situation. With a tape of relaxing nature sounds as background, this respite became a first inroad into the turning of attention to the self. It allowed me to establish the presence of art therapy at the shelter, as well as affording me an opportunity to make my first therapeutic contact with the abused women.

   I noted that most of the women thoroughly enjoyed the mask making and, in fact, a few became so relaxed that they fell asleep. On the other hand, some chose not to have their eyes covered and/or seemed to be fidgety. I felt it important in these situations to allow the woman to do only what she was comfortable with and to continue verbal contact through the mask-making process. A second session allowed time for painting, using their own creativity in this personal expression.

The masks revealed insight, as expressed by one woman who, as a finishing touch, added a ring in her nose as a reminder never to be led around by others in the future. The masks also allowed for processing affect. For example, one woman came into an art therapy session after a house dispute and chopped the looped yarn hair bangs she had made previously, giving the mask a frenzied appearance. She then proceeded to add yarn pigtails, creating the semblance of a young child. This provided a good point of departure for discussing her feelings of helplessness and anger.

A few women were disturbed at the frightening physiognomy and discovered they did not want to keep the mask or rework it. Some women chose to display their work proudly on a display board made of coreboard, painted gold, and hung in the living room. Others chose, after showing other residents and receiving positive affirmation, to keep them in their own rooms. Mask making not only established the presence of art therapy with residents, but also piqued the interest of staff.

Within a month of the start of the fledgling art therapy program, I gave a brief presentation on the nature of art therapy and its applicability to this particular resident population at a general staff meeting. This proved beneficial in removing some of the "mystique" of art therapy and resulted in better use of the program by the staff. Later in the year, I presented a full-day program to the entire staff. This program used slides of client work. From the beginning of my tenure, the staff was eager to learn about art therapy and willing to utilize art therapy adjunctively in their own work.

Throughout my stay at the shelter, art therapy was used specifically as individual primary and adjunctive therapy, as an assessment tool for establishing personal resources and motivation, as family therapy, as individual child therapy, as group therapy, and as a means of promoting house cohesiveness.

Given the crisis nature of this population, I found it awkward in the first stages of primary counseling to include the use of art. The women needed very practical advice regarding community resources, advocacy rights, vocational counseling, apartment hunting, and the resolution of other crisis needs before being able to consider artistic expression. It wasn't until the woman felt safe in her new environment, had settled her children in school, and had generally begun to set up her priorities of short-range goals that we were able to turn our attention to visual communication (see Maslow's Hierarchy of Needs, Newman & Newman, 1984).

The application of art therapy to mandatory weekly support sessions proved to be an effective tool in terms of education, identification of feelings, and, in general, an enjoyable engagement with the art-making process itself, oftentimes evoking hidden feelings as well as latent talents.

EXAMPLES

Characteristics of the Abuser

One highly successful project was a 4-week study of the general character and personality traits of both the abuser and the victim. The art project evolved out of an expressed and repeated concern of the women regarding their mistrust in their own personal ability to identify potentially abusive personal relationships in the future. Most women were resolved never to get into a repeat of abuse and felt the only assurance they had was to mistrust all men.

Week 1

We began by listing the traits of their abusers on a large posterlike sheet. Many commonalities were discovered, and such comments as "My husband and your boyfriend sound like twins," and "It sounds like you must have known my husband" served to strengthen the concept that there is a pattern.

This project was repeated with different groups, and those traits that freely came up were: aggressive, manipulative, intelligent, moody, easily irritated, secretive, childlike, easily hurt, selfish, liar, split personality, dependent, noncommunicative, charming, powerful, untrustworthy, lived in a fantasy world, sexually satisfying or aggressive, insecure, exploitive, kind, generous, unpredictable, penitent, lovable, addicted to alcohol, drugs, or work, demanding, demeaning, irresponsible, and can't seem to connect emotionally.

Week 2

The following week I brought back the trait chart and again placed in on the wall. In addition, I had come in prepared with a life-size body tracing of a male. This had been rolled up and, with the help of masking tape, placed on the wall next to the chart prior to the meeting.

I recapped what we had discussed the previous week and when the timing was appropriate, released the tape so that the full-size image stood among them. The impact was powerful and mixed, with the women expressing a sense of anxiety at having a "man" present in the room as well as a sense of longing in recognizing they had lost a significant person in their lives.

Each woman was asked to close her eyes and quietly think of one or two traits among all of those listed that she felt best described her abuser. They were then asked to express these symbolically in artwork. Then each was asked to place her symbol, which was either drawn or cut out of a magazine, in an appropriate place on the image.

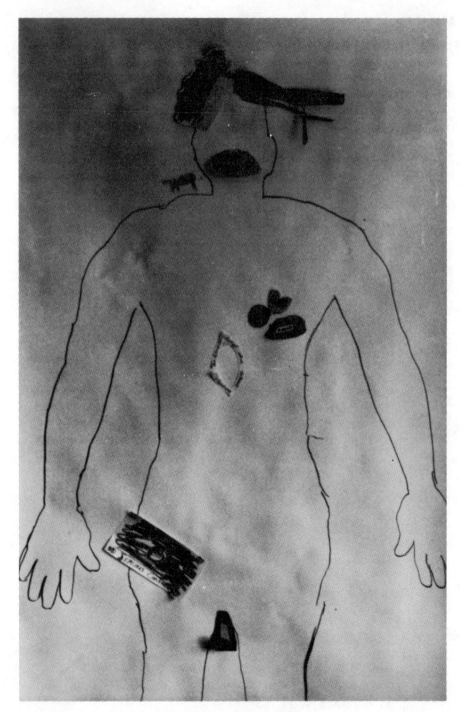

Figure 5.1. ''Noodle Brain.''

Figure 5.1 shows one woman's depiction of her husband as a "noodle brain," symbolizing his irresponsibility. Another woman had difficulty deciding where her symbol of the abuser's temper was to be placed on the figure. She put it first on his hands, then his brain, and finally settled on the mouth. Another group member placed a help symbol with an arrow pointing to the mouth. To her this represented the confusing dual nature of the abuser, who would first lash out at her and then solicit her help. This put her in the position of being a victim responsible for nurturing her own victimizer.

When this particular project was repeated later with other groups, I found that the slight variation of suggesting to the women that they work directly on the male image allowed for greater ease and freedom than making symbols separately and taping them onto the image. I have also found that in those groups whose abusers showed greater ability to be kind and sensitive as well as to be abusive, the women seemed more conflicted and offered reasons and excuses for the abusive nature. Such comments as "I know he didn't mean to do it," "He's really a nice person when he's not going crazy," or "He was really sorry afterward" were not uncommon.

Figure 5.2 shows evidence of a greater sense of freedom and spontaneity of symbols drawn directly onto the male image as opposed to being cut out separately and placed on the image. The two faces symbolize the angry–kind nature to be found in many abusers. The beanie with propeller placed on the head refers to his childlike quality of needing to be taken care of. Numerous question marks symbolize his unpredictability and inability to understand and control his own mood changes. The wristwatch symbolizes the abuser's selfish need to base his actions on his own timing, rather than the needs of other people involved. The black diamond-shaped heart is both jailed and bleeding, symbolizing to the woman his inaccessibility and hurt. The second heart and the bleeding hands again refer to the abuser's capability of being both good and bad.

Characteristics of the Victim

Week 3

During the third week, the chart showing the traits and the male image were placed again on the wall. Our agenda this week was to focus on the woman's personal traits. This focusing on the self was somewhat more difficult but proved beneficial.

The personal traits of the victims that appeared repeatedly were: passive, nurturer, afraid to rock the boat, hopeless, responsible, insecure, expectations of improvement, sense of humor, childlike, loss of confidence, fear of hurting others, wishful thinking, fear of being alone, lack of money, feeling of being used, afraid of him and his temper, off balance about his moods, naive, sense of guilt.

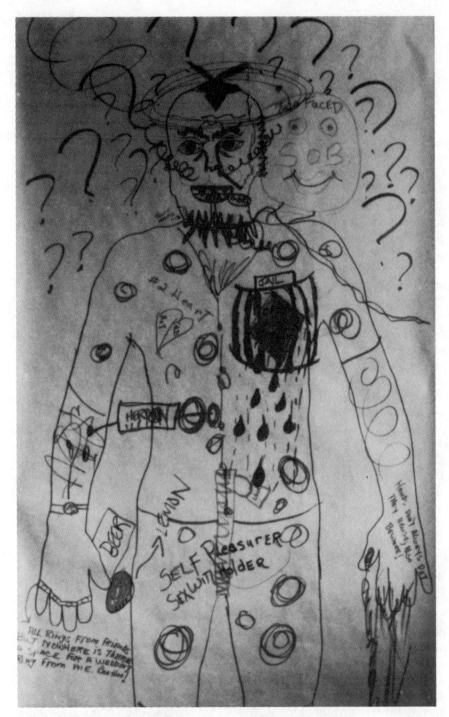

Figure 5.2. Abuser characteristics applied directly to figure.

Weeks 3 and 4

During our fourth session, after I recapped the victim characteristics, the women established a quiet time for centering, and they were asked to own one or two of the listed traits that they felt best applied to themselves. At the appropriate time, a female image was released from a rolled position on the wall and they created symbols for their own traits.

Figure 5.3 shows a smile the woman labeled a sense of humor, and later described as placating. A boat depicts the need not to rock the boat, and a female form was placed next to it with the comment that the woman had shown no backbone. A symbol for vulnerability was placed in the pelvic area and resembled ovaries.

Figure 5.4 shows a bleeding nose, downturned mouth, and long stream of tears, along with the somatic disorders resulting from being encased by the "all heart" symbol.

The next facet of the project was sometimes included in Week 4 and sometimes carried over into Week 5.

The project was brought further by discussing how the abuser and victim traits created a kind of lock and key situation. This was made visual by having each person select a piece of yarn and trace it from her trait to her symbol. She continued to carry the yarn to his symbol and trait. As these strands were put into place, there was created a tangled, enmeshed mess that graphically depicted the fettered, stuck, paralyzing aspect of the relationship (Fig. 5.5). While it was generally more difficult for the women to explore their own contribution to the dysfunctional relationship, the insight that eventually came as they viewed the correlation and enmeshment provoked much discussion.

During subsequent group sessions, it was not infrequent for the women to refer to the symbol that served as a quick reminder of all that the abuser represented.

The power of this art project to put abused women in touch with the reality of the situation was significant. Prior to this project, the women repeatedly expressed the desire and fantasy that "another chance" might make things better. After this, they seemed to be more in touch with the reality of the abusive personality. Whether or not they would return to their former situation or become involved in a similar situation would now, perhaps, at least have the dimension of an informed choice. A crack had probably been made in the denial system.

Confusion of Anger and Helplessness

The denial of anger and the minimization of the abusiveness directed at them have been well documented in the writing of Walker (1979, 1984). These repeatedly surfaced in the art expression of abused women.

In order to have some grasp of where the women were coming from, one of my initial projects was a guided imagery that invited them to recapture

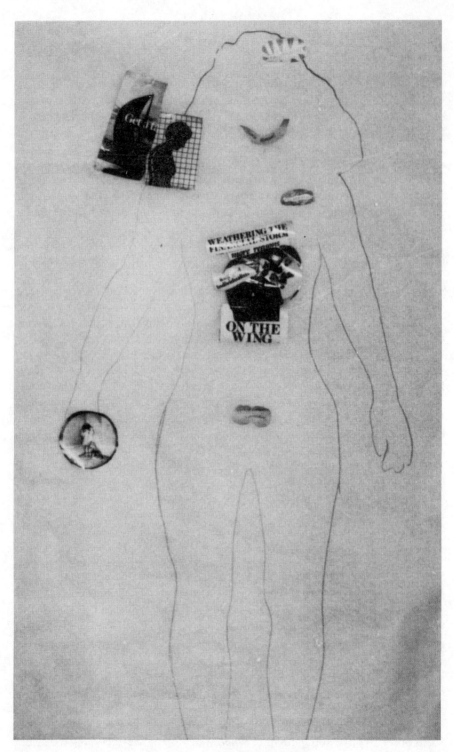

Figure 5.3. Victim characteristics.

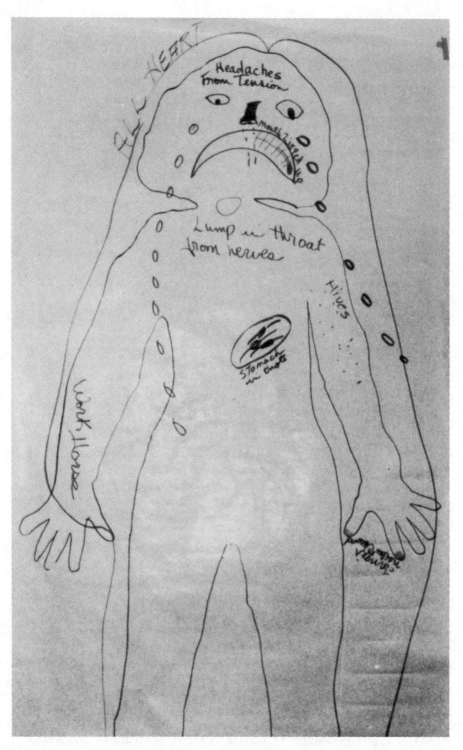

Figure 5.4. Victim characteristics.

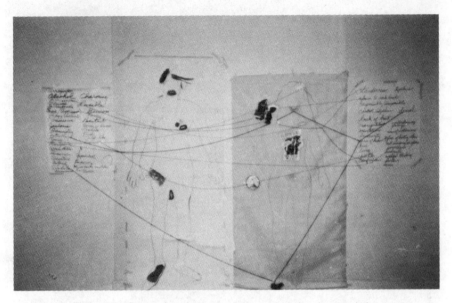

Figure 5.5. Connections between abuser and victim characteristics.

their earliest memory. The visualization continued in incremental 5-year blocks of time, and they were slowly brought back to the present moment.

The abused women were then requested to create a visual life line by using art to communicate the images that had come forth for them. The result was surprising to me. The artwork of the women depicted, with very few exceptions, the recollection of only pleasant memories. Yet, as we processed what their early family life had been like for them, it was obvious that most had experienced great anxiety, stresses, and traumatic physical or psychological abuse.

Anger

Generally, there was an inability of the women to get in touch with their anger. I came to recognize that there was a lack of understanding of what, in fact, had happened to them. Many believed that abuse was a part of life they would have to accept, that they must be failing in their role as women who can make their men happy. They had been, as one person said, "in a hell of a war, and didn't even know it."

Artistically, this expression was made clear. When situations occurred during the course of treatment where women expressed anger, they were encouraged to use art. In most situations, despite a wide range of art materials, the women selected pencil as their medium of expression. This in itself showed a timidity in expressing anger.

Denise, a 16-year-old, was angry about the many adult women residents who were, she felt, imposing their restrictions and judgments on her. She

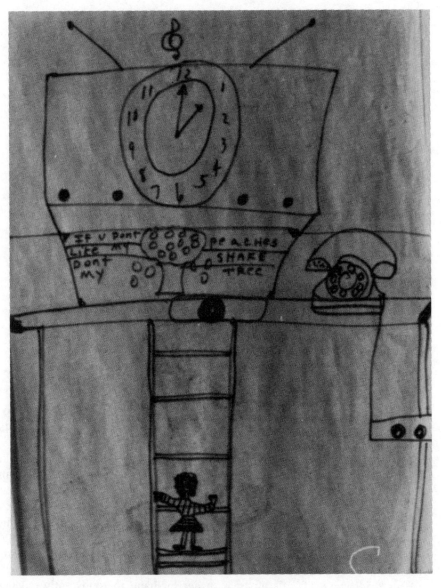

Figure 5.6. Lisa's anger.

reacted to the situation by throwing her books down to the floor and running up the stairs to get away from the residents. Her artwork depicted tiny, pencil-drawn hands on the lower left side of the large sheet of paper. Her sense of helplessness was apparent.

In Figure 5.6, Lisa's depiction of her anger also centered on her feelings of helplessness. She had recalled being furious with her husband because

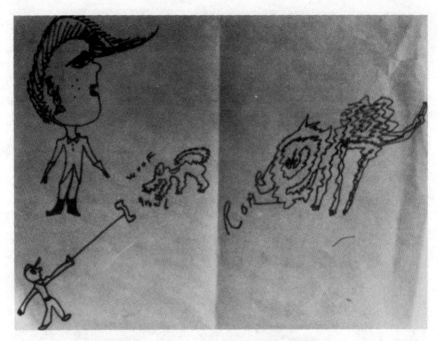

Figure 5.7. Lisa's identification with the family dog.

she was always subject to his needs and wants and oftentimes denied simple privileges of communal living, like a joint decision on which television program to watch, or the use of the phone without his permission. The objects loom large in Figure 5.6.

As we processed this anger, Lisa was asked to express what she would like to do to her husband. Her drawing depicted a ¼-inch black square in the center of a sheet of 18-by-24-inch paper. She stated "I'd like to put him in a real small box with no room for him to move. But I'd put some airholes in it so he could breathe, because he's human." Lisa's drawings and comments seem to confirm Walker's (1979, 1984) work, which describes the women as only wanting the abuse to stop, and not desiring retaliation or vindication.

Figure 5.7 shows Lisa's anger with her husband for constantly teasing the family dog. She identified herself as the dog on the far right, whose escape wish is to be like the rock star, upper left, who symbolizes the freedom to "do his own thing."

In Figure 5.8, Diane, who was angry about house issues and policies, drew herself as handcuffed and powerless. When asked if she could relate it to similar feelings from the past, she responded with Figure 5.9. In this drawing, Diane, as a child, was placed in a stuffed chair and forced to listen

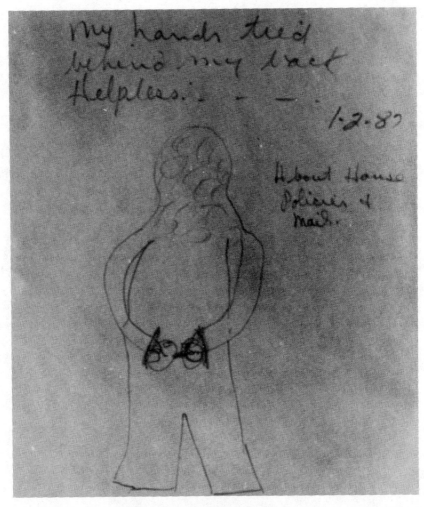

Figure 5.8. Diane's feelings of powerlessness.

to her mother's devaluating comments. It is interesting to note how much her mother's finger resembles a gun.

Two months later, Diane was frantically seeking housing for herself and children, and with only 10 days left in her shelter situation, she expressed her anger toward a landlord who had reneged on his promise of an apartment. This time, her art expression depicted the landlord on the road, hit by a car to his right (Fig. 5.10). Just to be sure of his demise, she had another car hit him from the left. She used bright colors now and, in fact, had green blood flowing from him to show how "rotten" he was. Diane was beginning to acknowledge her anger more openly through a safe medium.

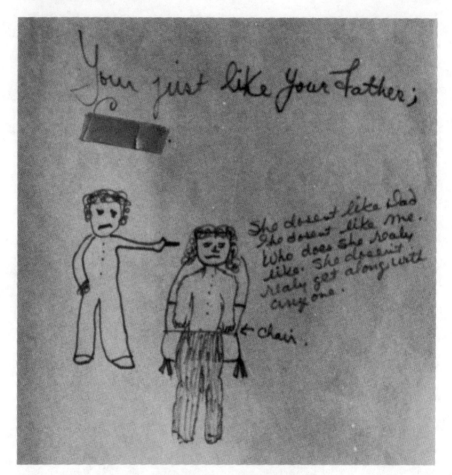

Figure 5.9. Diane and her mother.

Does a Woman Unknowingly Contribute to Her Own Victimization?

During a counseling session, Holly, who had been making great progress, expressed feeling "strange and uneasy." She was unable to express it more clearly, and I encouraged her as she left the session to take art materials with her and use them. The next time I saw her, she shared her "doodle" with me (Fig. 5.11). Her affect was somewhat silly and her verbal statement about the art was "It doesn't mean anything." This piece was unlike anything Holly had done before. It was a collection of random, disjointed parts. I thought it important to know something about the sequence of the piece and had her describe how it was made. It was only after a subsequent event took place that I recognized more completely what Holly was communicating. The shelter was structured around a system that imposed warnings for infractions of house policy. When a specified number of warnings were ac-

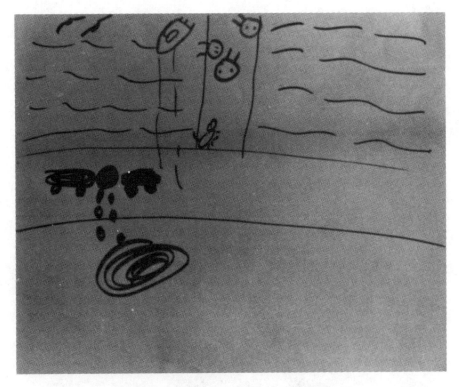

Figure 5.10. Diane's anger at her landlord.

crued, a woman was asked to leave. Holly's infractions for not doing chores by a specified time left her only one remaining warning with still 2 weeks to go in her 3-month stay. Apparently, not knowing when or whether she would be required to leave created unbearable tension for her, and shortly after expressing it in this picture, Holly, in a seemingly deliberate gesture, broke a rule and was asked to leave. Was there a relief in putting an end to the anxiety of the next 2 weeks?

Holly's artwork depicts a cigarette lighter just beneath a balloon and topped by an explosion. Nearby is a large wall clock, perhaps the most prominent object in the piece, like the clock that hung in the shelter living room. Although these elements had not been drawn in sequence, they somehow fell into meaningful place for me after her infraction.

Holly's work brought to my mind the words of Lenore Walker regarding the abused woman: "Sometimes she precipitates the inevitable explosion so as to control where and when it occurs, allowing her to take better precautions to minimize her injuries and pain" (1984, p. 96).

It was time for staff to examine and evaluate our existing system. Were we somehow recreating abuse in a shelter dedicated to offering the woman a safe place from abuse?

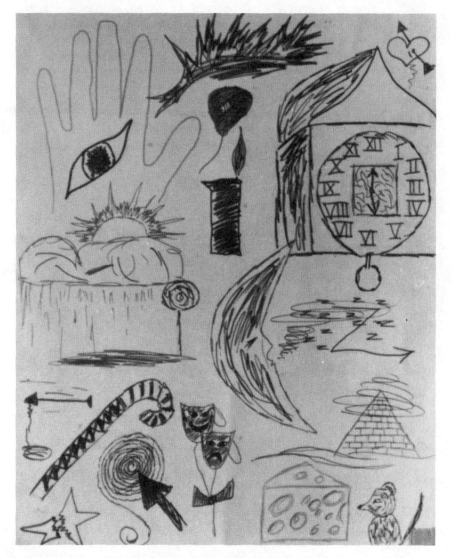

Figure 5.11. Holly's doodle.

Art Making Helps Abused Women Grow in Self-Esteem

As art therapy sessions continued, the women were able to review their progress over time. They began to identify existing strengths and capabilities and to recognize their capacity to take risks toward the unfamiliar. Upon leaving the shelter, each woman was asked to portray what she was leaving behind that she no longer wanted and what she was taking with her as a new-found strength.

Sharon's collage showed a man and woman hiding behind the theatrical masks depicting tragedy and comedy and bore the words "leaving behind gullibleness and taking self-confidence." It was a simple and powerful statement.

The Children's Art

A common element that ran through the artwork and counseling sessions was a naïveté about what constitutes abuse. Many mothers were not aware of the impact of environmental abuse upon their children. They would frequently continue to endure personal abuse in an attempt to provide the children with a father and sense of family. The children's art images and issues of concern regarding monsters, weapons, and identification with the aggressor or the victim were valuable tools in helping the women to understand this impact of abuse on the children.

Several cases of incest were revealed through the trust relationship established in art therapy. Once the incest was revealed, family art therapy sessions were started to make the entire family openly aware of the problem and to build on family strengths. Older teens, especially girls, utilized family art therapy to help in gaining an awareness and understanding of how victimization occurred and how it affected their present and future lives.

DISCUSSION

As is stated repeatedly in the literature, abused women need to let go of the fantasy of being able to change or control the abusive behavior, mourn the loss of their hopes and dreams for a wonderful family life, and experience the freedom from an abusive situation and have the opportunity to explore new personal strengths. The making of art and the processing of that art address these areas.

First, art making helped the women get in touch with the reality of their situation. By using art to explore abuser and victim traits and by creating a meaningful symbol for themselves, the abused women began a confrontation with the reality of the true personalities of both victim and abuser and a letting go of the fantasy of singlehandedly being able to change the situation. As stated by Walker (1984), "It may be that battered women do believe they can control their own lives. Battered women often manipulate the environment in order to minimize the opportunity for the batterer to find a reason to be angry" (p. 79). She continues:

> It may be this sense of internal control that is the hope which allows the battered women to believe she will be able to change the batterer or the environment in such a way that things will get better. . . . When in a violent relationship she becomes so involved in doing whatever it takes to keep the batterer happy

that she thinks this is being in control. The reality is that he does have control by keeping her in fear of receiving another beating if she doesn't keep him from getting angry.

Once the woman becomes aware of the futility of her efforts, she can begin to move away from the repetition cycle. Second, in addition to fostering feelings of self-worth, awareness, breaking of the denial system, and repressed affect and isolation, art helped the women to monitor their own progress over time. Third, communication expressed through the residents' artwork can help the shelter staff to monitor how effectively they are meeting the needs of the residents. Art evaluations helped staff to understand better the capabilities and motivations of clients so that pertinent issues could be addressed more readily. Art products confirmed and broadened staff findings and at times even heralded information that would become clear later in treatment. We learned together that art therapy is not only relevant but also important and empowering during crisis situations. Fourth, to make best use of the brief time women stay within the shelter, a series of structured and progressive art endeavors can be developed.

Norwood (1985), has developed progress and recovery cycles similar to the graphic curve that charts the alcoholic in his or her addiction and recovery. Just as art therapy has been successfully used in a structured way to break through the denial component of the disease of alcohol, I believe art therapists can structure a series of art tasks to break down the minimization of abuse that is part of the abuser–victim phenomenon. To continue with further possibilities, if funds and space allowed, another important facet of a comprehensive art program could be a drop-in studio. This would allow the women an opportunity to structure their own time, and most importantly, to find new creative ways of exploring themselves and their environment. With the presence of an art therapist, these drop-in sessions could act as an extension of therapy sessions. If using the studio unsupervised, the women could choose any form of art expression including craft work. There is an element of healing even in making ashtrays or wall hangings. They can be symbols for the preparation the women must make for the journey and resettlement ahead.

Abused women are struggling with issues of guilt, anxiety, anger, loss, and fear. Their personal art expressions, in or outside of therapy, can be helpful in processing these feelings. Their art products can serve as objects and reminders of a time when they heroically made the quantum leap to save themselves.

CONCLUSION

The problems of the abused women in a state of crisis are manifold. The resolution of her situation is not simple. The helping profession needs to be creative in its approaches for effective intervention.

The abused woman needs more than shelter if she is to break the repetition cycle. She needs to be educated to the identification and recognition of the devastating effects of abuse. She needs to be counseled, to be offered assertiveness training, parenting skills, vocational counseling, stress management, and personal health care information.

Art therapy can take its place in the shelter system by touching all of these areas. Art therapy can continue to assist the abused woman after she has left the shelter by patiently helping to guide her own personal center and life-sustaining spirit. In sum, art therapy can prove to be an effective educational tool, a vehicle for insight, a strong impetus toward self-affirmation and improved communication skills. It is a creative means for identification and expression of affect for the abused woman.

Research has shown that women frequently practice leaving an abusive situation from three to eight times before they actually leave permanently, unless effective intervention takes place. Ultimately, the woman must decide for herself, based on her own personal and situational needs and capabilities, whether to leave or return to the abuser. Whether she decides to stay or to leave, therapeutic intervention and the use of art can assist the woman in finding her own strength and resolve for self-concern and dignity.

This chapter is offered with the hope of challenging the creativity of those working with this newly recognized segment of society. It is another area in which art making can become meaningful in the lives of individuals and the structure of society.

REFERENCES

Aguilera, D., & Messick, J. (1986). *Crisis intervention: Theory and methodology*. St. Louis: Mosby.

Forward, S., & Torres, J. (1986). *Men who hate women and the women who love them: When loving hurts and you don't know why*. New York: Bantam.

Malchiodi, C. A., & Peterson, I. R. (1985). *Creative art modalities with children from violent homes*. Communications Art Department, Cardinal Stretch College, Milwaukee.

Newman, B., & Newman, P. (1984). *Development through life: A psychosocial approach*. Homewood, IL: Dorsey Press.

Norwood, R. (1985). *Women who love too much: When you keep wishing and hoping he'll change*. Los Angeles: Tarcher.

Puryear, R. (1979). *Helping people in crisis*. San Francisco: Josey-Bass.

Shainess, N. (1984). *Sweet suffering: Woman as victim*. New York: Bobbs-Merrill.

Spring, D. (1985). Symbolic language of sexually abused, chemically dependent women. *American Journal of Art Therapy, 24*, 13.

Walker, L. (1979). *The battered woman*. New York: Harper & Row.

Walker, L. (1984). *The battered woman syndrome*. New York: Springer.

Wohl, A., & Kaufman, B. (1985). *Silent screams and hidden cries*. New York: Brunner/Mazel.

CHAPTER 6

The Arts in Therapy with Survivors of Incest

This chapter reports the evolution of a sexual abuse group whose members moved from victim to survivor using the arts in therapy. The arts in therapy and the group process address directly the main dysfunction of the abused victim's psyche: disintegration. Victims have fragmented and isolated minds, bodies, and hearts[1] from themselves and others in an attempt to create safety through repression and denial: "What I don't know won't hurt me." When victims can no longer tolerate the pain of alienation from self and others and are ready to choose a more meaningful life, they may seek help. The arts in therapy is a process in which victims help themselves to unblock, to gather together fractioned parts and become whole.

In group, the arts in therapy process helps victims undergo the transformation process toward integration. The spontaneous act of seeing, hearing, and feeling themselves promotes catharsis, healing, and integration. The sharing of trauma through the arts process creates cohesion and safety leading to early group trust. Victim survival strategy includes extreme intellectualization, the numbing of emotions, and body rigidity as an early defense against intrusion. Enactment in the arts is a catalyst to bypass intellectualization. Victims gain a new sense and understanding of themselves through the relaxation of defenses and the reduction of anxiety in role playing, body work, visualization, drawing, and sculpting. The group sharing of the secret, the surrounding pain and anger, leads to validation from the group and eventual self-validation as the trauma victim begins to understand, "If this happened to her, maybe I'm not so bad."

---

[1]In this chapter, *body, mind,* and *heart* are used to refer to action and sexuality, reason and judgment, emotion and feeling respectively.

114

GROUP FORMATION AND STRUCTURE

This particular group had two leaders, a survivor of incest and a nonvictim. One therapist had a basic understanding of the arts in therapy but considered herself primarily a verbal therapist. I am an artist and expressive therapist with a working knowledge of psychotherapy. My co-therapist recognized many victims of sexual abuse on her normal outpatient caseload and offered group treatment. I proposed the use of the arts in therapy and offered to co-lead the group.

The group started with six members, adding a member in the fourth session. This member did not continue beyond what was for her a third session. The group met weekly for 25 sessions with each session lasting for 1 hour and 45 minutes.

The arts in therapy process was introduced the first session, and members were told it would be an integral part of the program. Most sessions began with a warm-up exercise, a middle working period with the arts and verbal processing of feelings of about 1 hour, followed by a time of wrap-up or ending. Because focus of the group was sexual abuse, we had an agenda with goals to help members move through the process. We checked in with clients and clients checked in with each other at the beginning of every session. If there were unresolved feelings from the prior group or ones that had come up in the interim that needed attending to immediately, therapists worked with those needs. Sometimes the planned arts process and thera- peutic goal for that session could be included and sometimes they could not. Most processes and all goals were attended to and worked within the natural evolution of the group by the termination date.

Most of the clients had experienced either exploitation or abandonment in their families. They brought this experience and continued expectation with them to the group. This initially caused collusion to suppress affect and gain control. Part of our earlier sessions' warm-ups included the formation of a circle where members could experience equality, safety, cooperation, protection, and nonthreatening touch.

Many sessions ended with a circle after group cohesion had been estab- lished. This, I believe, was a natural evolution of the group's progress. After having shared strong emotions intensively the group members needed to touch one another in sympathy and caring, and also perhaps to form a nonverbal symbol of containment.

At the closure of each session, we processed how the group was for each member, any new cognitive insights that had occurred, and the feelings and tensions in each person's body. The attention to mind, body, and heart at the end of each session helped to remind members of the integrating process as they moved in a cooperative venture toward wholeness.

THE MEMBERS

The ages of the six members in the group ranged from 19 to 36. All had experienced incest as an introduction to sexuality. The start of the abuse occurred for most victims between 3 and 5. Two members were first molested at the onset of puberty. The abuse for most victims ended when the woman left her parents' home. In one case this occurred at age 32, just 2 weeks before her marriage. The extent of the abuse varied from occasional incidents of breast fondling to digital and penal penetration of the vagina.

Two group members had experienced physical as well as sexual abuse. There were two cases of multigenerational abuse. For one woman, the sexual abuse was a "heritage" from her grandmother. All of the members were adamant about stopping the pattern with themselves and were vigilant protectors of their daughters. The women with the most intense and longest history of abuse were the most fragmented, defended, and powerless.

Along with fractioning of mind, body, and emotions, physical rigidity and tension, all members experienced nightmares and insomnia. Hypervigilance and a sense of extreme vulnerability included great fear of being alone in their homes to the extent of not answering a knock on their door. Many were careful of how they positioned themselves in bed to avoid repeating a position in which they had been molested.

While all had been their families' caretakers, they were extremely negligent in caring for themselves as they had a sense of being contaminated, "a bad person," and were therefore unworthy. It was easy for them to nurture others as this act allowed them some power and control, but they were unable to nurture themselves.

A commonality among victims is a distortion of body image. All of the women felt themselves to be ugly. While negation of self, actualized in bulimia and anorexia, is common for sexually abused victims, this condition was not an issue among the women in this group, though many reported problems with being overweight and had multiple hospitalizations for stomach and gynecological problems. One woman at age 36 had had 32 serious operations in these areas. Several members were overweight. Lacking the ability, because of poor self-esteem, to set limits with another's exploitation of them, they used their weight as a boundary. One woman had made three suicide attempts and all verbalized that if they could not get help, taking their life was an option they thought about.

Only one of the victims upon disclosure of the sexual abuse was believed by her mother. At 3 years of age, she was molested by a 19-year-old neighbor. She was taken to court where she was not validated by the male judge who, in fact, found her at fault for being seductive. In her teens, this same woman was approached and eventually molested by her mother's alcoholic boyfriend. Her mother did not believe or protect her this time. Not having their stories of sexual abuse believed by their mothers made all members feel inadequate, impotent, and lonely. They suffered from a sense of neglect and rejection. All had a deep yearning for an emotional reunion with their mothers, by whom they had been abandoned.

TABLE 6.1.   The Arts in Therapy as Integrator—Beginning Stage

Process—Action	Process—Verbal
Draw a group you feel safe in.	Group spoke of alienation, fear, lack
All members drew a *single figure* in a threatening natural environment.	of safety, and vulnerability.
Body work. Form a circle. Hold hands. Touch shoulders.	Spoke of body contact avoidance, fear of intrusion, relationships.
Some members tactually defensive, others intrusive.	
Clay. Represent yourself and your mother in clay. Can be symbolic or figurative.	Invalidation by mother. Invalidation of self. Abandonment. Blurred boundaries in family. Caretaker of family as child. Confusion.
Members struggle with process. Two refuse. Those that participate create caves, an imbalanced seesaw, a stern, towering, unapproachable mother and tiny, clinging child.	
Body work. Form a group of three. Middle person allows others to support arms—middle person is rocked back and forth. Exchange places.	Relationships—power and control issues. Some members comment on comfort of the session.
Initially some members very hesitant, rigid. Eventually, nearly all allow others to support them.	

GOALS

Self-stated goals in therapy were to reduce depression and anxiety, and to increase trust and the quality and quantity of relationships with both males and females. All of the members at the beginning of the group, with the exception of one woman, were married, had children, and were caretakers and homemakers. They lived quiet, isolated, and constricted lives in their communities, rigidly relating only within their families and within the contexts of their roles as wives and mothers, where they allowed themselves to be imposed upon and in some cases exploited.

Our goals included helping members to increase self-esteem, to empower themselves, to vent anger, to share their sadness, to grieve, and to integrate body, mind, and heart.

As the individual group members moved from the position of victim to that of survivor, they became much more aware of their entire selves, how dysfunctional they were, and how dissatisfied they were with the way they lived their lives. As the members gained strength from the group and began to empower themselves, they proposed and acted upon many new goals, most of which involved communication and interaction with others.

Tables 6.1, 6.2, and 6.3 describe a sampling of the activities that were incorporated into the group during the beginning, middle, and termination stages of the groups' development.

TABLE 6.2.   The Arts in Therapy as Integrator—Middle Stage

Process—Action	Process—Verbal
Draw walls around yourself. Walls of rock, brick, wooden fences. Most drawings of a figure. Most drawings showed ways to get through or around structure.	Spoke of isolation. Reluctance to leave house or allow others in. Feelings of inadequacy. Frustration in personal relationships. Body weight as boundaries or walls. Members help one another see and find ways to get through or around walls.
Draw yourself when you feel adequate or inadequate. "Adequate" generally represented by communication with others. Single figures tended to be sad, withdrawn, or "made of fluff."	Spoke of inadequacy, sadness, anger, and power. Formulation of individual goals. Support from group verbalized.
Body work. Choose a partner. Push gently back and forth with open hands. Use shoulders—push harder. Struggle with body weight against each other. Body contact in a tentative fashion in beginning. With more struggle, some removed selves, others worked hard.	Inadequacy, fear of being overwhelmed, feeling own power. New personal decisions of empowerment shared.
Psychodrama. Choose a partner. One will say "yes," and one will say "no." Exchange positions. Continue with "I want to," "I'm sorry, you can't."	Easier to say yes than no. Directly in touch with abuse and abuser. All share present feelings for perpetrator and much support for participant with empty chair. Members leave together after therapy session for the first time.

Note: A distinct change in group after above session. Next few therapy sessions centered on patterns of abuse and how to change them. Anger and impotency with mates. Suicide. Group and self-affirmation.

TOWARD INTEGRATION

As Table 6.4 shows, members moved from alienation and isolation as victims to an eventual place of empowerment as survivors. Using the arts in therapy helped members to understand and resolve unconscious conflict. Art produces a concrete visual image of the problem. The members of the sexual abuse group could see while processing artwork that they were separated from their bodies and that the parts were separated from one another. The members pointed out to one another that most heads were removed from the bodies by the use of either color or space. They drew attention to the fact that arms and legs were missing and asked one another the meaning of that. They questioned the blackness of genital and abdominal regions. Gradually, victims became aware of their fractioned parts. They realized the absence of arms and legs represented the helplessness they felt. Awareness became the first step toward recovery.

TABLE 6.3.   The Arts in Therapy as Integrator—Termination Stage

Process—Action	Process—Verbal
Guided Imagery to Drawing. Relax. Visualize body parts, find tension. Draw part that needs relaxing/attention. Drawings of backs, stomachs and abdomens, heads.	Body images, discomfort with illness, and somatization of emotions. Numbing of body parts.
Art (two sessions). Visualize color in body parts. Replicate body with construction paper. General anxiety. All members separate head from body either with color or in space. Many fractioned all body parts from one another. Many represented genital region as black.	Lack of integration of body—lack of integration of body, mind, heart, and how it is possible to integrate. All supportive of one another.
Guided Imagery—Art. Relaxation. Visualization of color in body as healing force. Draw color throughout body. General color flow throughout, no gap or separation of line.	General discussion of giving to self. Improved body images and positive feedback from others.
Draw your child self. Many spontaneous drawings of pleasure, joy: children on swings, playing together, etc.	Spoke of playfulness and spontaneity versus fear and blocking. Discussion of many selves and of risk taking.

As members of the group moved from the position of victim to the stature of survivor, the changes in body posture and chosen positions in the room were striking. In the initial stages of the group, members were very withdrawn, made poor eye contact with others, and displayed slouched, constricted, and avoidant posture. The victims with the longest history of abuse chose the far corners of the room.

Gradually this changed. As members felt the nurturing quality of the group, they relaxed their vigilant stance and allowed others in. Once they felt safe and less isolated, the constriction of body, mind, and heart lessened. They slowly freed themselves and simultaneously reached out to one another. Arts in therapy was an important part of this process. It allowed the women to see themselves as they created a concrete visual image, an image that was often painful but one that could be shared. The image of the pain promoted catharsis, and the group held out its loving arms to enfold and nurture. Many in this group space actually felt others' nurturing for the first time. The nurturing acted as a creative catalyst for change.

Each member internalized strength as she became able to receive and give to the group. The recognition, through the arts, of being "stuck" in old roles and patterns created dissatisfaction. As the women helped to empower one another, they started visualizing and trying out new roles for themselves.

The creative act of art calls forth a creative response to the act of living. As previous deadened responses to life were understood, energy was freed

TABLE 6.4. Stages of Movement in Group with Sexually Abused Victims

	Beginning Stage	Middle Stage	Termination Stage
Body: Seat of action and sexuality	Isolates self from others Isolates self from self: body—mind—heart Rigid, tense Tactilely defensive Hypervigilant Weight as protection Distorts body image Self-abusive	Allows others in—extends self to others Recognizing fractioning of body from heart and mind Relaxation of tension begins Decrease of vigilance More body awareness—weight loss begins	Become therapists for one another Integration of body with mind and heart begun Spontaneity Acceptance and appreciation of more positive body image
Mind: Seat of reason and judgment	Powerless Self-negating, judgmental Conflicted Controlled, critical Victim Extreme separation from body and heart Nightmares	Safety in group Establishing self-goals Confusion Recognition of strength in others Increase in self-esteem Letting go of mental anguish	Taking own power Ability to take risks Achievement of universality Commitment and working through goals Responsibility for self Move toward independence Survivor
Heart: Seat of emotion and feeling	Powerless, vulnerable Inadequate Depressed, guilty, sad Controlled, unresponsive Fearful and impotent Alienated Group collusion to suppress feelings	Trust with group established Accept nurturance of others Sadness increases Struggle with self and group: control vs. spontaneity Anger	Can love and nurture self Trusts self Absence of guilt Spontaneity of feelings

up for living in a new way. The enactment of new roles freed creativity further.

As previously mentioned, all members, with one exception, were caretakers and homemakers. This was the only role in which they felt safe and from which they were able to derive satisfaction. Through the process of the group, the women wanted to expand the range of talents they possessed and experience more of life. After having released some of the power of negative relationships, they were ready to deepen present intimate relationships and to seek out and begin new ones.

CASE EXAMPLES

EDNA

The mother of two children whose husband was confined to a wheelchair, Edna had dreams of running her own certified childcare center. Her husband, because of his disability, was often short tempered and intolerant of any noise or disruption. Before entering the group, Edna had relegated her desire to become more independent to the realm of fantasy. Through the group process, she was much more in touch with her needs and was empowered to act on them. She announced to her husband that she indeed intended to apply for certification and that he needed to make his own arrangements and plans as several more children would soon be occupying the kitchen and living room for a certain number of hours each week. Edna followed through with her plans and her husband outfitted their car to suit his needs and followed his own interests outside of the house. In follow-up sessions with her individual therapist, Edna reported that both she and her husband were much more satisfied with their life and with one another.

DEBRA

Debra's family of origin were very insistent on her remaining their caretaker even though she now had her own family with two children. Debra felt emotionally and physically drained by their imposition and especially angry with her father who still acted in a seductive manner toward her.

Debra described "Drawing of Myself as Inadequate" (Fig. 6.1) in poetry:

A feeling of incompleteness
A height that can't be reached
A soul full of woe
Ashamed for what you don't know
Trying is never enough
For those who are made of fluff.

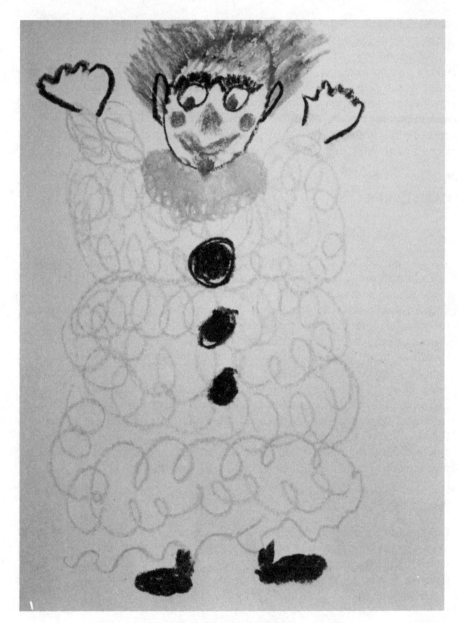

Figure 6.1. "Drawing of Myself as Inadequate," by Debra.

Her drawing is that of a clown, whom she described as presenting a laughing face for the world but who is made of nothingness, "fluff," on the inside.

Meeting everyone else's needs prior to the group made her feel adequate, but depleted and exhausted as her drawing (Fig. 6.2) depicts. She said the word *throb* that circles her head represents her heart's yearning for com-

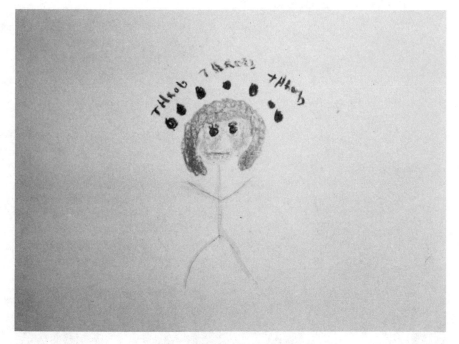

Figure 6.2. "Throb," by Debra.

pletion. Debra was able to get in touch with her feeling through the art process.

Gradually she put limits on her family's demands on her time and energy. She was able to establish firm boundaries with her father and by the group's midpoint would no longer allow him to enter her home without someone else present.

After setting limits with her family of origin, she turned her attention to her family of choice. She recognized that she found her relationship with her husband lacking and together they began to sort through problem areas and work to deepen their intimacy.

Simultaneously, Debra followed her desire to become a writer. By the end of the group, she had begun continuing education courses at the nearest university. She found that she now had a reserve of energy.

DIANNA

Dianna originally had come into couples therapy with her husband. He could not tolerate the new knowledge that she had previously been violated by her father, and he had begun an extramarital affair. After joining the group, she chose to leave the marriage as she could not tolerate further abandonment. Making this choice was extremely heart wrenching for her as she also left her children because she was afraid she could not support them.

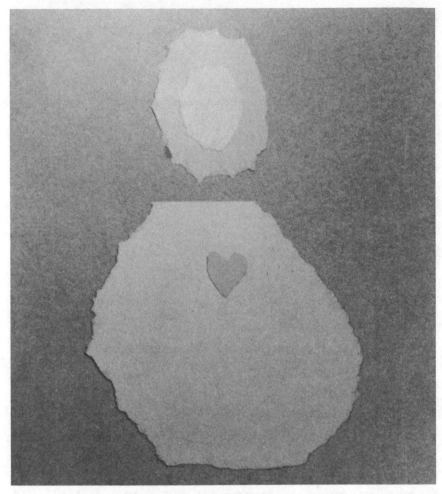

Figure 6.3. Dianna's body parts (facsimile).

Dianna's depiction of her body parts (Fig. 6.3) lacks arms and hands and legs and feet. She felt helplessly stuck. She was aware of her good heart, which is prominent in the artwork. The group commented on her choice of colors: a soft blue ground with yellow and pink trunk and head. Edna, who was involved in child care, asked if the figure represented a baby, as the head appeared to be wearing a bonnet and those color combinations were most often seen in infant wear.

Through the art process in group, Dianna was able to get in touch with her own need to be loved and protected. As she gained clarity and strength, she became increasingly unwilling to leave her children with her husband as she had evidence that they were not being well cared for. Dianna initiated a new court procedure to regain custody of her children and sued her husband for child support. She also found a higher-paying job and a larger apartment for her family.

SUMMARY

This is the history of one group of women: survivors of sexual abuse. They began the group in fear and trepidation; fearful of stirring up long buried terror, the memory of which may again threaten to poison their lives. They were able to grow through the arts in therapy group from victims to survivors.

Starting the group, they felt powerless, empty and vulnerable, impotent and isolated. At the end, although all members still had many issues of anger and sadness that came with the recognition of their losses, they had mastered their terror. Together, they had accepted and nurtured themselves as others had accepted and nurtured them; together, they had empowered one another and accepted their own power to take part in the world and to take risks.

Much of the work toward integration and healing happened through the arts in therapy. It was a living process through which the group members unblocked and opened to themselves. The arts helped them to unify their parts as they saw, heard, felt, and accepted themselves.

This is the story of one sexual abuse group. Every group is an entity unto itself as each member helps to form the whole. Because such work is a living process, the therapist must carefully attend to its pulse, going neither too slowly nor too quickly. Media and material to process must be selected to suit the group's stage of development. A group may be ready to meet the inherent goals and challenges in each working stage more or less quickly than this group. The therapist needs to judge with caution and sensitivity which art process will help the group to move and when to hold back so as not to violate the group's safety. Perhaps some of the processes used here could not be used at all in a particularly fragile group. Perhaps individual members may be well along through individual therapy or have participated in an earlier sexual abuse group so that more advanced body work could benefit its members.

The creativity of the arts helps people to experience themselves anew—it is a living and life-giving process. This particular group was a cooperative venture toward achieving wholeness.

CHAPTER 7

Making Art in a Jail Setting

ELIZABETH STRAIT DAY AND GREGORY THOMAS ONORATO

The correctional arena is one barely explored by art therapy. This chapter discusses art therapy applications to mental health problems typically found in jails. Such problems include adjustment to incarceration, depression, suicidal ideation, and a wide range of pathology as found in nonforensic mental health institutions. Formats for individual and group art therapy with inmates are presented.

LITERATURE REVIEW

The world of art therapy has scarcely penetrated the walls of correctional facilities. Few articles in the art therapy literature address matters particular to the forensic or criminal population. The criminology literature similarly contains a dearth of references to art as a treatment modality for inmate mental health problems.

The few art therapy references on the matter cite art as useful in promoting group cohesiveness and in alleviating stress (Levy, 1978; Marano, 1983; Rylander, 1979; Wadeson, 1987). Art therapy has been used with inmates in solitary confinement to provide a cathartic experience, allowing acceptable expressions of powerful emotions. These inmates were found to have a lower incidence of violent or disruptive behavior as compared to a control group (Rylander, 1979).

Though the art therapy literature is extensive on mental health issues pertinent to corrections, we found no further mention of treatment specifically within correctional facilities. Many mental health problems germane to a forensic population are identical to those found in most mental health facilities. It would be a mistake, however, to neglect the specificity of treatment within the context of the correctional institution. To find art therapy's niche within this setting we must turn to the correctional literature for its identification of treatment issues.

Incarceration is an experience that brings about a myriad of responses within one individual. Most inmates respond with anxiety, anger, hostility,

126

depression, and/or fear (French, 1981; Schneider, 1979). Given that the jail population generally contains individuals with inadequate methods of handling stress, incarceration only exacerbates problems already existing within the individual (Stone, 1984).

Suicide is one of the most prominent problems in correctional facilities. Inmates come from the most suicide-prone subgroup within the population at large (Stone, 1984). Contributing factors include the large number of inmates suffering from mental illness and/or substance abuse, and the low income and educational levels of the overwhelming majority of detainees. At Menard Psychiatric Center, the mental health facility of the Illinois Department of Corrections, an average of eight suicide attempts per month occurred between 1981 and 1984. More than half the institution's population has a history of suicidal behavior (Hardy, 1984).

Jails are pretrial holding centers. Prisoners who are awaiting transfer to prisons following sentencing in particular frequently attempt suicide. The accused offender experiences his or her first loss of freedom in the jail until such time as bail can be posted, or a trial concluded. Frequently, the jail inmate, that is, a pretrial detainee, experiences acute anxiety and depression as a result of his or her arrest and incarceration. Further, the jail inmate may be involuntarily going through drug and or alcohol withdrawal. Pretrial and posttrial anxieties are also stressors unique to the inmate. All these factors contribute to suicidal ideation. Though suicide remains a problem for prisons as well, most prison inmates have adjusted to incarceration by the time they are sentenced. Those who have not are more likely to commit suicide while still in the jail setting (Schneider, 1979).

Gang intimidation and homosexual rape are other constant stressors for both jail and prison inmates. Although the correctional literature refers only fleetingly to the impact of sexual aggressions upon the incarcerated individual (French, 1981), our experience with jail detainees was that these stressors were commonplace. In some instances they were responsible for somatic complaints or other regressive symptomatology including psychosis.

Deinstitutionalization of the mentally ill has resulted in a marked increase of disturbed offenders in both jail and prison (Hardy, 1984; Steadman, Monahan, Duffee, Hartstone, & Robbins, 1984). At Menard Psychiatric Center there was a 375% increase in average monthly admissions from 1975 to 1983. The chief administrator at Menard, Steven Hardy, said that projections indicate that these trends will not change significantly.

Typical personality types found in jail populations are antisocial, borderline, avoidant, dependent, compulsive, and passive–aggressive. These character disorders present a serious management problem to correctional staff as well as to other inmates. The very experience of incarceration may precipitate adjustment disorders or somatoform disorders as well as malingering (French, 1981).

A review of the correctional and art therapy literatures suggests that an integration of these two bodies of knowledge would benefit the inmate population. There are currently too few examples of implementation of art therapy programs within jail facilities to allow us to evaluate the potentials therein. This chapter is written with the hope of beginning to bridge the worlds of art therapy and corrections.

INTRODUCTION

As art therapy professionals venture into the world of the incarcerated client–patient they will face challenges unencountered in any other treatment setting. Initially, the therapist must understand fully the nature of the treatment setting. The jail is first and foremost a penal institution. Whether one considers its function to correct, to incapacitate (i.e., to separate, to make inactive), or to punish unacceptable behavior, penal institutions are only incidentally treatment settings. The therapist must recognize the context in which he or she is treating the client. One cannot conduct appropriate therapeutic sessions as though the correctional setting were any other mental health institution or clinic. Possibly the most important consideration in this regard is the fact that "clients" in jail are not there by choice. They are usually not seeking therapeutic intervention or psychic insight. They are being detained by the courts pending adjudication of the cases brought against them by the state.

Art therapy rarely, if ever, focuses on implementation or development of the therapeutic process with involuntary clients. Correctional settings thus present the mental health field with the challenge of motivating individuals who are not clients by their own consent. In fact, inmates are typically resentful, angry, alienated, and distrustful. If art therapists meet the challenge of reaching such individuals, they will be all the more prepared to motivate nonforensic clients who are merely "resistant."

As art therapists we have a certain advantage over other mental health personnel. Creative expression may be one choice an inmate does make. Where options are few and boredom is rampant, a piece of paper and a set of pastels begin to look pretty interesting. Art also becomes a safe place to exorcise some of the vulnerable feelings associated with incarceration: loneliness, sadness, guilt, and fear. The inmate may inadvertently find help and motivation to change via the discovery of the creative process.

A second challenge to the art therapist in a jail setting is to work in harmony with the correctional facility. The art therapist has the dual potential to help the institution while helping the inmates. Art making alleviates the urgency on the system to contain volatile individuals by providing inmates an appropriate vehicle for the expression of powerful emotions. Certainly, art therapy cannot transform every explosive situation into a therapeutic visual expression. It can, however, offer an alternative method for inmates to voice their feelings while still maintaining control over their own behavior. The institution's strict control over inmates can thus be lessened. For example, the necessity for restraints or isolation may be minimized as a result of fewer incidents of inappropriate verbal or physical behavior when art therapy techniques are used to allow emotional ventilation.

Most mental health institutions do not have as distant a relationship with their clients as does the jail facility. The correctional setting's primary purpose is to incarcerate individuals, not to meet their emotional needs. Its function is to keep potentially dangerous individuals "off the street." Correctional officers usually relate to jail inmates at arm's length. They often expect the worst from the pretrial detainees and are ever watchful for an escape attempt or violent episode. The jail personnel are not concerned about painful affect experienced by inmates. Therefore, the cornerstones of therapeutic treatment, that is, providing a safe environment, unconditional positive regard, empathy, and so on, may be viewed as conflicting with the jail's function to detain alleged criminals. If the therapist is not careful, she or he may develop a conflictual relationship with correctional staff and thereby fall into a splitting of the mental health and security personnel. This situation is most untherapeutic for the inmate–client. The labeling or identification of all correctional officers as insensitive and all therapists as compassionate does nothing toward helping the inmate adjust or deal appropriately with the experience of incarceration. If, on the other hand, the therapist can adopt a systems view of treatment within corrections, the security–therapist conflict is nullified. In such a framework the therapist accepts the jail setting for what it is. He or she focuses on helping the inmate deal with the reality of incarceration, rather than on establishing himself or herself in an adversarial role with the institution. In this way, the inmate does not become a confused "child" with quarreling "parents." Inmate attempts to play clinical staff against correctional staff are not rewarded.

As art therapists, we can gain much knowledge and experience from a jail setting that can help us in other less severe treatment settings. For in most facilities, problems arise concerning staff conflict, patient attempts at splitting, and maintaining consistency in treatment goals and policies. These concerns are magnified within a correctional setting. The resolution of these problems is crucial to establishing a successful treatment environment in any setting.

SETTING

The examples of art therapy that follow are based on the first author's experiences as an art therapy intern at a metropolitan county jail. All clients referred to in this chapter were housed for at least part of their incarceration in the acute psychiatric ward of the jail hospital. The jail also had a separate building with dormitories housing less acute mentally disturbed inmates. The acute psychiatric unit could hold 22 inmates. The population fluctuated constantly, as inmates were either admitted or discharged to other parts of the jail, or transferred to a Department of Mental Health (DMH) institution to await determination of competency to stand trial, or were sentenced, or released. Average length of stay ranged from a few days to a few weeks. In rare exceptions, inmates remained in the acute unit for several months.

The types of pathology found on the unit were diverse. Some admits had no previous mental health history and were admitted due to acute adjustment reactions, often exhibiting suicidal ideation, alcohol toxicity, or aggressive acting-out behaviors. Others had a long-standing history of mental illness and hospitalizations. These included chronic schizophrenics, major affective disorders, and severe personality disorders, especially borderlines.

THERAPEUTIC STRUCTURE

The professional staff on the unit included three part-time psychiatrists, one psychologist, one clinical psychologist, an art therapy intern, two nurses, and three correctional officers. The inmates were required to attend two therapy groups Monday through Friday. Inmates in restraints or those proving to be too disruptive were excused from groups. The morning group was structured as a community meeting. Each inmate was addressed individually by the group leader who asked about his general well-being and how the staff might help him. Suggestions and comments from other inmates were elicited. The evening group meeting focused on intrapsychic issues. Inmates were encouraged to share their problems with the group and to get help from their peers. Unfortunately, a vast majority of the evening sessions were spent arguing about the no-smoking rule for the unit. Only in rare instances was meaningful dialogue exchanged between group members. The wide range of pathology and the rapid turnover of inmates made it quite difficult for deeper levels of interaction to occur. Although sessions were rare in which the inmates "worked hard," that is, focused on their own and others' problems, benefits of group therapy were not to be dismissed. The staff had to remain realistic about which goals could be accomplished given the setting and the population.

GROUP ART THERAPY

Group art therapy was held one evening per week in place of group psychotherapy. A correctional officer and a psychologist participated as coleaders. Individual art therapy was offered to those who expressed an interest and were deemed "safe" by security. It was also suggested for inmates who appeared unresponsive to verbal therapy.

Goals

The goals of group art therapy are multifold. Primarily it is used in the overall treatment plan to help inmates adjust to incarceration. Specifically, group art therapy is used to build cohesiveness on the unit, prepare inmates for court, and relieve tension, rage, or other disturbing emotions. Art also provides a mechanism for "psychic escape." Inmates can go home, to tropical islands, or to outer space through their own visual images. In making art, they leave the stark and emotionally oppressive walls of the jail behind for a welcomed hour's respite. As a nonverbal modality, inmate artwork may provide clinicians with information that otherwise might not surface. Art might expose an individual's higher level of functioning, or shed light on relevant treatment issues.

Format

I began the group by introducing myself, and informing the members that the evening's meeting would be group art therapy. After everyone introduced himself, a veteran group member was asked to tell the others a little about art therapy. The important concept conveyed, either by an inmate or by me, was that talent isn't important. Inmates were to express themselves through a picture. I indicated that art can be a way to learn something about oneself and others. Inmates were asked to be respectful of others, to listen, not to interrupt, and not to ridicule. The art task for the evening was then introduced. I told the group that after people had finished with their drawings we would sit down again and each person would have an opportunity to share his picture. The inmates had the option of not speaking about their images. They also had the option of not actively participating. This, I felt, helped to neutralize feelings about mandatory attendance. Although they were required to come to art therapy, staff would not coerce them to draw or to speak. Finally, inmates would be given the chance to hang their pictures on the dayroom wall. Displaying the work was enormously important. It allowed for later reflection on the drawings. The art also helped to make the barren room more lively and personal. When new admits arrived, the displayed works oriented them to art therapy and served as a catalyst for their own creative expression. Before closing, the leaders invited comments from group members about how they thought the session went. Processing was thereby modeled for the inmates. Reflection and observation on an interpersonal as well as an intrapersonal level were demonstrated. Typical comments from the inmates were "I thought it was nice," and "I had a good time." It was difficult to tell from these comments whether they had gotten something out of the experience or were merely placating group leaders. Other typical comments were "This is stupid," or "I did stuff like this in kindergarten." I felt that those who did not offer observational comments or gave sarcastic responses were often those really most affected by the creative process. In these cases, I felt the individuals were publicly denouncing their possible enthusiasm for the group experience in order not to appear emotionally vulnerable or weak to others. According to the unwritten inmate code, to show weakness is to invite abuse of all kinds by other inmates.

Exposure of self to clinicians was similarly regarded as a potentially dangerous act. After all, clinicians are seen by inmates as part of the "jail staff." Talking to them implies that secrets will be shared with correctional officers. From an inmate's perspective, officers will use any piece of information against the individual. This sort of distrust is always present and is a prominent issue that must be confronted in any therapeutic relationship within a correctional setting. Art therapy as a nonverbal modality may enjoy more privileges of inmate disclosure. Inmates often did not consciously realize that their images reflected something of themselves. In such instances I shared my own impressions of the artwork with the inmate. I was not interpreting the "deeper" meaning of the image (as if that could be determined by anyone other than the maker), but rather I was giving the inmate a basis from which to begin to observe his or my impressions. Most importantly, group members were given a safe place in which to express and explore themselves through creativity. Each could choose the depth of his verbal expression and thereby maintain a sense of his own boundaries. In so doing the inmate could regulate his own vulnerability.

Immediately after the session, I met with the correctional officer and psychologist to process the group experience. We noted members' degrees of participation, congruency of verbalization and imagery, and interaction among members. Candidates for individual art therapy were evaluated. Appropriate treatment plans and communications to other shifts were established.

One frustrating aspect of group art therapy was the amount of time available to discuss each member's work. I felt it was important that every person wanting to share was given the opportunity. In order to make this possible, we often had to cut explanations short or minimize questions about important drawings. Unfortunately, we lost significant data about the meaning of the artwork.

Participation of Leaders

I frequently drew along with the group in order to demystify the drawing process for group members and to model appropriate self-disclosure. Active participation, however, required that I heighten my self-awareness on multiple levels. I had to keep tabs on the group dynamics at the same time that I was thinking of a constructive image to convey a therapeutic message to the inmates. I found it a very difficult task. On some occasions I opted not to draw. Art therapists, as artists, have to be especially aware of their tendency to get swept into the creative process. Inadvertently they may leave behind their responsibilities as therapists. This is a fine line to walk, as the engagement of the therapist in her or his own work may also appropriately model the creative process for the client.

Another point is that the art therapist cannot draw too superficial an image. Such a drawing may be seen as phony by group members, or may suggest that risks should not be taken in imagery. For example a therapist's drawing of a vase with flowers or a sunset on the beach might convey little to a group about the value of self-disclosure. A solution to the therapist's dilemma is to draw about an issue that is real for him or her, but has already been resolved. The therapist need not share with the group that the self-disclosure does not reflect a current problem. Another way to avoid the situation is for the art therapist and participating co-leaders to get their "creative fix" outside of group sessions. I found that making art on my own time lessened the possibility of unconsciously expressing personal issues during the group period. Although the authenticity of a therapist is important in a conventional treatment setting, it is even more important in a correctional setting. One of the most salient characteristics of the antisocial inmate–client is an almost uncanny knack for detecting falsehood or insincerity. Pretentious behavior on the part of the therapist results in his or her rejection by the inmates. Consequently, the therapist lacks the respect of his or her clients. Under these circumstances, no therapeutic process can take place. Therefore, an art therapist working in a jail setting must be appropriately transparent. However, the therapist must at all times be aware of his or her personal boundaries and be prepared at every turn to inform the inmate–client whenever he or she feels that these boundaries are being violated.

ART MATERIALS

Due to security precautions, art materials were greatly limited. Drawing and painting media comprised the primary supplies. At every group session, pastels, craypas, watercolors, colored pencils, and felt-tip markers were available. Scissors, glue, clay, and plaster were contraband and therefore never used. Security was concerned that inmates would use glue and clay to plug up keyholes. Plaster was suspect as a material that could be fashioned into a crude weapon. On some occasions I provided collage materials including magazines, tissue paper, and liquid starch. Tempera paints were used for a few sessions, these being limited due to budgetary restrictions. I felt that the limitations of materials in no way handicapped the art therapy process. If there is a story to be told, it will be told; creative expression is never contingent upon the availability of elaborate art supplies.

DRAWING TASKS

I identified a drawing task for each session. Group members were asked to respond to an identified subject that in some way related to their current experience of incarceration. The tasks were open-ended, leaving room for individual interpretation and self-expression. They were not gimmicks or contrived ideas, but rather a means to help inmates focus upon their emotional issues. Examples of drawing tasks include: "Draw a place you'd rather be," "Draw something you lost that was important to you," "Draw your

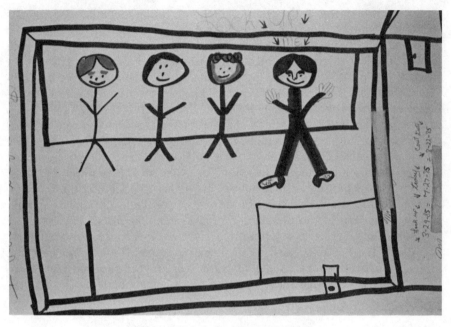

Figure 7.1. Jesus's self-portrait in jail.

expectation of your court experience," and "Draw your self-portrait in jail."
In large part, I specified these tasks in response to my own need to establish
structure within an unpredictable and multilevel group. I found that I was
anxious about the direction of the group when I did not provide a focus or
catalyst for the session. I also felt that individuals invariably draw what they
need to draw regardless of my instructions. The assigned task would not
prohibit them from making their own statements.

EXAMPLES OF GROUP ARTWORK

Self-Portrait in Jail

Inmates were helped to focus in a "here and now" sense on the reality of
their incarceration by drawing self-portraits in the jail setting. The activity
provided a vehicle for the inmates to relate their feelings and to find commonality with others. These drawings acted as a vessel, a container, for the
various painful emotions incurred as a result of the jail experience.

Jesus drew himself in the police lockup area where he was taken immediately after his arrest (Fig. 7.1). In his picture Jesus says loud and clear,
"I love to be free today." He includes others in the lockup with him. Only
Jesus is depicted with hands and feet. He is also the only one with a substantial body. On the right side Jesus listed his lockup date, the current date,
and his court date. Jesus's doors are clearly too small for any of the inmates

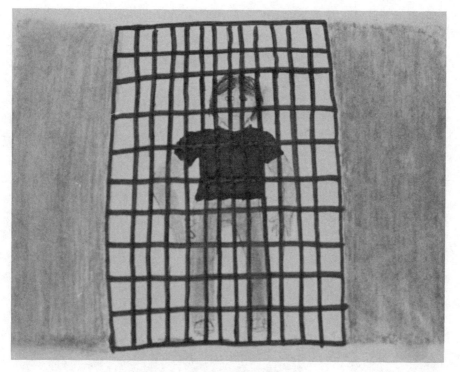

Figure 7.2. Eddie's self-portrait in jail.

to fit through. The drawing's mixed perspective is typical of an 8-year-old's work, and may reflect Jesus's emotional or developmental maturity.

Eddie shows himself behind bars (Fig. 7.2). In actuality these bars are not a part of the physical structure on the unit. The bars are more symbolic of incarceration than real. Eddie says that he can't wait to get out of jail. He says that he's made some dumb mistakes in the past. He wants to get a fresh start and put his life together. I pointed out to Eddie that his jail doesn't look too formidable. It looks as though he could walk around it or climb over the bars. I added that Eddie, as an 18-year-old, does have a chance to make some changes. He can get out from behind the bars with relative ease. He is young, and his theft charge is a misdemeanor. He would not have to spend a great deal of time in the penitentiary if he were to be convicted. Eddie's drawing seems to suggest that his appraisal of his chances to start a better life may be similar to my own appraisal. The drawing made clear for him that he has some options, but that he is the one responsible for his coming out from behind the bars.

Leonard's self-portrait in jail (Fig. 7.3) seems to reflect accurately his experience of incarceration. He portrays himself in full leather restraints. Due to his out-of-control behavior Leonard was frequently in restraints. The

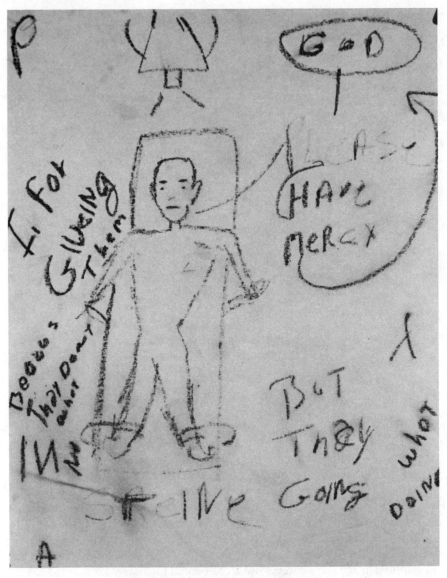

Figure 7.3. Leonard's self-portrait in jail.

triangular shape at the top of the page seems to be an overhead light. The mark on the right side of the torso is an "L," referring to the letter on his T-shirt that indicates the jail dorm from which he came. The written message appears reminiscent of what Christ is reported to have said in the Garden of Gethsemane the night before he was to be crucified. Leonard writes, "I for Giving Them—Because thay don't what—But They going what Doing—God Please have mercy." Perhaps Leonard sees himself as a Christ figure who is unjustly persecuted. His image may be viewed as a crucifixion pose. However, Leonard declined to share an explanation about his drawing. As he was actively psychotic, I was extremely gratified that Leonard partici- pated in the art making at all and did not push him for verbalization.

Draw Yourself as an Animal

One task I felt was unsuccessful for the most part (largely because of its unrelatedness to the here and now) was to have each inmate imagine himself as an animal and then draw that animal. The drawings, not surprisingly, did not generate significant data or interaction among group members. Tom's drawing (Fig. 7.4) was a notable exception. It was an extremely powerful image. His animal appears to be the human animal. This is my interpretation, not his. Tom had nothing to say about his picture. The head is clearly a skull, the hands are barely attached to the body, and the fingers have what appear to be claws. The drawing was very disturbing to me. I had trouble connecting it to the small, quiet man sitting before me.

I later found out that Tom had killed his father's lover. He dismembered her body and put the many pieces into small plastic bags, which he then laid out on the street. I suddenly became aware of the connection between Tom and his drawing. Apparently his quiet demeanor masked an enormous amount of rage.

INDIVIDUAL ART THERAPY

Client Referrals

Candidates for individual art therapy were referred to me by the clinical staff and Security. Some were self-referrals and others were selected by me. Individuals were often referred to art therapy when they were nonverbal, exhibited somatic dysfunction, were anxious, depressed, suicidal, or had an approaching court date.

Format

I introduced myself to the inmate and usually asked a number of background questions. I inquired as to how long the inmate had been in jail so that I could better assess the degree to which he had adjusted to incarceration. I asked whether the inmate had ever previously been in jail or a mental health institution. The information elicited also provided clues to the nature and extent of the inmate's presenting problem. I asked what precipitated the inmate's transfer to the acute psychiatric unit. Often, I explained that this unit was for inmates with the most serious mental problems. I asked the individual what he thought his mental problems were, if any. I sometimes

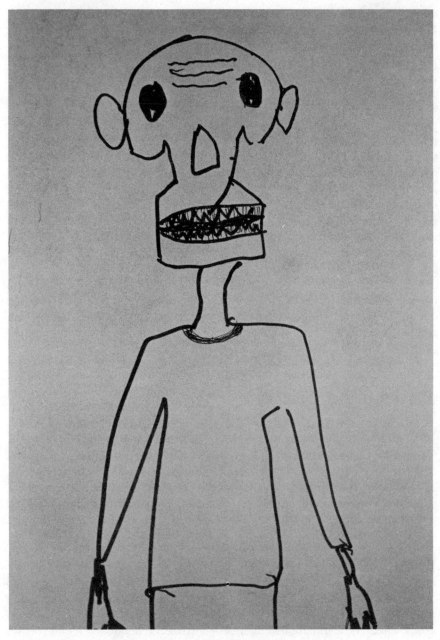

Figure 7.4. Tom's animal.

asked what the inmate was charged with. Frequently I found out the inmate's charge ahead of time because I wanted to have an awareness of the individual's capacity for violence before walking into a session with him. On occasion, the inmate volunteered information about his alleged crime. In other instances, the inmate did not bring up his charge. At times I felt that my inquiring about the charge or alleged crime only put the inmate on the defensive. In these instances, I did not pursue a discussion regarding the details of his arrest.

Occasionally the inmate immediately picked up art materials and began to draw. When art making began so spontaneously, I did not bother gathering background data. This information could be elicited later, and I did not want to obstruct the invitation to make art. It was more important that I support the inmate's natural creative drive by attending to his unfolding image. If the artwork did not unfold spontaneously, I introduced the process of art therapy by explaining that art could be used as a different way of expressing one's self. I conveyed that it wasn't important how well the individual could draw or paint. What mattered was that the individual used art to say or to learn something about himself. If relevant, I added that many people feel "funny" or self-conscious about drawing when they haven't made art for many years. I suggested using stick figures, if that would make things easier to express. I emphasized that I wouldn't be analyzing the picture—only the individual would do that. The meaning the creator found in his image was important—not what I interpreted his work to mean.

In contrast to group art therapy, I found no purpose in defining a drawing task. Inmates were rarely at a loss for something to draw. On the few occasions when an individual had difficulty getting started, I told him that sometimes it takes a while to get an idea, and that it was all right if he took his time. If he continued to have trouble, I suggested just trying out the various materials to see how they would work.

The length of the sessions was between 45 and 75 minutes. Obstacles to consistently timed, ongoing sessions included court dates, transfers within the jail, inadequate security coverage, or the inmate's placement in restraints. I met on a weekly basis with each client when this was feasible. Some inmates were seen only once. Others attended sessions over a number of weeks.

Confidentiality

Information gathered from art sessions was considered confidential in the same manner as that gathered in any nonforensic therapeutic relationship. I had an obligation, however, to share information relating to suicidal or homicidal intent with the clinical staff. I advised the inmate of my responsibilities in this regard so that he could gauge how much he was willing to disclose. It was also important to inform the inmate that the content of art sessions, as with any other therapy, would be documented, and that the possibility existed that the court would subpoena these documents. This, too, allowed the inmate to gauge the extent of his disclosures.

Setting

Individual art therapy sessions were held in a medical exam room. We worked at a desk 60 by 30 inches in size, making it very difficult for me to participate in the art making. The room provided for limited privacy and was readily accessible to the officers' station, which stood approximately 20 feet away. Though an officer was not present during sessions, one passed by the doorway occasionally to make sure there were no control problems. This arrangement allowed the inmate to be more relaxed without an officer present, yet it ensured my protection. When an inmate's behavior was unpredictable, I worked with him in an open hallway, approximately 30 feet away from the officers' station. The officers had full view of the inmate and myself, yet were far enough away to allow for verbal privacy.

CASE EXAMPLES

Matthew

Matthew was charged with setting a fire and pulling a knife on a young girl with the apparent intent to force sex upon her. He initially denied his guilt about the knife incident and expressed anger that anyone would accuse him of doing something so horrible. He set the fire in retaliation for being wrongly accused.

During one session Matthew told me an important story. The night before he had been snoring very loudly. A nurse woke him and made him move to another bed as he was disturbing the inmate next to him. Apparently Matthew had been dreaming when he was awakened. Therefore, he remembered his dream quite vividly the following morning. His dream was a reenactment of the incident with the little girl. Through the dream, Matthew realized that he had, indeed, pulled the knife on the child. He was very shaken by this realization.

Matthew then told me numerous stories about his childhood. His mother had forced him to stand naked in front of her. He remembered wanting to jump through her window, trying to kill himself. He also gave me what amounted to accounts of incest, though it appeared Matthew was not aware that there was something wrong in the acts that were demanded of him. He simply recalled these incidents with sadness and anger.

Matthew continued to communicate verbally, but he showed little interest in the art materials. I encouraged him to pull something out of our discussion that could become an image for him to draw. He suddenly said, "It's my hands! My hands get me in trouble!" I suggested to Matthew that he draw

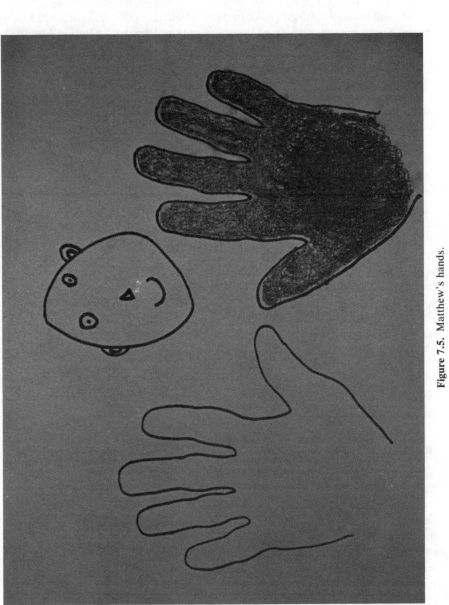

Figure 7.5. Matthew's hands.

his hands. At first he protested that he couldn't draw his hands because it was too difficult. I suggested that he put his hands down on the paper and trace around them. Matthew picked up on this idea (Fig. 7.5). I directed him to identify one hand as the "bad" hand, and the other as the "good" hand, and to select a color for each. I was hoping to convey to him that he has both good and bad aspects, just as all people do.

Matthew chose to draw the "bad" hand first. He colored it red. He began at the fingertips, using the pastel in tight circular motions. While drawing, Matthew again reexperienced his crime. He appeared to have gone into a trance. He began to rock back and forth. He applied more pressure to the pastel and the circular motion became larger and more aggressive. The density of the pastel in this area is readily apparent in the drawing. All the while he spoke about the incident with the little girl and how he had meant no harm. Matthew made no eye contact with me while he was in this trance-like state.

I became quite anxious. I had no idea how to close the session, which was now approaching an hour and a half, nor did I know how to help Matthew use his art to deal with the feelings that resulted from the realization of his crime. Somehow, Matthew found it within himself to bind the immediate experience. By the time he finished coloring his "bad hand" he had stopped rocking and was again able to look at me. I asked him if he would like to color the "good" hand but he declined. I then asked him if he would like to put something in his hands. He decided he would like to put his mother in his hands.

The art was an important cathartic holding place for all of Matthew's feelings. He was owning his crime for the first time. This was a very frightening acknowledgment. By giving form to his guilt and fear, Matthew was able to contain them to some extent.

WILLIAM

William attended only one individual art therapy session. He immediately picked up a marker and began to draw. The picture is a floor plan of William's apartment (Fig. 7.6). He told the story of his alleged crime with his marker, moving it from room to room, describing the details of movement and conversation. William's son was 15 minutes late from school. His son had been late before, and this had made William very angry. He showed where his son entered the apartment. Then he explained how he had spanked his son, while drawing the boy laid out on the couch. William said after that he went out on the porch, leaving his son inside. When he came back in, his son was vomiting. William was worried about his son and sat him in a chair. Then the child began to choke on his vomit. William tried to give him mouth-to-mouth resuscitation. Suddenly there was an ambulance outside. The paramedics tried to save his son, to no avail. William then drew his son on the ambulance stretcher in the living room. The next thing William knew, the

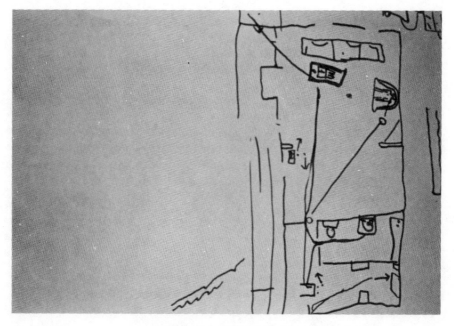

Figure 7.6. William's story.

police came and arrested him for murder. He kept saying that he hadn't done the mouth-to-mouth resuscitation the right way, but it wasn't his fault that his son had died. It was all a misunderstanding. He hadn't killed his son; he had only tried to save him.

In actuality, the police report indicated that the son had been beaten to death with a baseball bat. It appeared that William was responsible. His use of art was similar to Matthew's. William expressed powerful emotions relating to his crime through his artwork, thereby helping himself to contain the feelings. However, he used the art in a manner that helped him deny the truth he was currently unable to accept.

BRAD

Brad had been transferred to the acute psychiatric unit as a suicide precaution. He had originally been admitted to the jail's medical unit as he claimed that his legs were paralyzed. This problem proved to be a conversion disorder. Brad repeatedly said, "Don't let them hurt me." When asked what he meant, Brad tearfully said that he had been in the penitentiary and had been gang-raped by five men. It appeared that the conversion disorder was Brad's way of protecting himself within the all-too-familiar penal setting. Once he let go of his "paralysis," Brad claimed that he was hearing the voice of his Aunt Ever (pronounced Eve-er), who told him to join her in

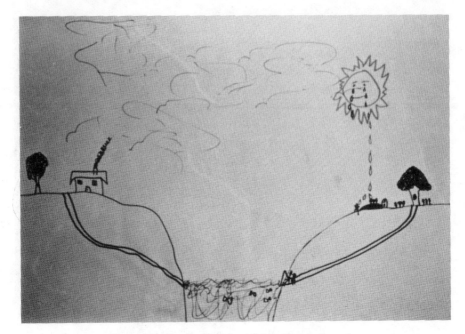

Figure 7.7. Brad's depiction of Aunt Ever's funeral.

heaven. The auditory hallucinations, like the paralysis, were very real for Brad. They became another defensive reaction to his incarceration. By being "crazy" Brad was taking care of himself. He remained too vulnerable and weak to be sent to the general population, where the possibility of being raped was quite real.

Brad drew a picture of Aunt Ever's funeral (Fig. 7.7) on his first day on the unit. He cried openly as he drew. He picked up the markers without hesitation and worked steadily in silence. After the drawing was finished, Brad described his image. He drew himself beside Aunt Ever's grave. The sun's tears fall onto the grave and Brad as well. Brad shows himself again down at the creek fishing with his papa (grandfather). I asked him how deep the creek was. Brad told me that it only had a little water in it and that one could see the bottom and walk across it. His grandfather's house is on the left side of the picture. At first, Brad did not draw the pathways on either side of the creek. I asked Brad how he and his papa got from the house to the other side of the creek; it seemed very steep to me. Brad said it was easy because there was a path. I asked him if he'd like to draw the path, and he then did so. I hoped to use the "paths" as a metaphor for the way to get from one side of a crisis to the other. I didn't want Brad to be without a means to move forward from his current dilemma. If he had not chosen to draw these paths, I would not have taken the idea any further.

Brad added that the truth was that he had not attended Aunt Ever's funeral. He felt terrible about his absence and continually chastised himself

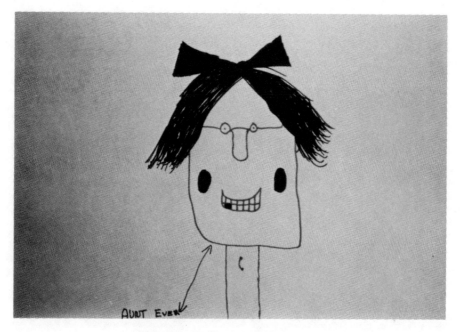

Figure 7.8. Brad's portrait of Aunt Ever.

for it. This self-imposed guilt was unwarranted, as it appears Brad was only 4 years old at the time of Aunt Ever's death, and he lived several hundred miles away.

I was struck with the depth of Brad's "creek." Compared to the scale of the human figures, the creek looked anything but shallow. Brad might have drowned had he tried to walk across. The chasm itself seemed quite steep and perilous. I wondered to what extent the picture reflected Brad's previous painful experiences. Primarily, exploring this first picture with Brad served to help me establish an empathic, therapeutic relationship with him. I took his hallucinations about Aunt Ever seriously. I accepted his reality as true for him, rather than challenge the validity of his experience.

In a later session, Brad drew a portrait of Aunt Ever (Fig. 7.8). He again became tearful. Brad found solace in the memory of Aunt Ever, and used her image to escape the reality of jail. Unfortunately, his identification with Aunt Ever included suicide plans for himself. I hoped that my continued dialogue with his inner world would help Brad finally recognize how he was using Aunt Ever to avoid his present situation, which included the possibility of being raped again.

I began to wonder, however, whether I was helping or hindering Brad. By focusing him on his hallucinations, perhaps I was inappropriately reinforcing Brad's delusional belief that Aunt Ever actually visited him from the grave. I decided to try a more grounded strategy. Perhaps he needed more directive therapeutic interventions. In following sessions, I helped Brad

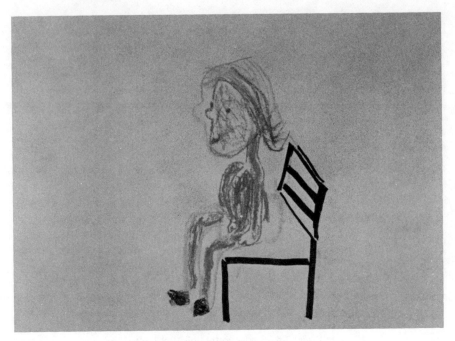

Figure 7.9. Brad's posture.

concentrate on his self-image. As he drew self-portraits, Brad began to place himself in the world—to take up space, to claim existence, and to find his identity (Fig. 7.9). We worked on breathing and posture awareness in conjunction with the self-portraits. Eventually Brad was discharged to a less acute psychiatric dorm. He apparently had little difficulty adjusting to the less protected environment. His self-image had improved tremendously, and he was no longer hallucinating or having suicidal ideations. Though Brad still had a fear of being raped, he could talk about his feelings without clothing them in "craziness."

CONCLUSION

The examples of artwork from both group and individual art therapy sessions illustrate art therapy's ability to meet the needs of the inmate as well as those of the jail facility. Group art therapy provides a much needed method of building appropriate cohesiveness on the unit or tier. Through the specified drawing tasks inmates share common experiences, thus promoting feelings of universality and belonging. Group cohesiveness is paramount in alleviating inmates' feelings of isolation and desperation. The consequent emergence of a social network results in fewer episodes of violence among inmates.

Though in many instances, inmates may be seen by the art therapist only once or twice, each art session, in and of itself, can be helpful in alleviating immediate crisis situations. This swift therapeutic effectiveness is in sharp contrast to the many traditional types of interventions in which transference or other kinds of phenomena must occur before real change can be realized. Art is able to engage withdrawn and depressed individuals who might otherwise feel too frightened by the jail environment to respond well to verbal therapeutic modalities. As such, it can provide an immediate cathartic experience in which the art object becomes a container for powerful, potentially destructive emotions. The creative process can, therefore, help detect, prevent, and treat crisis situations such as suicide. For instance, making art may act as a catalyst for discussions of suicidal ideation. The verbalization of such self-destructive feelings may be viewed as the first step in suicide intervention.

Art therapy can make important therapeutic contributions to jail settings, as it addresses the inmates' "here and now" issues of incarceration in a nonthreatening manner. Though art therapy is frequently a pleasurable experience, it does more than distract inmates from the monotony of jail life. By valuing the inmate's creative process, the art therapist makes emotional contact with the individual. The inmate's experience is thereby validated, and he or she has the opportunity to move forward emotionally. Tendencies to become disruptive, destructive, or overwhelmed by the experience of incarceration can be replaced by creative expression.

REFERENCES

French, L. (1981). Clinical perspectives on crisis intervention in jails. *Prison Journal, 61*(1), 43–53.

Hardy, S. L. (1984). Dealing with the mentally and emotionally disturbed. *Corrections Today, 46,* 16–18.

Levy, B. (1978). Art therapy in a women's correctional facility. *The Arts in Psychotherapy, 5,* 157–166.

Marano, R. (1983). *Art therapy as part of a psychiatric program in a jail correctional facility.* Unpublished.

Rylander, B. (1979). Art therapy with prisoners in solitary confinement. *Proceedings of the Tenth Annual Conference of the American Art Therapy Association,* Washington, DC: AATA.

Schneider, M. A. (1979). Problems in short term correctional settings. *International Journal of Offender Therapy & Comparative Criminology, 23,* 164–171.

Steadman, H. J., Monahan, J., Duffee, B., Hartstone, E., & Robbins, P. C. (1984). Impact of state mental hospital deinstitutionalization on United States prison populations, 1968–1978. *Journal of Criminal Law & Criminology, 75,* 474–490.

Stone, W. (1984). Jail suicide. *Corrections Today, 46,* 84–87.

Wadeson, H. (1987). *The dynamics of art psychotherapy,* New York: Wiley.

CHAPTER 8

Fighting Cancer with Images

The intimate connection between mind and body, psyche and soma, becomes increasingly apparent when exploring the imagery and artwork of an individual with cancer. While this interconnection is certainly not a new concept, it has attracted renewed interest in recent years with the advent of biofeedback and the increasing knowledge that we may be able to influence our physical state through our minds. The use of guided imagery and art plays a central role in this endeavor. Guided imagery, also called visualization, allows individuals to create a set of images or pictures in their minds that, it is to be hoped, establish the climate for these images to grow in reality. Unfortunately, while individuals may wish to harness their imagination for healing purposes, often unconscious attitudes can undermine these attempts, leaving a sense of helplessness that pervades their entire mental state. In this context, art therapy can be an invaluable tool in providing an avenue for exploring those attitudes that may be blocking the healing process. Art becomes a way of capturing and recreating the images seen in one's mind and provides a concrete picture that often reaches beyond the images originally envisioned to tell a story about cancer patients' lives including their feelings toward their illness, their treatment, and themselves.

THE USE OF GUIDED IMAGERY FOR HEALING PURPOSES

The use of images and symbols for healing purposes is an ancient art. In the book *Imagery in Healing: Shamanism and Modern Medicine,* Achterberg (1985) describes the role of shamans, possibly the world's original healers, and their use of the image to treat a variety of diseases. Achterberg explains that the shaman's ritual work creates a direct therapeutic effect on the patient by creating vivid images and by inducing a state of consciousness conducive to self-healing. Archeological evidence dating as far back as 20,000 years ago in the form of painting and carving suggests that shamans may have existed and utilized masks and representations of animals to invoke a healing spirit in their followers (Achterberg, 1985).

Although it is evident that imagery has played a powerful role in both health and disease through the ages, the question we now face is how we can understand this ancient process in modern terms. What role has the image played, and what role does it continue to play, in our overall physical well-being? This is a crucial question, for as art therapists we interpret and manipulate images and symbols, profoundly affecting those with whom we work. How can we use images so they most benefit our patients?

Progress has been made in our understanding of how a thought or image gets translated into a physiological response. In the 1960s, biofeedback studies demonstrated that bodily functions under the auspices of the autonomic nervous system, long thought to be out of our conscious control, could be brought under control after only a few biofeedback sessions. Individuals with no prior training could consciously influence their heart rate, muscle tension, sweat gland activity, skin temperature, and a wide range of internal processes normally considered involuntary (Simonton, Simonton, & Creighton, 1978). In the 1980s, an entirely new area of study has been developed, called psychoneuroimmunology, combining the fields of psychology, neurology, and immunology, so that the links between the body and mind could be investigated on a scientific and in-depth level (Hurley, 1983). Yet with all the advances that have been made in tracing a mental impulse to its logical conclusion within the body and watching for the neurological and immunological effect, much still remains to be discovered. The artwork and imagery of the cancer patient provide needed clues to individuals' attitudes and the subsequent effect these attitudes may be having on their present and future physical state.

In 1971, Carl and Stephanie Simonton began their pioneering work of utilizing guided imagery and drawing with cancer patients (Simonton et al., 1978). They reported dramatic results with their first patient, a 61-year-old man with advanced throat cancer, who responded positively to utilizing the imagination to help fight his disease. Carl Simonton, a radiation oncologist, suggested to this patient that three times a day, for 5 to 15 minutes, he imagine his radiation treatment as a stream of energy. As tiny bullets, they would destroy his cancer cells but not his normal cells. His body's white blood cells would swarm over his cancer cells, picking up and carrying off the dead and dying ones, and flush them out through his body's normal elimination processes. Finally, he was to visualize his cancer decreasing in size and his health returning to normal. This patient went into an extended remission of more than 6 years, showing no evidence of his original throat cancer; nevertheless, when the Simontons utilized the same program with other cancer patients they were unable to produce similar dramatic results consistently. This raised a series of questions as to why one individual could utilize imagery to influence the course of illness while another individual could not, even though there appeared to be no negative side effects and many possible benefits.

The Simontons initially neglected a body of literature dating back several hundred years that documented the role psychological factors play in illness and in cancer (Kowal, 1955). This literature makes it evident that, in order for an individual to think positively about the possibility of overcoming cancer and getting well, the cancer patient's life outside the illness cannot be ignored. What is happening to an individual prior to illness at work, in relationships with other people, and in the capacity for handling stress needs to be investigated along with the images and symbols used for depicting the cancer. The imagery and drawing of the cancer patient do not exist in a vacuum, nor can they be changed through mere suggestion. The colors an individual chooses, where symbols are placed on the page, and the intensity with which illness is drawn have roots deep in the individual's psyche.

EMOTIONS AND CANCER

The physicians of the eighteenth and nineteenth centuries in Europe were impressed by the frequency with which certain life situations tended to appear prior to the development of a neoplasm (Kowal, 1955). For example, they noted that loss of a significant life goal (economic, political, professional) became a common denominator underlying the diverse situations the cancer patient presented. In most cases the reaction was the same, and a sense of hopelessness and despair prevailed. In 1846, a treatise on cancer was published by Walter Hayle Walsh, a physician in London who wrote one of the definitive works of that time on this subject (Kowal, 1955). He discusses in this work the relationship of mental affliction to cancer and goes on to state:

> Much has been written on the influence of mental misery, sudden reverses of fortune, and habitual gloominess of temper, on the deposition of caracinom-atous matter . . . it would be vain to deny that facts of a very convincing character, in respect to agency of the mind in the production of this disease, are frequently observed. I have myself met with cases which the connection appeared so clear and decisive, that to question its reality would be a struggle against reason. (p. 220)

Twentieth century physicians and health professionals have formed conclusions similiar to those of medical men during the eighteenth and nineteenth centuries. Lawrence LeShan, a psychoanalyst, published the results of a 12-year study carried out on 450 cancer patients, where the feeling of hopelessness once again emerged as significant. Those in the study were administered the Worthington Personality Test to gain an in-depth picture of their lives. The study found a specific life history pattern emerged encompassing 72% of the cancer patients and only 10% of the controls. This pattern points to specifics such as damage to an individual's development within the first 7 years of life that often was accentuated by the loss of a significant member of the family. A sense of guilt resulted from these early childhood experiences. In adulthood, these individuals did find some extended periods of their lives enjoyable, though a sense of having failed gradually began to predominate their entire existence (Achterberg, Simonton, & Simonton, 1976).

Arnold Hutschnecker (1951), a physician, also observed the role the mind plays in our well-being. He believes that a healthy individual, one sound in body and mind, holds enormous resources for sustaining health. He cites a study conducted at Sloan-Kettering Cancer Institute in 1956, where human volunteers were implanted with live cancer tissue. Their healthy bodies responded with a vigorous inflammatory reaction that fought off the transplants, which subsequently disappeared. Judith Glassman (1983), a reporter, researched what mental qualities might be present to cause an individual's physical defenses to rally most effectively. She defines "survivorship qualities" as those attributes often found in patients who recovered from their illnesses against great odds. Glassman points to hope and a positive attitude, an ability to fight back and express anger, a sense of responsibility and involvement in one's healing process, a strong life purpose, and a tremendous determination to live as some of the vital elements essential to a survivorship attitude.

PSYCHOLOGICAL AND SOMATIC IMPLICATIONS

Glassman's research and the research of the others mentioned are supported by a steady and flourishing body of information on survivorship connecting the mind and body. The artwork of cancer patients can be most poignant in helping us understand this connection. From a holistic perspective, the artwork provides art therapists with a much deeper level of understanding and the possibility to participate more fully with clients in their healing process. This whole perspective will reach beyond the physical and emotional states of individuals to encompass their intellectual and spiritual sides as well.

Carl Simonton (Simonton & Simonton, 1975) observed the importance of one's personal beliefs and their subsequent impact on the imagery process:

> If I had nothing but one tool to use in looking at my patient's attitude it would be how regularly he is relaxing and what his imagery is. This tells me so much more than what he could tell me consciously, because he isn't even aware of what he is telling me. (p. 33)

Carl Jung utilized dreams to investigate his patients' psychological and somatic states in much the same way that the Simontons looked at the imagery processes of their patients. Russell Lockhart, a Jungian analyst, discussed how dreams were used by Jung to investigate organic functioning. Lockhart related that "dreams may not only anticipate the development of somatic involvement, but may also reflect bodily disturbances in the process" (1981, p. 22). Lockhart concluded that "bodily organs and processes have the capacity to stimulate the production of psychic images, meaning-fully related to the type of psychic disturbance and its location'' (p. 24). If we extend this hypothesis to art, a symbol becomes a representation of a symptom. What is shown in a drawing, therefore, is also happening or may happen in the client's body.

Susan Bach, another Jungian psychoanalyst, studied the relationship of body and psyche through the use of drawing with terminally ill children (Kübler-Ross, 1981). After years of work reviewing these children's pictures, she concluded that the physical condition of the child was revealed in his or her art and that the drawing served as a record documenting the child's current body–mind state. She believed, if these pictures were read properly, one could see that the child unconsciously used the drawing for self-diag-nosis. Additionally, she noted, these images held the child's unspoken wants, needs, and anxieties as well. According to Gregg Furth, who has incorpo-rated Bach's methods into his own practice, ''adults' pictures reflect the psyche/soma condition no less than children's pictures'' (Kübler-Ross, 1981, p. 68).

Drawing has also been used as a predictor of future disease states. In 1975, a research effort was conducted in which 870 medical students were asked to draw a human figure. Findings suggested that the position or stance of the figure is a reflection of a subject's attitude toward the outside world and can be correlated to the development of certain types of illnesses (Har-rower & Thomas, 1975). For example, those students who went on to develop hypertension or coronary diseases had a high percentage of drawings with an outgoing or demanding attitude, while those individuals who developed malignant tumors had drawings characterized by ambivalence or an uncertain attitude. It was concluded that psychological precursors may exist for future disease states.

Work in the area of projective techniques has also sought to link an individual's body image to one's internal physical state. In 1957, Klopfer reported on his work with cancer patients using the Rorschach as a way of understanding the personality factors present by comparing a patient with a fast-growing tumor to a patient with a slow-growing tumor (Klopfer, 1956). In 1956, an article published by Fischer and Cleveland described work done with the Rorschach and its value in determining the site of an indivdual's cancer. Using subjects' projected body image fantasies, it was concluded that psychological data alone could determine where on the body the can-cerous mass would be located (Fischer & Cleveland, 1956).

In these studies it appears that physical processes, present and future, are represented in projective tests, as well as the symbols of one's dreams and artwork. Because the art therapist is accustomed to reading a symbolic language, he or she has the opportunity to cue into these messages and to play a central role in their understanding. In the cases that follow, I wish to illustrate how guided imagery and art were used not only as a reflection of an indvidual's existing psychological and somatic state, but also as a source of encouragement for the patients to experiment with a new attitude toward their immune systems and illness in general. Using individuals' artwork to improve their emotional outlook and rally the body's defenses, the art therapist advances the patients' potential to participate more fully in their own health.

CASE EXAMPLES

KAREN: DENIAL AND BENEFITS RELATED TO CANCER

Karen, a 31-year-old woman with advanced lymphoma, gives us a chance to consider how the defense of denial may affect one's artwork. Denial often acts as a buffer after unexpected shocking news (Kübler-Ross, 1981). Karen had known she had cancer for many months, and her medical prognosis was growing progressively grim as one drug after another failed to slow the course of her illness. Her response to this news was to maintain an outwardly cheery face, possibly to buffer the news from her loved ones as well as from herself. During the cancer support group Karen attended, she presented herself as a model patient. She held back her tears and stated her desire to think positively, defending the benefits of guided imagery, protecting the group's leader, and utilizing her artwork as a source of encouragement for other group members. This patient's denial of her serious prognosis was not a totally negative factor since this defense at times gave her the strength and hope to go on living in the face of painful treatments, multiple hospitalizations, and increasing pressures at home. Karen's drawing, though, points to a level of denial that may have undermined her healing process (Fig. 8.1).

This woman drew her tumor as an energized, yellow mass that extended out toward the lower right corner of the page. It almost reaches three celebrating individuals, each holding a flower. The treatment, chemotherapy, is symbolized by three arrows. Immune system cells in the form of men carrying shovels are actually digging into healthy pink cells, rather than touching the tumor. We also see a piece of yellow tumor broken off at the bottom, with arrows marking its path, which ends at the celebrating men. Karen described with great joy how the picture symbolized a victory celebration of her cancer being eliminated.

As group leader I remember my own feelings of denial, wanting to see the drawing as depicting a joyous event rather than a bleak one. This woman's enthusiasm influenced my feeling that I had overreacted to her drawing and projected my own fearful feelings onto it rather than seeing her strong desire to live, which might have influenced a positive change in her physical condition. Yet as the group progressed over the next weeks, Karen discussed her great relief at being ill and having been able to leave a career and job situation that placed her under large amounts of stress. In addition, she described her life since becoming ill as a "continuous birthday party" where

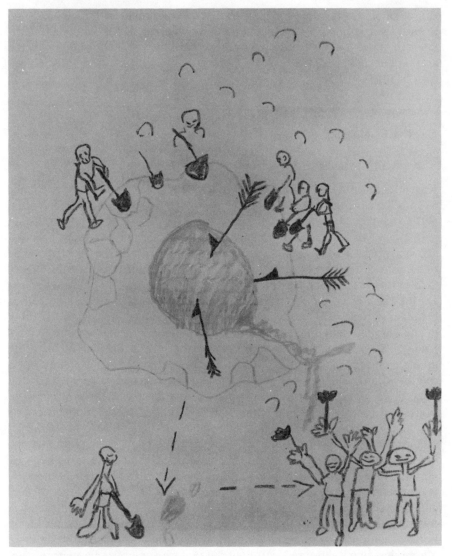

Figure 8.1. Karen's image for her tumor (center), chemotherapy treatment (arrows), and immune system (men with shovels).

there was an endless stream of cards, phone calls, and gifts from family and friends. It is far more likely that the celebration depicted in her drawing reflected her life with cancer, rather than her life without cancer, which prior to her illness was exceedingly difficult.

BILL: USE OF POSITIVE ENERGY

When Bill, a middle-aged professor at a local university, first came to see me he was clearly overwhelmed by his medical diagnosis, measuring time

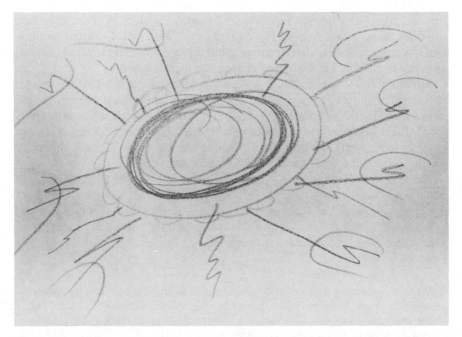

Figure 8.2. Bill's image for his cancer (center), radiation treatment (zigzag lines), and white blood cells (curved and straight lines).

and events "pre and post" his diagnosis of cancer. Physically he felt fine, but emotionally he was drained. Our first meeting together, less than a month after this news, was spent discussing the possibility of utilizing guided imagery, positive thinking, and drawing to involve his mind in the healing process. After being led through a relaxation and guided imagery process, art materials were made available for him to draw what he had imagined.

Figure 8.2 illustrates Bill's feelings about his cancer, his radiation treatment, and his immune system. A large, inward-spiraling blue circle appearing to have a thin outer barrier around it depicts his cancer. Also in blue are his white blood cells, which are symbolized by thin lines. Most reach only the cancer's outer edge but one fully penetrates the outer barrier and touches the inner core. Bill's radiation treatment represented as a bolt of loud and crashing lightning is drawn in orange with more jagged lines than those symbolizing the immune system. The lines respresenting the radiation treatment appear only slightly more effective than the white blood cells in reaching the inner core. Seven orange half-circles representing the immune system are shown around the perimeter of the drawing. He saw his cancer as strong and powerful. This clear and dominant feeling comes through in his art.

During a follow-up review of his drawing Bill focused on how he might reduce the intensity of his cancer and increase the impact and effectiveness of his immune system. Often patients need some basic information on the functioning of the body's immune and defense system. This information provides them with a rich set of visual images. With Bill, I wanted to guide him toward creating positive feelings about the body's ability to regain health. In order to do this I encouraged change through his images.

Utilizing Bill's symbols, on a separate piece of paper, I drew several smaller blue spirals representative of his cancer and several orange, jagged lines indicating his immune system. In my drawing, each white blood cell made direct contact with a cancer cell. Using his colors, shapes, and lines I sought to illustrate how his imagery and subsequent drawings could convey a more powerful feeling for eliminating the cancer.

Because it was impossible for me to enter into this patient's mind and manipulate his thoughts in a more positive direction, I combined my own imagery with his to convey a more positive feeling for mobilizing his defenses. I believe in this instance the therapist's artwork permitted entry to an area where purely verbal exchange may have been less effective. According to McNiff (1981):

> When the therapist and client are finding it difficult to relate directly to one another, the art work may be a bridge between them, a third object, or what the psychoanalysts call a transitional object, which gives them a safe middle ground through which they can be together. (p. xiii)

My drawing was a bridge to a belief system with which Bill was not yet acquainted.

The concept that his immune system could be rallied through the use of imagery and positive thinking was new to him. It was not until several sessions later that he was able to begin thinking of his body's own healing potential. Drawings made at that time show a much more pulsating and energized immune force in direct contact with his cancer cells.

Figure 8.3, drawn 4 weeks after Figure 8.2, incorporates his new attitude. What is most striking about the immune system, now drawn in yellow and green, is its energized quality and ability to reach out to all cancerous areas. Gone is the earlier feeling of cancer as an overwhelming implosion. Here the cancer is shown in six different red areas that appear to be equally matched to the immune system's strength. Each tumor has the immune system coiling around it or being touched by it on the outer edge. Large yellow immune system cells appear throughout the body, especially in the forehead, pelvic area, and chest cavity. Three of these yellow areas appear almost as suns, with their rays shining out into Bill's body.

Yet while this patient was experiencing many physical difficulties in his life, he had drawn his face to be relaxed and at peace. We discussed the meditative quality of the picture and the deep changes that might be going on inside of Bill, since he had never taken so much time for himself before to relax and use his imagination.

Over the next weeks we discussed other aspects of Bill's life outside his

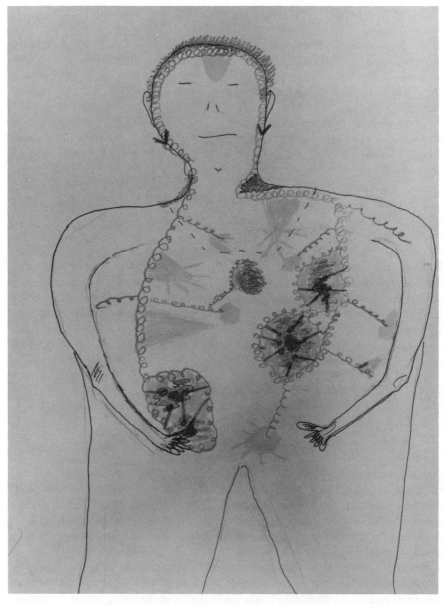

Figure 8.3. Bill's second image of his cancer and immune system.

illness, emphasizing areas that might be causing him the most stress. The Simontons found that their patients tended to experience a cluster of stressors 6 to 18 months prior to the onset of their cancer and that these stresses contributed to the weakening of the immune system's normal functioning (Simonton et al., 1978). Bill seemed to be a prime example of this hypothesis.

Eight months after witnessing the accidental and traumatic death of his grandchild, he had been diagnosed with three different types of cancer, one of which was considered fatal. Bill clearly lacked sufficient outlets to release his deep feelings of mourning and to complete the grieving process. This loss coupled with a series of career disappointments may have left Bill in a state similar to that of individuals cited in studies earlier, with a sense of hopelessness.

During those weeks where therapy sessions focused on Bill's stress, he was faithfully engaging in the imagery process at home. At least once a day he would quiet his mind and review the elimination of his illness and imagine his body's full recovery. This helped him gain a sense of control over his life and had the added benefit of allowing him to relax and be less anxious.

Six weeks after we had begun work together, Bill had lost his voice almost totally. I recognized that our entire session would be channeled through imagery and art, except for an occasional whisper. Because I knew there would now be much time for the imagery and art process, I decided to lengthen the imagery process from our usual 20 minutes to 30 minutes and focus much more intently on the concept of the immune system becoming active. Bill had made great strides in understanding the concept of his body having its own set of defenses, but there were still many passive features ascribed to his white blood cells.

Figure 8.4, entitled "Throbbing," shows the drawing Bill made directly after this lengthened imagery process. What was most noticeable was the intensity with which he portrayed the immune system. Whereas Figure 8.3 shows carefully coiled lines that were well thought out, here Bill has aggressively used a brown crayon and literally attacked the pink outline that was the cancer. This was the first time his white blood cells had totally covered his cancerous tumors. The activity of his immune system was the most visible. Bill was unable to say much about this image. Each word was a strain. He felt pain around his throat represented by a blue line that cut across this reddened, irritated, and throbbing area. Bill said he was frustrated that he could not speak with other people. Colleagues that he encountered shied away from him while he shied away from social engagements. These frustrations came out in his drawing, which may have been a release for that week's feelings.

In the 3 months that have passed since I began work with Bill, both his physical condition and mental attitude have continued to improve. With his radiation treatment completed, his voice is returning along with his energy. He is walking around a track (instead of jogging) and taking on a small number of speaking engagements. Bill feels that the imagery process and keeping a positive attitude helped him tremendously. He said he needed someone "to bring from inside me what I already had." I believe by combining the imagery process with art therapy, Bill had a tangible tool that he could use daily and an outlet for his emotions even when he had no voice.

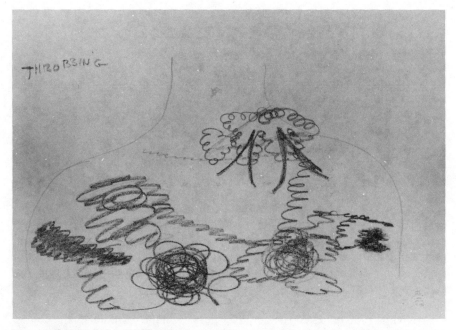

Figure 8.4. "Throbbing," Bill's third image of his cancer and more activated immune system.

While Bill's overall prognosis remains serious, he is living each day more fully and focusing on spending time with family and friends.

Regarding Bill's intense feelings of grief over the loss of his grandchild, as he reached the 1-year anniversary of his 21-month-old grandson's death, his white blood cell count plummeted and his doctors feared he might need to be placed in isolation as protection against contracting an infection. Our session that week focused on this great loss, and Bill found overwhelming feelings of grief welling up in him. Tatelbaum (1980) has discussed the intensity of anniversary reactions and states: "Anniversaries are all the more potent when our feelings about the loss were supressed. We may be caught by surprise at a time that may feel inappropriate" (p. 52). After acknowledging these strong feelings and releasing some of them, Bill appeared more at ease physically and emotionally. The following week his white blood cell count had risen to normal and he was making plans to attend several workshops. I believe Bill's intense physical reaction to his grandson's death points to the deep connection between the mind and body. This child had died in his home, leaving Bill and other family members with unresolved guilt over not watching the toddler more carefully and therefore "allowing" the accident to take place. This 1-year anniversary seemed to be a line of demarcation for Bill, after which he appeared much more clearly focused on the goal of living.

FRAN: POSITIVE IMAGING OF CHEMOTHERAPY

Fran, a musician in her fifties, immersed herself in drawing and the problems contained in her artwork rather than plunging into the problems in her life. Working out her feelings concerning her illness on paper first, she emerged from the art process with greater clarity and insight into her body's own resources and the conflicts she was facing.

When Fran first came to see me, she had recently been told she was ill; however, her reaction was quite different from Bill's. While Bill's symbol for cancer was seen as a large implosion, Fran's cancer was portrayed as gray and brown dots. The drawing made during our first session together showed her cancer as light, small, and contained in one area. Her immune system, in the form of large, yellow white blood cells, was heading toward the cancerous area. What contrasted with an otherwise optimistic picture was that the white blood cells stopped just short of the cancer. This is not an unusual initial reaction, and in Fran's case, she showed her denial and desire not to touch these abnormal cells. What was also clear was that Fran believed she possessed a powerful immune system that could be harnessed to work for her. Fran described her immune system as a cross between a "housecleaner and a doctor."

Yet while Fran believed she could harness her mind to influence the course of her illness, she was greatly distressed at the forthcoming operation to treat her cancer. We discussed what might make the operation easier to face, and it was decided that a relaxation and imagery process focused on her body healing after surgery could be a reassurance. During our next session later that week, I led Fran through an imagery process where she saw herself undergoing successful surgery and experiencing a smooth convalescence. The drawing she made directly after that imagery showed a series of four small pictures of her scar tissue being healed by her immune system. In the last frame of this series, the scar tissue was totally gone. Even as Fran created the picture, she appeared to be healing herself. She made flowing movements with a yellow crayon to indicate the immune system "oozing" out onto her scar tissue. When I asked her how long this healing process would be, she wrote at the bottom of the page: "In 6 weeks the scar tissue will be back to normal, not inflamed or red, just flesh colored."

Six weeks later Fran was, in fact, greatly healed from surgery. At this time, almost 2 months after our first session, she entered a support group that I led and began to explore some major issues in her life around the topics of stress, career, relationships, and goals. What came out of group sessions during those few months was the large amount of stress Fran had placed herself under due to career pressures and outside obligations. Her drawings and collages were often crowded, and Fran worked on the concept of leaving more space in her drawings and in her life. She depicted the pressures 6 months prior to her illness as a yellow flower being crowded out by gray, brown, and black waves of energy that were encroaching on the flower's petals. Fran's strength was that she could conceptualize how things could be different. She might start out the group session by doing a heavy drawing, then portray the opposite feeling in a much lighter picture. She was able to use the art to represent opposing viewpoints.

Fran's image of her cancer had also changed. While her initial drawing showed many positive elements, the drawings she made after recovering from surgery were far more vibrant. Her immune system was shown as flowing out over the page from four directions, instead of just one, and large pink healthy cells appeared as well. Craypas replaced crayons, all lines and shapes were thicker and fatter, yellows were more gold, and light pinks became dark pinks. Over the course of the next 6 weeks, as a group member and at home, Fran did several of these vibrant pink and gold pictures illustrating her immune system's potency. Not one of these drawings showed a cancer cell going astray. I noted to Fran that she never included her chemotherapy treatment in these drawings. She replied that she wanted to accept the chemotherapy better but worried about the side effects.

The following week, Fran and I had an individual session where she discussed this aversion to her treatment. After exploring the pros and cons of undergoing chemotherapy and her ambivalence about this issue, she spent the rest of the session making another, even more detailed and vibrant drawing of her immune system and cancer, this time conscious to include a symbol for chemotherapy. Fran first drew the medicine as green, entering the body and going right for the cancerous area. Later, she drew more of this green chemotherapy going into areas of healthy tissues, saying these chemicals might "go out of control" and affect good cells. She titled this picture "Chemotherapy I," which became the first in a series of pictures that explored her feelings about treatment.

The next week Fran arrived with three more pictures made at home since our last session. The first of these pictures, "Chemotherapy II" (Fig. 8.5), a sequel to "Chemotherapy I," showed a progression in Fran's thinking in reference to her treatment. Her chemotherapy was now shown as pink, wavy lines, no longer flowing into healthy pink tissues where it had not been directed. Fran seemed to have come more to terms emotionally with her treatment, and at the bottom of this picture she wrote:

Chemotherapy II-Pink   flood of chemo, White
Blood and Red Blood Cells being made in the bone
marrow . . . white blood cells spilling out to go after cancer, standing
guard   so that the chemotherapy doesn't get out of hand and do
what it is not   supposed to
   -W blood cells attack cancer along with chemotherapy. . .
   -W blood cells carrying out dead cancer cells to get rid of them
   -cancer nearly obliterated

"Chemotherapy III" (Fig. 8.6), seemed to move into a later stage of the healing process. Fran again showed a petallike diaphragm in red at the top

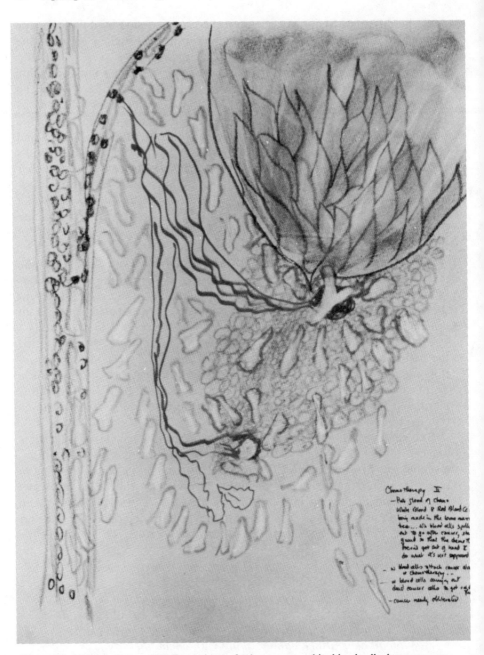

Figure 8.5. ''Chemotherapy II,'' Fran's image for her cancer, white blood cells, bone marrow, chemotherapy, healthy cells, and diaphragm.

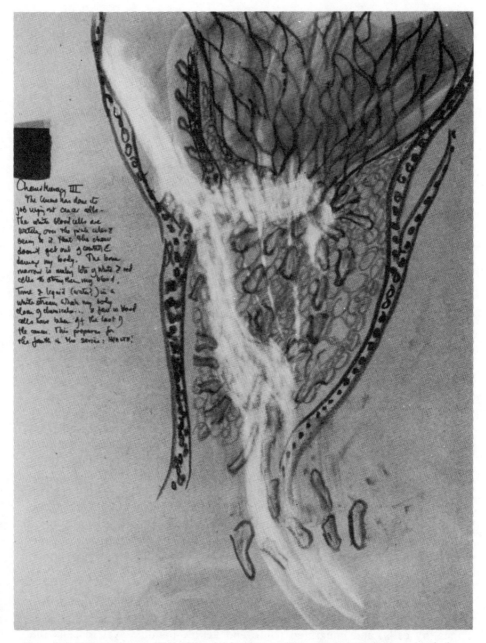

Figure 8.6. ''Chemotherapy III,'' ''Time & Liquid (water?)'' washing chemotherapy chemicals from Fran's body.

of the page and a fantasized inside view of her chest and stomach cavities on a cellular level. While "Chemotherapy II" appears to be an image of organization and activity, "Chemotherapy III" appears to be an image of cleansing and great stability. This later drawing allowed Fran to see her treatment being washed from her body after it has done its job, giving even fuller control and connection to the type of results she would like to envision. At the side of this drawing Fran wrote:

> *Chemotherapy III—The chemo has done its job wiping out cancer cells—The white blood cells are watching over the pink cells and seeing to it that the chemo doesn't get out of control and damage my body. The bone marrow is making lots of white and red cells to strengthen my blood. Time & liquid (water?) in a white stream wash my body clean of chemicals . . . a few W blood cells have taken off the last cancer.*
> *This prepares for the fourth in the series: HEALTH!*

As previously mentioned, Fran had the ability to use her mind and imagination to think positively. Even though she experienced many side effects from her treatment, such as nausea and exhaustion, she was able to discuss her feelings on this issue and depict a more positive outcome through art. While she discussed her medical treatment negatively, on paper it appeared mostly positive. Her drawing allowed her to see concretely that medication might help her body, rather than harm it. Because she spent several hours working out the details of her "Chemotherapy Series," Fran became the symbolic director of her treatment and, I believe, gained some sense of control. While in reality Fran was a passive recipient of her medication as it dripped into her arm, it was now up to her to move the chemotherapy along, seeking out cancerous cells and avoiding healthy cells in her drawing.

This series of pictures did not totally eliminate Fran's conflicts around treatment; nevertheless, she had the chance to confront feelings and fears concerning chemotherapy, the result of imaging something positive entering her body rather than negative. This is a significant shift in thinking and was especially important for Fran, who was starting a macrobiotic diet to support her body's recovery in a more natural way. To continue to imagine her treatment as negative or poison was clearly undermining a basic desire to love and nourish herself back to health.

The last picture of this series, in many ways, speaks for itself. Fran's drawing "Health" (Fig. 8.7) had been given tremendous care and artistic expression. She took the time to draw meticulously more than 100 pink, healthy cells, and integrated white and yellow immune system cells that stand guard "watching out" over her body. "Health," the last of four pictures, explored the issue of chemotherapy and also represented 3 months of work and more than a dozen pictures, exploring, visualizing, and detailing her body's recovery from cancer. This rich image projected onto paper showed deep inner changes for Fran as she utilized art to perceive health.

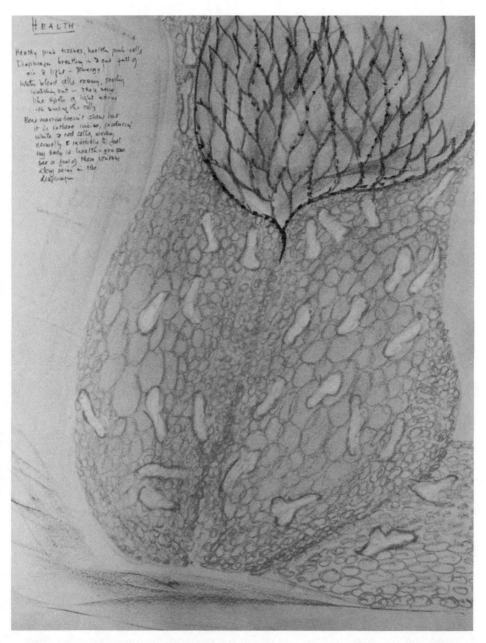

Figure 8.7. "Health," white blood cells "watching out" among Fran's healthy, pink cells.

Fran used art making to leave the "now" and perceive her body as she would like it to be. Drawing was a way to move into the future and stay focused on recovery. She is an excellent example of using the creative process to help oneself heal, not so much by analyzing one's finished artwork as by becoming totally involved in the forms created and perceiving through these productions an alternate way to view cancer and treatment. Through many more months of struggle to regain her energy and vitality, Fran remembered the images and words from her drawings. These pictures were a powerful reminder of Fran's own healing potential. Together, over the next months, we reminded each other of the words and ideas captured in Fran's description of the drawing "Health."

> *Healthy pink tissues, healthy pink cells. Diaphragm*
> *breathing*
> *in & out full of air & light—Energy! White blood cells,*
> *rooming, soothing, watching out—they seem like spots of*
> *light coming in among the cells Bone marrow doesn't show*
> *but it is there inside, producing white & red cells,*
> *working*
> *normally & invisibly to fill my body with health—you can*
> *see a few of them coursing along veins in the diaphragm.*

FUTURE CONSIDERATIONS: UTILIZING IMAGERY AND ART IN HEALING

Helping professionals are placing increased significance on an individual's imagery and art as a way of recognizing and following physical conditions present in the patient's body. The art therapist, who is trained to speak the language of art, is in an optimal position to utilize these messages to influence attitudes blocking the healing process.

The individuals discussed in this chapter used imagery and art as a way to experiment and reinforce beliefs around self-healing that were new to them. Imaging proved to be a useful tool to both Fran and Bill. When Fran wanted to consider that undergoing surgery could be a positive experience, she imaged that first in her mind and then drew her scar tissue being soothed by the immune system. When Bill wanted to ascribe less power to his cancer and more power to his immune system, he also imaged that first and then made a drawing to reinforce that imagery. What was envisioned in one's mind and on paper had an impact on unconscious feelings that might run contrary to the positive images presented. These individuals were able to confront their beliefs that they might not get well or could not possibly play a role in their own recovery. The size, shape, color, and density of one's white blood cells became representational of how individuals viewed their body's healing resources. Likewise, these qualities were investigated in the individuals' images of their cancer with special emphasis placed on whether or not the cancerous cells were actually being directly contacted and affected by the white blood cells.

Once individuals had the experience of completing an imagery and art process centered on eliminating their cancer, an entirely new set of possibilities lay ahead. Here was a tool that could be used daily to participate in and possibly take control of physical functions previously thought to be out of conscious control. Just the mere repetition of a structured relaxation and guided imagery process is not always healing, however. Individuals using imagery need direction. Images can harm as well as heal. In this role, the art therapist's skills are called into play to point out how individuals may increase the positive power of their symbolism and grasp its negative ramifications. It is vital not to rely on verbal reports of one's imagery process, but rather to use subsequent drawings, as illustrated throughout this chapter, to observe that an individual is shoring up defenses through imagery, rather than tearing them down.

The recent scientific research from the new field of psychoneuroimmunology shows the deep and far-reaching connection between the body and mind. The image is reemerging to take its central place again in the healing process. The extent to which the altering of an individual's imagery will concretely change the course of the disease still remains to be seen. Enough evidence does exist, however, to warrant forging ahead with imagery and art as powerful catalysts to stimulate the outlook of cancer patients in a more favorable direction. It is my hope that in the future individuals' treatment programs will be considered incomplete if they do not include art therapy to allow patients to investigate their outlook toward their illness, their immune system, their medication, and their goal of regaining health.

REFERENCES

Achterberg, J. (1985). *Imagery in healing: Shamanism and modern medicine*. Boston: New Science Library.

Achterberg, J., Simonton, C., & Simonton, S. (1976). *Stress, psychological factors, and cancer*. Fort Worth, TX: New Medicine Press.

Fischer, S., & Cleveland, S. (1956). Relationship of body image to site of cancer. *Psychosomatic Medicine, 18*(4), 308.

Glassman, J. (1983). *The cancer survivors*. Garden City, NY: Dial.

Harrower, M., & Thomas, C. (1975). Human figure drawings in a prospective study of six disorders: Hypertension, coronary heart disease, malignant tumor, suicide, mental illness, and emotional disturbance. *Journal of Nervous & Mental Disease, 161*(3), 191.

Hurley, T. J., III. (1983). Psychoaneuroimmunology: The birth of a new field. *Investigations: A Bulletin of the Institute of Noetic Sciences, (1)*2, 1.

Hutschnecker, A. (1951). *The will to live*. Englewood Cliffs, NJ: Prentice-Hall.

Klopfer, B. (1957). Psychological variables in human cancer. *Journal of Projective Techniques, 21,*

Kowal, S. (1955). Emotions as a cause of cancer: 18th and 19th century contributions. *Psychoanalytic Review, 42,* 220.

Kübler-Ross, E. (1981). *Living with death and dying.* New York: Macmillan.

Lockhart, R. (1981). Cancer in myth and dream. In J. Goldberg (Ed.), *Psychotherapeutic treatment of cancer patients.* New York: Free Press.

McNiff, S. (1981). *The arts and psychotherapy.* Springfield, IL: Charles C. Thomas.

Simonton, C., & Simonton, S. (1975). Belief systems and management of the emotional aspects of malignancy. *Journal of Transpersonal Psychology, 33,* 7.

Simonton, C., Simonton, S., & Creighton, J. (1978). *Getting well again.* New York: St. Martin's.

Tatelbaum, J. (1980). *The courage to grieve.* New York: Harper & Row.

CHAPTER 9

Engaging the Somatic Patient in Healing Through Art

MARI MARKS FLEMING AND CAROL THAYER COX

Martha reluctantly sat in the art therapy group and said she didn't belong there. "The only thing wrong with me is my headache." Always difficult to engage in the group, Martha showed no interest in the art media, nor the group discussion.

"Could you draw your headache?" I asked. Martha picked up red and orange and with intense strokes drew a head with a band of color around the forehead. Lines and bursts of color surrounded the head.

It is often difficult to engage the patient who experiences unspecified anxiety or distress localized in the body. Clients seen as resistant or not yet available to psychotherapeutic intervention may be referred to the art therapist. Increasingly, among these clients are those who initially present physical complaints, although hospitalized on a psychiatric unit.

Art therapy with clients who present physical concerns emphasizes the art process, the client's interpretations, and growing awareness of self. Patients can then be assisted in focusing on their physical pain in making connection between their physical distress and their experience and feelings, and thus begin to own and express disowned aspects of the self.

Psychosomatic illness provides an extremely effective defense against awareness of underlying anxiety. Art therapy with these patients requires an approach that will integrate physical and affective experience.

PSYCHOSOMATIC ILLNESS

Ramsay, Wittkower, and Warner (1976) state that psychosomatic patients' insistence that their problems are solely medical makes them a major challenge for even the most proficient psychotherapist.

Exposed to stress—feelings of threat, loss, gain, or insignificance—psychosomatic patients defend against feelings they consider childish or threatening. This warding off of painful emotions leads to lack of awareness of body warning signals and to cutting off of spontaneous emotions. Stressed by physiologically experienced danger and autonomic nervous system responses that are consistently ignored or inhibited, vulnerable systems of the body are eventually affected, leading to physical pain or distress. The resultant illness can be life threatening.

The term *psychosomatic disorders (psychophysiologic disorders* in DSM-III) is generally used to describe a group of disorders characterized by physical *symptoms* that are affected by emotional factors and that involve a single organ system, usually under *autonomic nervous system* control (APA, 1980). Illnesses generally agreed to be within this category include: bronchial asthma, rheumatoid arthritis, ulcerative colitis, essential hypertension, neurodermatitis, thyrotoxicosis, peptic ulcer, diabetes mellitus, migraine, and coronary artery disease, as well as eating disorders (Ramsay et al., 1976).

Possibly resulting from disturbance in the early mother–child relationship, the development of a psychosomatic disorder occurs only following an interplay of many factors. These include:

1. An inherited or early-acquired organ or system vulnerability
2. Consistent emotional arousal that therefore affects that organ system
3. Early maladaptive patterns of conflict and defense; sustained emotional arousal resulting from stress, dependent upon the kind of stress and the individual's perception of it
5. Precipitating life situations
6. The individual's tendency to focus on the physical disturbance
7. The society's attitudes concerning stresses (Ramsay et al., 1976)

In treating these patients, the complex physical and psychological interrelation must be considered. Constant therapist availability, good advice, a positive transference relationship, improving object relations, and the patient's developing the ability to deal with the problems are advised (Freyberger, 1973). Although generally resistant to psychotherapy, patients who can learn to recognize the relationship between their somatic disorder and the emotional difficulty are most likely to respond to treatment (Dunbar, 1943). The art process described in this chapter provides a way of facilitating this recognition.

REVIEW OF ART THERAPY TREATMENT

The majority of art therapy work with physical distress focuses on medical illness and emphasizes expression of the experience and feelings concerning the illness and hospitalization. It includes working through and accepting the physical condition and losses inherent in the illness (Landgarten, 1981; Ravenscroft, Bruhn, Sims, Datel, and Jensch, 1979).

In contrast, the psychosomaticizing patient represses underlying affect, protecting him or her from unacceptable dependency needs. The limited art therapy literature in working with psychosomatic illness usually suggests a focus on the presenting problem. Landgarten (1981) proposes art as a tool for insight into attitudes toward pain. Her focus includes depiction of the pain and autogenic training including relaxation and reinforcement of pleasant feeling (Shapiro, 1985). For example, by asking patients to draw their feelings of pain and then use the same colors to create something more satisfying, pain can be symbolically transformed through the creative act.

Fleming (1985) stresses the importance of the client's becoming involved in the art process and using the art in self-exploration. This was found to be successful in increasing fluidity of control and self-awareness.

According to Wolf, Willmouth, and Watkins (1986) in their review of the literature, art therapy was used with eating disorders to increase the patient's awareness of unrecognized and unacknowledged feelings, to promote controlled expression and self-awareness, and to use the art therapist as a self-object. Art therapy is occasionally found to be a bridge to verbal therapy, and the concrete and kinesthetic nature of the art process can be a container for early, intense, and painful affect, supporting the patient's experience of gaining control.

Art therapists working with patients who have somatic concerns offer support, open discussion, and reassurance concerning the presenting problem. In addition the positive consistent relationship provides gratification of dependency needs as does the provision of art supplies and satisfying activity.

Yet despite the art therapist's empathy and support, the psychosomatic patient generally resists treatment and sees the physical illness as the only problem (Lachman-Chapin, 1979).

Can art therapy also provide that necessary step for awareness of underlying factors, for making the connection between the somatic distress and the affective domain? Can the making of art provide experiences of healing? Theories of development, including the role of sensory experience and of creativity, provide models for an art therapy process as an integrating dynamic. This process connects into a new whole what has previously been split into two: the awareness of bodily discomfort and the repressed emotional need.

DEVELOPMENT OF THE SOMATIC–AFFECTIVE ART PROCESS

The somatic–affective art process I developed to use with the psychosomatic patient first encourages the depiction of one's physical concerns, that is, one's known and accepted view of oneself. The second phase of the process involves the patient in an affective use of color and form in developing an image from these colors and lines. As patients are invited to alter or modify this image to make it more satisfying or complete, they in some sense change or attempt to heal it. Reflecting on their experiences, patients explore the relationship of their images to their experience, thus reintegrating cognitive awareness and affective experience.

When Martha insisted that her headache was the most meaningful fact about herself, the communication of this in art provided the possibility of involving her in the materials, giving her an experience of membership in the group, and validating her observations and experience.

While others could better see and empathize with the tightness and intense pain as pictured in the drawing, Martha became only minimally involved in the materials and allowed no new experience or idea. Therefore, I suggested she look at the lines and colors she had drawn in and around the head and see if they suggested an image. After looking at the drawing for several minutes, Martha changed the color in the forehead to a headband and the lines emanating from the head to a feather headdress. Pronouncing it an Indian, she labeled it "On the Warpath!" In discussion, others wondered whether the Indian was mad, and whether Martha ever got angry. Looking at the drawing, she laughed and agreed that maybe she was feeling a little mad. The group talked about when they got headaches and related their head pain to events and feelings in their lives.

This process proved to be useful in finding a relationship between physical ailments and instances of stress or tension. The process was later modified into two drawings. First, a drawing of a human body with lines and colors denoting physical pain or distress localized within the body outline was requested. Then a second drawing was made with only the lines and colors for the physical sensations reproduced on the page. These lines and colors were used as the foundation for projection of an image (similar to Ulman's [1977] diagnostic use of the scribble), and finally the image was completed. The image was then explored in relation to the experience of physical distress.

A further modification of the procedure came about as I participated in a group led by a student intern. I used black to show neck and shoulder tension and upper back pain. The resultant image, an ink bottle filled with intense and vibrant colors, was tightly closed. The colors needed to come out! The inhibiting of productive aspects of the self seemed to lead to physical sequelae, just as did repression of negative emotions.

We introduced the suggestion that images could be modified or changed to make them more satisfying for the artist. Following the inclusion of this step, individuals appeared to experience increased identification with their images (owning them) and increased awareness of their ability to make changes in their personal circumstances.

Certain patterns in the use of color and line began to emerge while using this process with patients. Patterns appeared to relate to diagnosis, incidence of earlier trauma, and the developmental stage at which any trauma occurred. The projected image usually reflected a feeling state needing acceptance or expression. The way in which the image was modified, helped, or healed reflected the patient's defensive or coping style and whether the patient might seal over or integrate the experience (Wadeson, 1980).

The somatic–affective process is similar to other art therapists' emphasis on recording perceived pain, particularly in the relationship between color, physical distress, and targeted areas of the body. It differs in its emphasis on the process and the patient's independence of choice in creating and modifying the image.

INSTRUCTIONS FOR USE OF THE SOMATIC–AFFECTIVE PROCESS

This process was developed for use within an art therapy group, but may be used in individual assessment and treatment.

First Drawing

1. "Draw a simple outline of a body, filling the page." This body outline provides diagnostic information. If clients are resistant, for example, stating they can't draw, you may add, "Just a general outline, it doesn't need to be of you." If further encouragement is needed, connecting circles or shapes may be mentioned.
2. "Use colors and lines to indicate physical pain or discomfort you experience and where you generally feel it. Fill all of the area where you experience the pain or discomfort. Differentiate between kinds and intensity of physical sensations by your use of color, line, or intensity."
3. If there is sufficient time, the patient may use this as a body history, including previous physical distress, surgery, and accidents, giving dates and written details.

Second Drawing

1. "Do not include body outline. Use the same colors, lines, shapes, and intensities that you used for pain and distress and transfer them to the second piece of paper in the same [spatial] relationship to each other. You may enlarge them or eliminate minor areas."
2. "Place your first drawing out of sight. Using your lines and colors as the beginning of your drawing, complete any image it suggests. [pause] You may extend the colors and shapes, add to, or change them." After picture is completed, instruct patients to title their picture.

Third Procedure

"Look at your picture—take your time. What would make this image better for you? Work on it, change, simplify, add to it. You may add new colors to soothe or comfort it. You may soften, change, or intensify it. Bring it to a place that is comfortable for you."

Final Procedure

"Compare your two pictures. Do you see any connections between them? Any differences? [Leave time for this self-investigation.] Do the drawings suggest any relationship between your physical distress and your feelings? Do you see any relationship to how you cope with stress?"

Discussion

The following comments are suggested to encourage discussion focusing on communication and the process.

What was this like for you?
Did you discover anything?

(If in a group, have all show the first picture at the same time.)

Discussion of the Second Drawing

What was it like to use the colors or to complete the image you found?
Did you find the picture or image changing as you worked on it?
How did you want to change or modify it?
What did you discover?
Do you see any relation between your image and feelings?
Is there a change you could make in yourself or your life circumstances that would reflect the change you made in your picture?
What could you apply to your life from the changes you made in the picture?
Would this change take care of your physical needs?
Your emotional needs?

Modifications

The process may also be used with psychiatric patients who focus on physical symptoms. It can provide a more inclusive view of the patient, through acceptance of the presenting symptom and an experience of the art therapy process.

The beginning exercise incorporates the clear boundaries and reality-focused orientation useful in work with the very fragmented or psychotic individual. With such patients, however, the instructions to project an image onto the colors and lines may be experienced as supporting hallucinatory or regressive material and therefore not advisable in early or short-term treatment. In step two, suggest that the patient draw a picture of some way to help the physical discomfort feel better, thereby encouraging a reality-oriented response.

CASE EXAMPLE

We have used this process in a variety of settings with psychosomatic patients. The case material will describe the process used within an inpatient eating disorder unit, in a clinical setting.

CISSIE

This 26-year-old woman was admitted to an eating disorder unit in a small private urban hospital. The multidisciplinary treatment included medical monitoring, a nutrition program, verbal individual and group treatment, family therapy, and body image group (art therapy). The body image group met three times weekly.

The somatic–affective process was usually used early in treatment, generally following an evaluative group that focused on depicting liked and disliked aspects of the body. This picture was also explored in relation to age of puberty, experiences of developmental change, and any similarities to areas of body disliked or familial patterns of illness, especially those stress related. The drawing of physical distress provided a way to communicate physical experiences and sensations related to bulimia or anorexia, including satiation, purging, starvation, or distress accompanying refeeding and changes in food consumption.

Cissie, a delicate blonde woman, was increasingly unable to eat. Admitted to the hospital because of her family's concern, she was diagnosed as having bulimia. Sweet, compliant, and vague, she avowed complete cooperation with the program. In the first group meeting, she tremulously told the group of a recent rape by an unidentified assailant. Her initial marker pen drawing of this scene demonstrated skill with the materials but had confusing overlays and was restricted to the center of the page.

At the next group meeting, to ascertain the level of pathology as well as give a concrete reality-based assignment, she was asked to depict areas of the body she liked or disliked. Cissie identified her hands and face as positive areas, the sexual areas as very negative and other areas of the trunk as disliked.

When asked to draw her family, Cissie made a circle with sunlike spikes emanating from the periphery. Within the circle family members merged in a sketchily drawn, faceless mass. Cissie depicted the shared projections, distorted relationships, and rigid boundaries of her bulimia family (Raven-scroft, 1988).

In the next phase of treatment, the group focused on family issues and experiences. An abstract family drawing assisted Cissie in differentiating between family members. A picture began to emerge of a depressed, poorly differentiated mother and a negative dominant father with enmeshed children who were to bring happiness and purpose into the parents' lives. Cissie had known more closeness with her father, but in family therapy the family secret, her father's bulimia, was discovered. Cissie's paternal grandmother had been anorexic, and the family pattern continued as Cissie's mother controlled and restricted access to the kitchen and food. In the hospital, Cissie called her family daily. When this was stopped as a family interven-tion, her mother became ill and the family wanted Cissie discharged. They felt that the hospital wasn't helping!

Throughout childhood Cissie had been a good child, popular and pretty. Having been a dancer as well as anorexic as a teenager, she had sought more productive individuation by entering art school. The family was not sup-portive and encouraged her to become a stewardess. At 19 she became engaged to the son of a neighbor. This boyfriend, idealized by Cissie's mother, alternately needed and physically abused Cissie. She was able to break free of this destructive enmeshment, ended the engagement, and sought work as a commercial artist. This change was probably facilitated by her brother moving back to the parents' home. Her fragile individuation was stressed by the rape and her brother's recent marriage and move from the parents' home. The world and sexual relationships were dangerous; her parents in their depression needed her. In response to the pull to parents who needed her, Cissie regressed to a fragile childlike self, alternately unable to eat, then secretly bingeing and purging.

On the surface, Cissie appeared to eat and cooperate with treatment. In her artwork she created cute childlike animal and people figures using marker and pencil or simplistic pictures storytelling about the group themes. Yet she did not gain weight and others suspected her of hiding food and vomiting. This was confirmed. Her only authentic liveliness appeared as she created a happy memory—a childlike plasticene horse with herself as a child, riding. She told of her years before puberty when she was left to ride free as the only time of pleasure, competence, and freedom in her life.

Following this experience of mastery, we introduced the drawing of phys-ical–somatic distress to provide an occasion where Cissie might safely iden-tify negative feelings and experiences. She told us about childhood abuse, verbal teasing, and fondling of her large breasts and buttocks. She pictured her painful churning stomach in red, using black for pressure in head, eyes, and lower back and in two painful pressure points in temple and hip. A scar was on her forehead as a result of the rape (Fig. 9.1).

Elaborating these colors and shapes in the next drawing, Cissie expanded them, picturing a child's horse on wheels. Although exhibiting her charac-

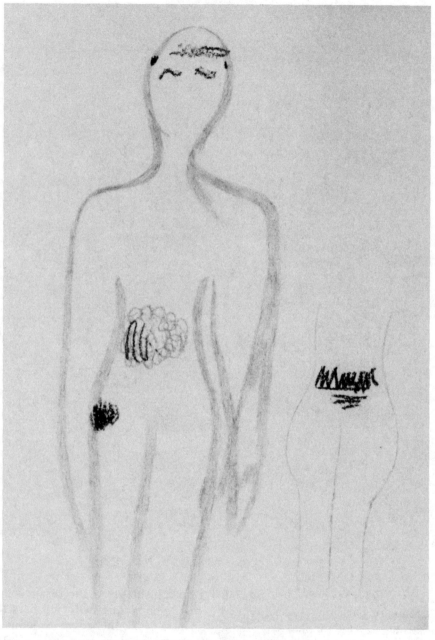

Figure 9.1. Cissie's drawing of somatic distress.

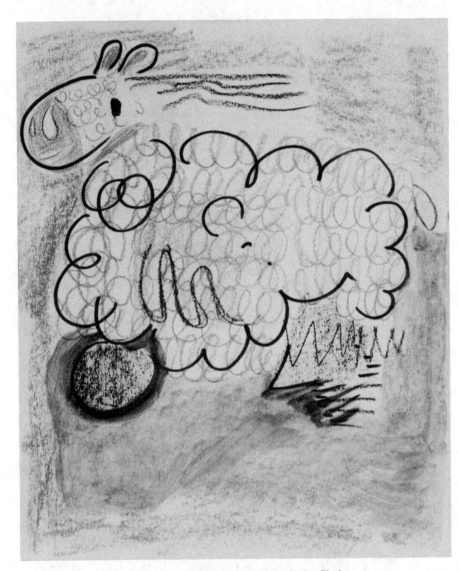

Figure 9.2. A child's horse on wheels, by Cissie.

teristic defenses of humor and childlike denial, she seemed to regain some feeling of pleasure. As she worked to make the picture better for herself, she added medium blue surrounding the image. She rubbed and smoothed this color and intensified the speed at which the horse moved (Fig. 9.2). Cissie began to recall her childhood on horseback, her adventures and independence. Through this image she identified her need to stay a child and to please others, as well as her family's need for her to deny or keep secret hurt and distress. In the next group meeting, Cissie began to experiment with materials and memories, new behaviors, and recognition of herself. As she tore paper and used intense paint, she pictured feelings and fantasies. She began to exhibit openly her hunger and her noncompliance with other patients and the staff, experiencing conflict between her needs and her striving toward life and independence.

DISCUSSION

Cissie's first attempt at individuation as an adolescent had taken place as a beginning dancer and focused on control of her hunger. Within a family where the mother rigidly restricted access to the kitchen and father alternatively binged and vomited, Cissie's denied needs for nurturance were expressed in somatic preoccupation. She embarked on a recurrent cycle of attempting to individuate; starving as she sought to control her needs; returning to enmeshment reflected in her family's choice of boyfriends or career; resulting dependence and victimization; then renewed attempts to launch herself. The focus on the body, denying her hunger with resultant secretive voracious binges, followed by expulsion of this regressive appetite (often experienced as a blank period), defended against the feelings of pain, neglect, and lack of authentic caring or support for her individuation. Within the therapeutic relationship, trust and participation had been stuck at this defended level until the experience of focusing on the physical experience of pain and distress. Given permission to project her own image and modify it, she experienced freedom within boundaries, and feelings within control.

As the nurturing image was experienced within the caressing and soothing experience of the media, Cissie experimented with modulating and intensifying colors and image, gaining an experience of trial action and affecting the outcome. Intense voracious hunger and vigorous action could now be experienced within the art materials and process, supporting awareness of rejected and internalized feeling states and part objects. Cissie found she could contain and experience her feelings within a new, more authentic whole.

CONCLUSION

Trained to empathize and support expression and self-understanding, art therapists often experience helplessness in the face of the psychosomatic client's intractable lack of awareness of feelings. Encouragement or requests for expression and involvement in the art process may elicit only resistance or incomprehension.

The drawing of somatic distress within a body outline conveys the client's experience and provides an alphabet of color, form, and pressure. Enlargement of these areas and elaboration into an image make use of this language in a personal expression.

The somatic–affective process can assist in assessment. The most significant information gained from our observations related to the high proportion of red, black, and gray used to depict painful areas of body, especially when coupled with early object loss or separation (Fleming, 1982).

Recombining experience and self-perception into a new representation prepared the patient to meet new experience (Blos, 1962). Art and the creative process can provide the connection between somatic concerns and underlying feelings. The crisis of psychosomatic illness creates an opportunity for acceptance and integration in coping with the stresses inherent in life.

REFERENCES

American Psychiatric Association. (1980). *A psychiatric glossary* (5th ed.). Boston: Little, Brown.

Blos, P. (1962). *On adolescence*. New York: Free Press.

Dunbar, F. (1943). *Psychosomatic diagnosis*. New York: Hoeber.

Fleming, M. M. (1982). Early object loss and its relation to creativity as expressed through art therapy. In Di Maria, E. (Ed.), *Proceedings of the Thirteenth Annual Conference of the American Art Therapy Association*. Philadelphia: AATA.

Fleming, M. M. (1985). *Body image therapy with groups of anorexia and bulimic patients*. Unpublished manuscript presented to Sixteenth Annual American Art Therapy Association Conference, New Orleans.

Freyberger, H. (1973). *Supportive psychotherapy in the medical clinic*. Paper presented at the Second Congress of the International College of Psychosomatic Medicine, Amsterdam.

Lachman-Chapin, M. (1979). Kohut's theories on narcissism: Implications for art therapy. *American Journal of Art Therapy, 19*, 3–9.

Landgarten, H. B. (1981). *Clinical art therapy, a comprehensive guide*. New York: Brunner/Mazel.

Ramsay, R. A., Wittkower, E. D., & Warner, H. (1976). Treatment of psychosomatic disorders. In B. B. Wolman (Ed.), *The therapists handbook, treatment methods of mental disorders*. New York: Van Nostrand Reinhold.

Ravenscroft, K., Bruhn, M., Sims, V., Datel, K., & Jensch, K. (1979). Art therapy with life-threatened medically ill children. In L. Gantt (Ed.), *Proceedings of the Tenth Annual Conference of the American Art Therapy Association*. Washington, DC: AATA.

Ravenscroft, K. (1988). Psychoanalytic family therapy approaches to the adolescent bulimics. In H. J. Schwartz (Ed.), *Bulimia: Psychoanalytic treatment and theory*. New York: International Universities Press.

Shapiro, B. (1985) All I have is the pain. Art therapy in an inpatient chronic pain relief unit. *American Journal of Art Therapy, 24*, 44–48.

Ulman, E. (1977). A new use of art in psychiatric diagnosis. In Ulman & Dachinger (Eds.), *Art therapy in theory and practice*. New York: Schocken.

Wadeson, H. (1980). *Art psychotherapy*. New York: Wiley.

Wolf, J. M., Willmouth, M. E., & Watkins, A. (1986). Art therapy's role in the ﹍reatment of anorexia nervosa. *American Journal of Art Therapy, 25*, 39–46.

CHAPTER 10

Severe Head Injury and Its Stages of Recovery Explored Through Art Therapy

JUDITH WALD

Fifty thousand Americans die each year as a direct result of traumatic brain injury, while another 50,000 to 60,000 survive severe head injury with varying degrees of disability. It is the leading cause of death in western nations for ages 1 to 44; two-thirds of the survivors left with physical, intellectual, or behavioral deficits are below the age of 30. Male victims outnumber females by four to one.

It is frightening to realize that a head injury can happen to any of us. Most head injuries occur in motor vehicle accidents, often alcohol related. The mishap of one moment can change an entire lifetime. Working for 5 years on a head trauma unit in a rehabilitation center, I also have encountered patients injured by motorcycle, bicycle, and snowmobile accidents; sports accidents involving skiing and boating; industrial accidents such as falls from a scaffold, window, or roof; a fall down an elevator shaft; a fall off a banister at a fraternity pledge party; falls and kicks from a horse; injury in a barroom brawl; injury from being pinned under a fallen tree; and gunshot wounds. Patients were also treated who suffered a hypoxic ischemic episode (loss of oxygen to the blood) following such incidents as cardiac arrest, stroke, strangulation, drowning, and drug accidents. Predominance of daredevil, sociopathic tendencies in males may account for the higher incidence of head injuries in males. Patients ranged in age from 14 to 70; the average patient was a 24-year-old male.

The art therapist who works with a head-injured population may be somewhat at a loss in a facility where physical medicine and rehabilitation are the prime focus, for our training has traditionally centered around psychiatric illnesses and psychological issues. Our knowledge of neurology and physical medicine is often nil. While physical injury has its psychological sequelae, which are indeed the art therapist's area of expertise, it is most important that the art therapist working with a head-injured population have a basic understanding of how the brain works and what happens morphologically during and after an injury. Injuries to specific areas of the brain have specific impacts on speech, movement, sensory interpretation, intellect, and behavior. We need a working vocabulary of medical terms to understand case presentations and to gain acceptance as part of the treatment team. The following section will describe what happens to the brain during traumatic brain injury.

MEDICAL DESCRIPTION OF HEAD INJURY

Head trauma may be divided into two main groups; open and closed head injuries. A gunshot injury typifies an open head injury, where the skull and dura (outmost membrane covering the brain) have been penetrated. Consciousness is often preserved; brain damage is localized and general brain damage may be minimal or even absent. Except in war conditions, the closed head injury is more common.

In closed head injury, the dura is not penetrated, but the type of blow, its situation, its velocity, and whether the skull was mobile at the time of impact are important factors. Brain movement and deformation within the skull occur in two ways: by acceleration and by deceleration injuries.

In an acceleration injury, the head is suddenly accelerated, as in a boxing impact when the head jolts back. Inertial forces strike the still unmoving brain against the accelerating skull.

In a deceleration injury, the rapidly moving head is suddenly stopped, as in an auto–tree collision. Though skull movement is arrested, the gelatinous and visco-elastic brain continues to move during a 20-millisecond time interval. The brain may rotate in the skull around the axis of the brain stem. Different loci of the brain substance become deformed to different degrees. Internal shearing and stress forces can traumatize and disrupt cells and their processes in the depths of the brain. Deep lacerations can cause subarachnoid, subdural, or intercerebral hemorrhage, leading to loss of function in affected body parts. Immediate loss of consciousness results from the deformation affecting the brain stem and its reticular activating system, which control sleep and wakefulness.

Contre-coup injuries result from the impact between the accelerating brain and the decelerating skull. Those parts of the brain most distant from the blow receive the most damage.

In closed head injury, changes of consciousness range from confusion, concussion, and semicoma to coma. This chapter will deal with severe head injury that occurs when the brain cells have been severely traumatized, resulting in at least 20 minutes of unconsciousness.

Following the initial brain damage, further damage may be caused by secondary hypoxemia (deficient oxygenation of the blood) from respiratory embarrassment, due to airway obstruction or circulatory disturbance. Forty percent of severely brain-injured patients have cerebral ischemia (deficiency of blood due to constriction or obstruction of a blood vessel) from elevated intracranial pressure (ICP), or brain shift from accumulation of intracranial hematoma (growing blood clot) or brain edema (swelling). When the brain swells, it has nowhere to expand within the solid skull. Surgery is usually required to evacuate the mass lesion and expanded swelling in order to prevent permanent brain damage to healthy cells.

Another complication of brain injury may be seizures, which occur when excessive and abnormal messages are released from damaged brain cells. A focal seizure affects one part or side of the body without change of consciousness. In a grand mal seizure, the patient loses consciousness, the body stiffens and jerks; the patient may secrete from the mouth or lose control of urine or feces, loses memory of the seizure, and needs to sleep afterward. In a petit mal seizure, there is no change of body movement, little behavioral change, and brief lapses of awareness. A psychomotor seizure results in changed behavior, patterned body movements, and brief lapses in consciousness or purposeful activity. The art therapist will frequently encounter patients who have setbacks due to seizures, and needs to understand what they entail as well as report back to the team their manifestation in artwork.

Brain injuries produce various degrees of pathological damage, ranging from cellular and subcellular reversible injury to shearing and tearing of brain cells, as well as disruption of brain tissue by contusion, brain hemorrhage, or laceration. The lesions vary in location and degree from patient to patient. The lesion of head injury is a combination of diffuse white matter disruption, contusion, and hemorrhage.

Contusions and lacerations occur mostly on the anterior and inferior surfaces of the frontal lobes and in the anterior and middle portions of the temporal lobes and limbic structures. This accounts for the deficits and alterations in intellect, memory, and behavior that characterize the head-injured patient. The art therapist must be aware of each patient's area of injury to clarify performance expectations.

The frontal lobes are the centers for initiation, foresight, judgment, and formulation of ideas. Frontal lobe injury causes personality changes, especially with bilateral injuries. The patient characteristically lacks insight into his[1] behavior and is disinhibited emotionally, especially sexually. Judgment is impaired, and the patient lacks ability to plan ahead. Mood is euphoric, without drive. Intellectual ability is diminished.

Temporal lobe damage results in explosive outbursts of rage and aggressive behavior, which can occur in a formerly placid individual due to seizure activity. Memory deficits and impaired capacity for new learning also result. The temporal lobe is also concerned with smell, balance, hearing, and sexual drive.

---

[1]Since most head injury patients are male, the masculine pronoun is used throughout this chapter.

The parietal lobe is primarily responsible for the interpretation of sensations of touch, pain, temperature, and proprioception. The occipital lobe is the area responsible for vision. Physical defects that frequently occur following head injury include the following eye signs: nystagmus (involuntary rapid movement of eyeball), ataxic eye movements; paralysis of eye muscles; widely dilated pupils that don't react to light; partial or complete blindness; color vision loss; and perceptual disorders (inability to understand or interpret what one sees).

Other physical defects can include: spastic diplegia, or paralysis affecting like parts on both sides of the body, causing difficulty in speech and swallowing, loss of movement and volitional control of limbs; hemiplegia, or paralysis of one side of the body; ataxia, failure of muscular coordination; apraxia, total inability to produce volitional movement; and dyspraxia, or partial loss of ability to perform coordinated tasks. The art therapist can avoid humiliating a patient who has physical, manipulative limitations by taping down the paper and placing the crayons on the patient's unimpaired side. Due to fiber crossover in the medulla (at the base of the brain), functional hemispheric dominance is opposite its locale.

One cerebral hemisphere is dominant in language, so a right-handed person who has left hemisphere damage has impairments in speaking, writing, and verbal memory. Language impairments range from aphasia (loss or defect in expression or comprehension of spoken or written language) and dysnomia (partial inability to name or recognize objects). Comprehension of speech is a function of the dominant temporoparieto-occipital cortex linked by neurons with the anterior part of the frontal lobe where further processing leads to sequencing of ideas and language. The nondominant hemisphere is concerned with visual memory, spatial relationships, body image perception, music, emotional response, and realization of wellness or illness.

It should be noted that, while certain parts of the brain are responsible for particular functions, the brain normally performs as a whole. Therefore, after brain damage, clinical deficits result not only from loss of localized brain function, but also from the healthy parts of the brain trying to perform without the normal inhibitions and interactions from other centers.

In assessing the severity of head injury after the acute comatose phase has passed, two measures are used; the duration of retrograde amnesia (RA) and post-traumatic amnesia (PTA). RA is the time elapsing between the last clear memory before the injury and the accident, ranging from seconds to 5 minutes. PTA, anterograde memory impairment, is the time elapsing between injury and the first clear memory the patient experiences. Most important is PTA, whose duration is correlated with measures of severity, with length of time away from work, and with residual psychiatric disability. For instance, with a PTA of under 1 hour, work can be started 1 month after injury; with PTA under 7 days, 4 months; more than 7 days, 12 months. Children recover more quickly. However, with open head injury, RA and

PTA may not occur (Leigh, 1979). The art therapist's awareness of the severity of injury can prevent him or her from encouraging false expectations in the patient.

Location and extent of initial and secondary brain injury determine the quality of the ultimate outcome. Prognosis is largely related to evidence of brain stem injury. Most persons who lose consciousness suffer some irreversible injury to brain cells. Although most of the traumatized cells rapidly regain normal function, some recover only after a protracted period of time, and others never recover. Most recovery occurs in the first 6 months. Some further neurologic improvement can continue for 12 to 24 months. Improvement thereafter is usually due to retraining or learning of special skills. While cell death and white matter destruction cannot be remedied, other pathways take over and the individual may learn in rehabilitation training to compensate for deficits. Plasticity and ability of the brain to develop alternate circuits decrease with advancing age, underlying disease, alcoholism, and after repeated injuries to the head. According to statistics, only about one-half of men over the age of 50 are able to return to their preaccident employment, while two-thirds of men below 20 can.

Recovery processes also depend upon the preaccident personality, constitution, intelligence, life situation at the time of injury, and the standard of medical care during the acute phase. A patient who demonstrates a wide range of interests and subjects in art therapy can draw on these past interests for renewed strength, and often has a better prognosis. Few patients with severe brain injury fully recover their neurological or psychological faculties. Psychiatric sequelae occur in approximately 25% of the survivors of head injury, far exceeding the physical sequelae. Early mental and physical stimulation and active rehabilitation are believed to promote greater eventual recovery.

ART THERAPY GOALS

As part of the rehabilitation team, the art therapist sees the head trauma patient after the acute phase has passed, when the patient is out of coma, physically stabilized, and transferred to a rehabilitation facility for intensive physical, occupational, speech, and recreational therapy, a neuropsychological work-up, and social work intervention. The art therapist may work through a therapeutic recreation department, through occupational therapy, or on his or her own. I worked through the inpatient therapeutic recreation department and on my own with outpatients. My therapeutic goals were largely drawn from Landgarten (1981):

1. To assess the patient's physical and cognitive abilities and reality orientation, manner of handling media, and the artwork itself to determine

manipulative abilities and self-image, which give clues to diagnosis and prognosis.

   a. To work through perceptual inaccuracies.

   b. To assess gains.

   c. To help patient gain maximum autonomy within the boundaries of the disability.

2. To deal with change in body image and to help the patient institute a compensatory means of accommodation.

   a. To acknowledge former strengths.

   b. To delineate new modes of adaptation.

   c. To accept limitations along with new body image.

3. To work through the trauma of change of body image by insight, catharsis, and resolution.

   a. To eliminate defense of denial by concretizing disability.

   b. To ventilate fear.

   c. To release rage against bodily assault.

   d. To mourn losses.

4. To give patient a means to record overt thoughts and emotions, as well as unconscious covert mechanisms.

   a. To reveal guilt or punishment fantasies.

   b. To discover clues to personality and psychological style of functioning.

5. To initiate and/or maintain a motivation for self-acceptance and adjustment.

   a. To regain sense of identity.

   b. To increase self-esteem.

   c. To activate motivation for recovery.

6. To give a nonverbal, visual means of communication, self-expression, and interpersonal exchange, especially with speech impairment.

7. To allow patient to experience a measure of success and to be in a situation where he is in control of decision making.

   a. To gain awareness of ability to be productive and to problem solve.

   b. To carry over into future trust in himself.

8. To clarify prognosis for self-management.

9. To deal with discharge anxiety.

   a. To rehearse for termination of treatment.

   b. To rehearse for home reentry.

Incidentally, I presented this list upon request to the neurologist in charge to introduce this new therapy, and his reaction was: "What are you, a shrink?

I don't want any catastrophic reactions!" "Don't worry, I go easy," I replied. Over time, my input in treatment plan meetings was appreciated. The neurologist said he was never quite sure what I did, but whatever it was, he thought it was great. Here again one sees the necessity for the art therapist to understand the medical aspects of head injury when working in a "medical model" facility. We need to translate our clinical observations into a vocabulary that the treatment team can understand and accept. We also have to understand what stage of recovery the patient is in before we attempt any insight therapy.

The stages of recovery from head injury can be broken down into (1) the initial stage, or reawakening stage; (2) the middle stage, or adjustment stage; and (3) the reentry stage into the outside world. The first two stages occur during inpatient hospitalization, when the most rapid improvement may be noted. In the third stage the patient has returned home and is seen on an outpatient basis. Physical, cognitive, perceptual, and psychosocial impairments are explored in each stage through art therapy.

INITIAL STAGE

The art therapist first encounters the head trauma patient in a rehabilitation setting after he has come out of a coma. Morphologically, the brain is beginning to heal, and internal swellings are subsiding. The mental state of the patient is characterized by personal confusion and disorganization. At this time the patient is not responsible for his behavior, which may be agitated, labile, aggressive, impulsive, inappropriate. Like a frightened animal, the patient is uncooperative, out of control. Range of behavioral symptoms may also include fatigue, hyperactivity, restlessness, distractibility, and hypersensitivity to any and all stimuli. Poor memory and short attention span make relearning difficult. The frontal lobe patient exhibits personality changes. A premorbid personality disorder can reappear, magnified.

In this early stage of rehabilitation, the patient is assessed to determine the extent of loss of function, particularly in the areas of manipulative skills, reality orientation, attention span, reasoning abilities, judgment, planning, as well as capacities for integration and organization, emotional stability, and motivation to engage in therapy. If the art therapist cannot assess the patient in a one-on-one session, an overall impression can be obtained from the patient's initial art production as well as from behavioral performance in a group session.

Physical disabilities that cause impairment of normal function are noticeable and measureable. Are there physical impairments that limit manipulative abilities: spasticity, apraxia, ataxia, hemiparesis, tremors, motor retardation? Is there loss of grasp, injury to the dominant side of the brain so a right-handed patient must use his nondominant left hand or adapt to minimal

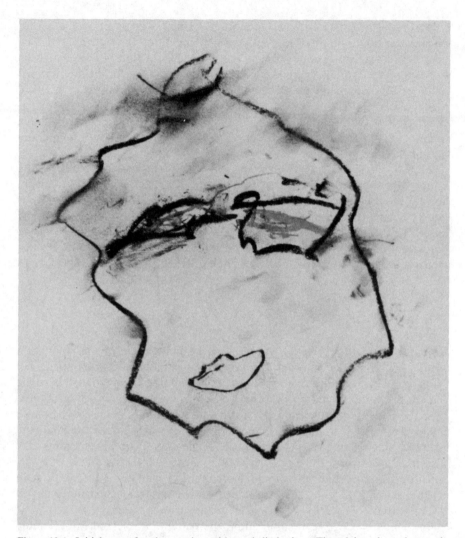

Figure 10.1. Initial stage: face by a patient with ataxic limitations. Though it took much struggle and effort on his part, the end product was recognizable.

use of the dominant hand? How does a patient compensate for a physical loss? If he cannot take the top off a magic marker because both hands won't work together, will he use teeth to hold the top and pull with the stronger hand? Can he figure out compensatory means? Is he self-motivated to relearn basic manipulative skills? Does he respond to the therapist's suggestions in these areas, such as using the nondominant functioning hand to stabilize the paper? The therapist can minimize frustration by taping the paper to the table. Physical pain from associated injuries may be so severe that the patient cannot concentrate on an activity. One alert, calm, but ataxic patient demonstrated patience and persistence in drawing a recognizable face (Fig. 10.1).

Physical impairments cannot be isolated from their psychological impact

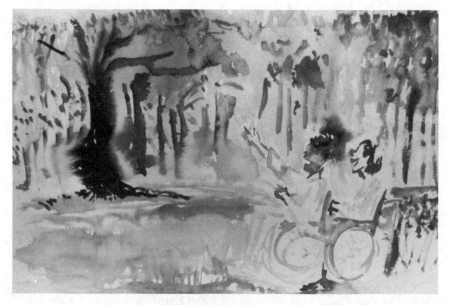

Figure 10.2. New body image includes a wheelchair.

on the patient's self-image. Though physical gains are visible from week to week, the patient has to deal with the psychological ramifications of his disabilities. The patient awakens from a coma to find an overt change in his body—facial distortions, such as external skin lacerations and skull indentations, eye distortions such as crossed eyes, a lazy eye, double vision. Hair is shaven, often unevenly (at locus of the injury or for surgery). Often body injuries—broken bones, paralyzed extremities, injured internal organs—cause pain, physical disabilities, and the patient suddenly finds himself with an altered body image. The psyche takes longer to heal than the body.

Art therapy is an excellent area to explore the patient's reaction and adaptation to his new body image. The assignment "Draw a person" gives the patient a safe distance from himself that may be necessary at this time. The patient often eliminates or emphasizes the area of injury (hands, feet, legs). Behavioral regression may appear in a childlike "person" drawing—simplified, without clothes.

The task "Draw the person sitting across from you" also gives the patient some distance from himself; to get a general idea of the patient's perceptual skills, the therapist asks the patient to notice the color of the hair and eyes, the shape of face and features. Finally, the patient may now be asked to draw himself, visualizing what he looks like in the mirror. Does his self-portrait acknowledge or deny an altered body image? How does he feel about the way he looks, about the way his body functions?

One patient clearly drew herself in a wheelchair, together with her hemophiliac brother who was also in a wheelchair, visiting a familiar vacation spot (Fig. 10.2). While she illustrated some acceptance of her disabilities,

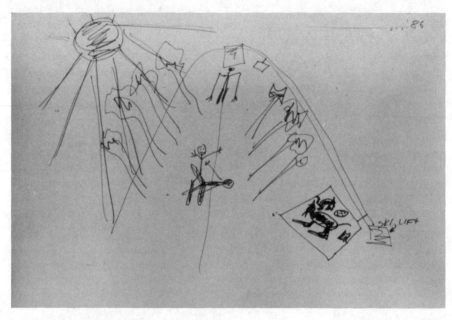

Figure 10.3. Initial-stage patient demonstrated cognitive–perceptual difficulties in organizing ideas from stimulus cards into a logical picture.

she also portrayed her desire to be mobile like other people. Another picture that she entitled "Joy of Expectation" contained a sky with many birds, a large bird in the lower left corner looking up to the sky "thinking of flying like the other birds," and a young child on the ground standing on one foot, reaching to the sky, "wishing she could fly." This patient had frontal lobe damage and often confabulated in an elated manner; art therapy helped her focus her thoughts. Despite her injury, she retained a high level of skill in art.

Perceptual skills can be assessed through such art therapy tasks as painting a simple still-life setup. Neurovisual impairments include visual field cuts, visual perceptual deficits, tracking disorders, defects in color vision. Paper-chopped elements, in the case of head injury, may be neurologically based. Perceptual and perceptual–motor deficits such as reduced motor speed, reduced eye–hand coordination, poor depth perception, and figure–ground problems may be measured by having patients copy two-dimensional and three-dimensional shapes and drawings.

Cognitive assessment includes specific assignments to evaluate a patient's ability to concentrate and follow directions, such as "Draw three blue triangles," or "Draw a clock that shows 10 o'clock." Can the patient remember the directions? Can he remember what he drew in the last session? When does the patient start remembering what he drew in the previous sessions? Communication disturbances include aphasia, word-finding difficulties, confabulation, slurred speech, and diminished writing skills.

The Rawley Silver Stimulus Drawings (Silver, 1986) test for deficits in processing and sequencing information and ability to make choices and organize visual stimuli and ideas into a picture that makes logical sense. An example of confused thinking at this stage may be seen in Figure 10.3, inspired by the stimulus cards. It is a ski scene, including cats on a picnic blanket. The patient gave the cats skis "so it makes sense." The picture was quickly drawn in a few minutes—the patient's attention span was very short.

The House-Tree-Person Test is another graphic assessment battery. Most patients draw the classic "trauma hole" in their tree drawing; the psychological impact is inseparable from the cognitive and perceptual areas as well. In this initial stage of recovery, House-Tree-Person drawings are frequently drawn impulsively, resulting in simplistic, regressed, primitive, and incomplete renderings. Decreased abstraction is apparent in an interpretive assignment, such as "illustrate a saying," which is usually portrayed in a concrete manner at this time.

Psychosocial changes in the patient's behavior, as well as his reaction to his hospitalization, can be further explored in art therapy. Behaving appropriately in a group is practiced in a group pass-around picture; silly, childlike behavior can be controlled by group pressure from higher-functioning patients. A scared, withdrawn patient may be paired with a friendly, helpful patient in a two-person painting to encourage social interaction and participation. Patients are encouraged to express how they feel in "Draw how it feels to be in this hospital." Aggressive, impulsive behavior had caused one patient to be physically restrained, and she drew herself restrained to her bed, shielded behind a curtain, describing graphically and verbally how humiliated and imprisoned she felt.

Hostility, aggression, and confusion appeared in a drawing of a face with two open mouths, many sharp teeth, and a tongue thrust out (Fig. 10.4). This patient also impulsively kissed the therapist. Inappropriate sexual disinhibition and regression can occur in an early stage, and a patient may masturbate or urinate while in a group. Sexuality appeared in a former bartender's picture of a large-breasted woman at a bar saying, "Hey, let's love each other." This patient later had no memory of doing this painting, showing poor short-term memory while in this stage of sexual disinhibition.

Premorbid personality disorders reemerge in the initial stage of recovery from head injury. A quote was interpreted in a socially inappropriate manner with a drawing of a deer with feces—premorbidly this patient had sociopathic tendencies. A personality disorder was evident in a "person" drawing that the patient entitled "Person and Brick Wall," drawing a man (head to shoulders) hidden behind a brick wall, grinning provocatively, with no clothes. Possible psychotic and morbid thoughts appeared in another patient's bizarre drawings and stories of a priest, Dracula, and a coffin.

To summarize the initial stage of head trauma in art therapy, the patient portrays confusion, disorganization, poor memory, short attention span,

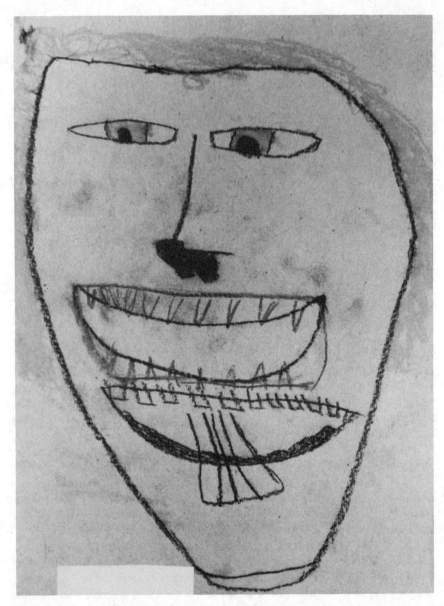

Figure 10.4. Psychotic ideation and confusion in a patient with frontal lobe damage. Also note sharp, aggressive teeth and tongue.

agitation, lability, and inappropriate behavior. At this time, the patient is dependent upon others for care. The therapist assesses the extent of the patient's injury in physical, perceptual, cognitive, and psychosocial areas, to determine "where we go from here." The patient reacts to the injury, often drawing the extent of impairment, and begins a program of adaptation

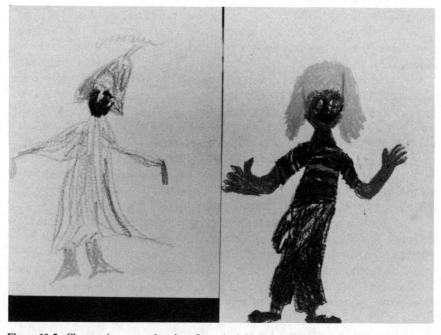

Figure 10.5. Changes in person drawings from the initial stage (left) to the middle stage (right): stronger crayon application, delineation of hands, feet, clothes, all indications of improved physical dexterity, reality orientation, cognitive thinking, and self-confidence.

and rehabilitation. While a patient may vent feelings about the accident and hospital treatment in art therapy, poor memory often prevents productive insight therapy at this time.

MIDDLE STAGE

The middle stage is usually the second half of the patient's inpatient hospitalization, particularly when the patient still needs extensive physical rehabilitation. At this time, the patient's behavior is appropriate, attention span is lengthened, and he can follow directions. Learning takes place at a slow rate, and memory shows improvements. However, insight is limited and judgment is impaired. Problem-solving ability has improved, but the patient can not plan realistically.

An example of the change from the initial stage to the middle stage can be seen in the "person" drawings done at each stage, (Fig. 10.5). Physical issues dominated the early drawing, lightly drawn due to manipulative problems. Body confusion or omission pointed to injured areas—no feet, drooping hands, confused facial features, overly large hairdo that covers the brain area. The patient said the hands drooped "because I had no room, I don't plan ahead"; they also convey a feeling of helplessness. Color choices lacked reality orientation—blue hair, yellow body parts. Her middle-stage "person" drawing, though still somewhat childish and disproportionate, showed improved manual dexterity in application, and physical gains (fingers, strong shoes) as function was improved or regained. The figure stance was stronger as the patient became more self-confident. Colors and clearer details, such as striped shirt and pants of the same color the patient wore, pointed to better reality orientation, improved cognitive thinking. However, the patient drew in a curious way, first drawing part of the face, then part of the feet, and then the middle; though the patient was original and creative, she was still somewhat confused and admitted to memory problems. She described the second "person" as a "10-year-old girl" who had long blond hair as she used to have; 10 was probably appropriate to the mental and psychological age she felt herself to be at that time.

A cognitive exercise in art therapy demonstrates the patient's ability to present a problem logically and think of steps to work out a solution in a four-box cartoon drawing. In this context, one patient described her frustration at the hospital staff and her family for not listening to her because she was head injured. Her leg was put in a brace to help her to relearn to walk; however, the brace caused so much pain that it in fact prevented her from making physical gains. She begged the therapists, to no avail, to take off the brace. The staff had not yet recognized that she was past the initial stage of impulsive outbursts and emotional lability, and did not respond to the patient's open signals and real complaints. When they finally listened to her and removed the brace, she made rapid progress. While the patient illustrated this problem and verbalized how it made her feel in this four-part cartoon exercise, her graphic presentation showed impaired sequencing; the order of the pictures was incorrect, indicating some difficulty in following directions and organizing thoughts.

Concrete thinking may still persist in some patients; a patient has reached a higher level of functioning when he begins to think abstractly. One patient chose to interpret a self-portrait assignment in a manner that demonstrated good abstract thinking. A former beach club director, he symbolized his recovery in terms of rising once again from low tide to high tide as he regains his abilities. He expressed optimism that his former strengths would pull him through these hard times.

In group art therapy, patients can share their problems, discuss alternative solutions, work on solving practical problems that may also affect them. In a group picture, patients practice social skills while trying to make a cohesive picture of their choice. They help each other make appropriate additions that meet group approval. A group of four patients overcame their embarrassment at their manipulative problems by concentrating on working together to make a cohesive spirited painting (Fig. 10.6).

This intermediate stage is an important time to work on feelings that the patient is going through; emotions can be dealt with more controllably and rationally at this stage. In a two-part drawing showing on the left how the

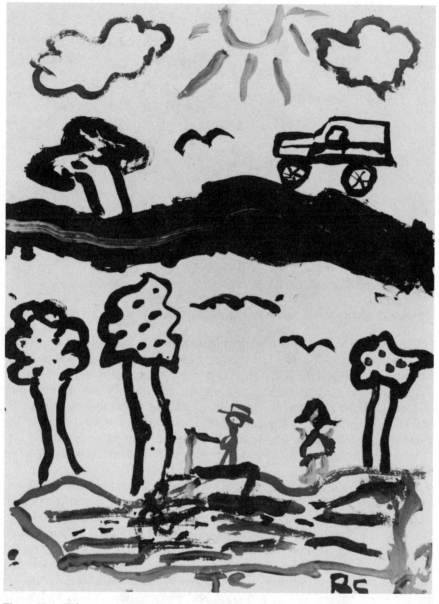

Figure 10.6. This group painting aided patients in socializing and overcoming embarrassment regarding manipulative problems.

patient felt at the beginning of his rehabilitation, and on the right how he felt at the middle stage (Fig. 10.7), a patient showed how his confusion lessened and optimism prevailed through the facial expression, stars, and question marks going around the head. This patient admitted that confusion, though reduced, was still a problem.

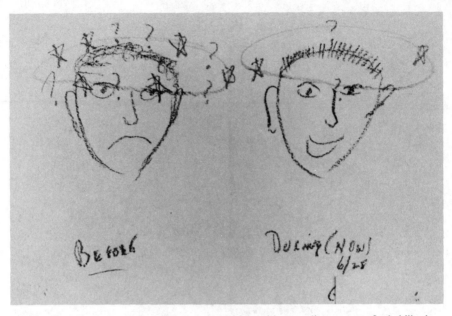

Figure 10.7. Confusion and optimism during initial and intermediate stages of rehabilitation.

Patients can also deal with feelings in a somewhat indirect way by writing a feeling on an index card. The therapist collects these cards and asks the patients to pick a different card. Each patient illustrates the emotion he picked, and the group tries to figure out the emotion. Presenting emotions in a gamelike way softens the tensions of dealing with them directly or by oneself. The therapist can encourage a discussion about who feels or felt sad, happy, confused, or frightened. With the emotion generalized and surfaced through art and discussion, the patient no longer feels so alone or overwhelmed.

As the patient readies for discharge to outpatient therapy or reentry phase, a before–after feelings picture can help in the transition. A realistic patient showed her mixed emotions upon discharge: happiness, sadness, and fear. She said she was happy about her good hospital treatment and improved abilities, and happy that she was leaving. However, she also expressed worries about her residual physical and cognitive disabilities, and was appropriately fearful of her ability to function in the outside world. Another patient drew smiles, question marks, and exclamation marks, and wrote "Hurray!!" "Questions, questions, questions," "Yeah!!!" and "Freedom Sort of."

To summarize the middle stage of head trauma recovery, the patient's physical condition is generally stabilized and no longer of primary concern. The patient has progressed from the initial period of confusion and disorganization, a stage he rarely remembers, to a more workable stage of appropriate behavior, longer attention span, and improved memory where learning can take place. Keeping in mind that the patient's insight may be limited and judgment still impaired, the art therapist can explore with the patient his reaction to his injury and altered body concept. Cognitive art therapy exercises provide him with a creative challenge for his memory and thought processes. He is given an opportunity to express his feelings and group support to deal with them, particularly with regard to preparation for discharge to the "real world."

REENTRY PHASE

The art therapist now encounters the patient in a new setting, the outpatient department. This is the last phase of active rehabilitation before returning to school, work, or vocational rehabilitation. At this time, the patient needs to learn to live with and work around his remaining deficits in physical, perceptual, cognitive, behavioral, and/or psychosocial areas.

Physically, the patient must learn to cope with a wheelchair, casts, and crutches in nonhospital settings, and if and when they are no longer needed, he must learn to accept such permanent disabilities as walking with a limp or restricted arm movements. His first outside experience as a disabled person may be transportation in a special van, together with other physically and mentally disabled people, to the outpatient therapy program. While he may find some comfort in being in the company of other people with similar problems, it is also quite a shock to realize that he is one of them. The humiliation increases with realization of dependency on the van for transportation, especially when he is often kept waiting for pickup; he is no longer in control and is often lost with regard to how, where, or when to they go somewhere. Places with wheelchair or disabled access are limited. One patient always drew himself in a wheelchair; it was as though it was an extension of his body, which indeed it had become. He and his wheelchair were always drawn isolated from the surroundings, which was how he felt.

What has occurred in the interim from inpatient discharge to outpatient entry?

As noted at the end of the middle stage, the patient left the hospital with mixed feelings. On the one hand, he was glad to leave behind the feelings of confinement, of being a dependent person. He looked forward to being home with his family and pets in a familiar surrounding. On the other hand, he left the security of the hospital, of being taken care of by skilled professionals, of intensive therapy and its pattern of setting goals and noting gains. The progress was visible, exciting, and promising.

Returning home, the honeymoon is short-lived. Usually a patient who has sustained severe head injury cannot return to a living situation where he is alone. The patient who had lived on his own pursuing an independent lifestyle before the accident now needs to live with a parent or relative, or hire an aide. He needs to adjust to a different role in his living situation. Not only does the patient have to contend with an altered self, but he has to relate in new ways to his family, who may behave differently in reaction to the patient's new behaviors.

One patient had moved to another state before his accident to get away from a negative family situation. His accident forced him to return home, where the preaccident destructive situation was further complicated by personality changes caused by his head injury. He frequently drew himself sitting on top of a hill looking down at the rest of the world, and entitled the picture "Fool on the Hill."

The hospitalized patient has had some opportunity to practice his relearned skills and adaptations to his injury during intermittent home visits when he and family members were usually on their best behavior. However, the actual reentry home is quite different, for the brain-injured person will never be the same person he was before the accident. The patient has begun to come to terms with his new self, and relatives are coming to terms with this altered loved one. The patient, parents, spouse, and children are all subject to denial, and if not properly counseled, may still harbor hopes that the patient will return to his former self. The family's early optimism at the survival of the patient and joy of progress in physical rehabilitation are replaced by shock at the patient's behavioral changes. A number of my patients were engaged to be married at the time of their accident—marriages are postponed or called off when the future spouse fears that he or she cannot deal with marriage to an altered or disabled person.

Relatives of head-injured patients observe the most common behavioral changes in the patient to be irritability, slowness, tiredness, anxiety, impatience, and depression. As is not the case with other physical injuries that improve over time, emotional symptoms of the head-injured patient often worsen. Twelve months after injury, reports indicate that bad temper and mood swings rise significantly. Depression, general personality changes, childish behavior, complaining, and disturbance of sleep habits are great burdens on the relatives who, along with the patient, need to adapt to the residual deficits of the injury (Bond, 1979).

Awareness of this problem was expressed in one patient's self-portrait. This patient was discouraged by his seemingly endless rehabilitation and setbacks from recurrent seizures. He was older than most patients (45), and his prognosis was not good enough for him to return to work. On one side he drew himself lightly in profile, facing a strongly colored profile of his wife. He colored the background in lightly with a blue crayon, going over his face as well. The patient said he was weaker, blended in with the sky, not on his own, a shadow of his former self. Asked to cut out words from a magazine that described himself, he chose "next thing" and "o"; "hopes." He said he really "felt like zero." Asked to write a wish for himself, he wrote, "I wish that I could get back to my wife in good shape, with mind and body."

A key goal in reentry rehabilitation is to eliminate or reduce behavioral problems. The patient is reeducated in new behavior patterns to facilitate successful reintegration into family, education, and employment situations. Maladaptive behaviors frequently encountered in an outpatient program include uncontrolled impulsivity, temper tantrums, negativism, and physical and verbal assaultiveness.

Murals give the opportunity, through group dynamics, for the patients to reinforce each other's gains and discourage disruptive or inappropriate behavior. At first they appear frustrated, at a loss, when the art therapist removes herself from the group and leaves the mural completely in their hands. Group roles form according to skill and confidence levels. A leader and assistant leader usually emerge. The leader may get carried away with the role and act bossy, and the others may react.

The most isolated patient is usually the last to participate in a mural. Lack of connection from one part of the mural to another illustrates each patient's feelings of isolation. One shy man connected his part of the mural with the others, showing his desire to integrate and communicate with them. (Similarly, his house drawing from the House-Tree-Person Test had shown great interest in the surroundings while his behavior demonstrated difficulty in participating in it.) Roles change as the patients regain their strengths. After repeated murals, the quietest may eventually become the leader. The patients learn coping strategies and work out behavioral problems through group interaction. Mural themes that the patients choose often include the desire to do what they used to do and no longer can (ski, drive), symbolically climbing steps or a mountain to regain their former selves, and taking one's own road in rehabilitation.

Any brain-damaged person feels some degree of anger, denial, and depression as his residual deficits become more apparent. It was interesting to note the frequent choice of a barking dog with sharp teeth from the Rawley Silver Stimulus Drawings by outwardly docile patients; their underlying anger was apparent. One such patient, a female taxi driver, whose injury resulted from a violent hold-up involving rape, knife slashes, and being run over, exhibited post-traumatic syndrome, a state of continuing fear following exposure to a frightening situation. She developed phobias about crossing a street and about driving a car. Original fear symptoms of anxiety, tremulousness, and tension became mixed with feelings of resentment, anger, self-pity, and uncertainty about the future. She also expressed her anger in paintings of bursting volcanos and whales spouting water. She relaxed as she worked on paintings of peaceful nature scenes. Art therapy became a wonderful emotional release for her and a source of new self-confidence as her formerly untapped art skills became apparent. She was gradually transformed from a shy, withdrawn group member into a clear-spoken leader.

Anger may also be directed at the weakest member of the group. One patient, brain injured by drugs, made no effort to help himself, despite constant group and individual encouragement. Though premorbidly this patient had also shown minimal effort in school and work, he was more severely impaired than the others. It was hard for the other patients to accept the extent of his injury, for they saw a part of themselves in him. They reacted by writing curse words about him, scribbling on his picture, making fun of him. One patient wrote on his own self-portrait, "You think I have it bad, look at Phil! He makes me look good." Even after his outpatient discharge (due to lack of progress), they included him in a group mural by putting him in a wheelchair atop a hill, slanted toward a body of water, holding a kite that was struck by lightning, with the caption, "Wee, here we go! Roll em, Phil." Even though he was no longer in the group, they seemed to need to kill him off, as well as that part of themselves that prevented their successful reintegration into the world of work, education, and family. The rest of the mural had someone rowing across the water, an airplane and a hot air balloon crossing to the other side, a person in a wheelchair looking up at another person climbing a mountain on the other side—all symbols of efforts to "reach the other side."

Cognitively, past memory is usually good at this stage, but short-term memory may still be impaired. The patient can learn new information, but at a slower rate. Speech and cognitive deficits are now relatively fixed. Decreased abilities to reason, to tolerate stress, and to use good judgment limit problem-solving skills. To help cope with remaining memory problems, the patient needs to simplify each task and situation, eliminate distractions, and concentrate on the task at hand.

Putting ideas together in a picture is one way to help organize ideas. A four-part solution to a problem, described in the middle stage, helps the patient structure and organize a problem. One patient portrayed a problem in making a meal—the vegetables, meat, and rice all came out at different times; she pictured eating three different meals from three different plates. She worked out a solution in this step-by-step form: (1) read directions; (2) use a clock to time each food—finally, it all came out on one plate at the same time. Incidentally, when I asked her several months later how she was doing in sequencing her cooking, she said she had bought a microwave oven and now quickly "zaps" her food all at once!

Another patient described a residual visual–perceptual problem of tending to drive in the center of the road. To solve this problem, he drew himself looking first to the yellow mid-road line, then to the side of the road, and finally carefully watching both these markers.

In another cognitive exercise, patients were given wire, a block of wood, and nails and asked to construct a standing figure. Later they were to cover the wire figure with plaster strips, and finally paint it. This exercise challenged their manipulative, cognitive, and organizational skills. One patient patiently redid his wire three times until he made a proportionate figure. He even animated the position of the arms and legs. Problems again arose in making the figure stand once the wet plaster strips were applied. This patient had a slowed rate of processing information and organizing ideas, and often asked for clarification of directions. The slowest to start, he was the most persistent once involved, and the last to finish, perfecting his work with special final details. Despite his cognitive deficits, his preinjury adaptive abilities helped him work through a problem at his own pace. Another patient attached the arms to the legs, not noticing what was wrong until another patient asked if he were making a chicken. We were able to get around his striking conceptual deficit with humor. A patient who had made the wire figure carefully lost patience with the plaster and made his figure into a mummy. Some patients didn't understand to wrap each leg separately with plaster strips.

Another patient, a big, strong pipe welder, made his figure into a muscle man, lifting weights. Loss of peripheral vision prevented him from returning to his job, but his mechanical skills were still intact, as evidenced by his carefully and sturdily constructed figure. He added a pot belly, which he had developed from lack of exercise, and said he was determined to return to his fit he-man self. He utilized this project to work on problems with his physical self-image.

Adaptation to an altered self-concept can also be directly explored in self-portraits. One patient was in an outpatient group due to maladaptive behavior patterns and cognitive disabilities; he had missed the middle stage as an inpatient because he had no physical or speech problems. An attractive adolescent, he drew himself (Fig. 10.8) in a childish, regressed manner that bore no resemblance to himself—large, round head, ears inside edge of face, long, thin neck, boxlike body. Though he always wore contact lenses, he drew glasses, saying he used to wear them. Though his hair was curly, he drew it as straight. Asked then to choose words from a magazine that described his traits, he picked "contents," "the difference between good and great," "he's some piece of work," which went along with his grandiose self-presentation. Asked to write a wish for himself, he revealed more appropriate reality testing in his wish "for my brain to work right, at least as good as before accident." Some patients are ready for direct insight therapy, but other patients need more time and group support before they can be confronted directly.

Another patient, a former special education teacher, was left with severe facial deformity and speech and cognitive impairment and walked with a limp. Her impulsively drawn, primitive sketches, particularly of people, revealed psychological regression. Her self-portrait was of a lopsided, deformed figure, which did show some insight into her altered self. She was aware of her severe disabilities, and her behavior was sluggish and depressed. She cut out a picture of a baby in a diaper to describe herself further. A sign of hopefulness was in her underlying wish "to be married." Unfortunately her prognosis for recovery was limited to reentry into a sheltered workshop.

At the turn of the year, a double picture depicting the last year on one half and hopes for the new year on the other half can help the patients pull

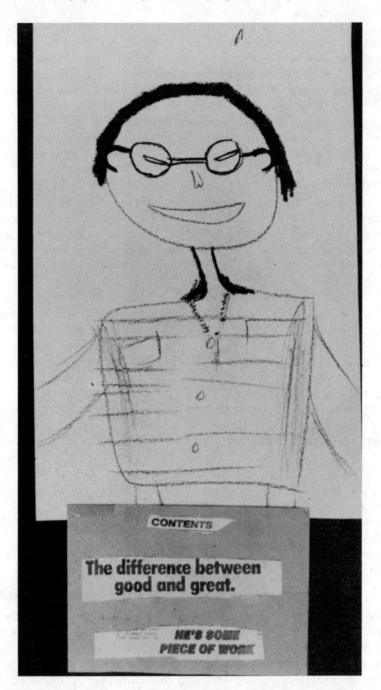

Figure 10.8. Self-portrait shows disparity between patient's verbalized self-concept, graphic physical portrayal, cognitive–behavioral disabilities, and actual physical appearance.

together their ideas of where they are. For the past year, the patients often drew their accident, confusion, and symbols of their close brush with death (a coffin, unfilled grave, crossed-out R.I.P. [Rest In Peace] on a gravestone. For the new year picture, patients drew hopes for growth, clarity, regained skills, or a question mark for the future. It is important for patients to have a clear idea of where they are and what they can and cannot do, without false optimism.

The process of emotional and psychological healing involves assessing and understanding one's deficits clearly, and learning to live with and work around these deficits. In the process, patients need to build up enough self-confidence not to see themselves just in the role of handicapped persons. Patients unable to return to former employment can be retrained through vocational rehabilitation for another job in accordance with remaining skills. Gradually they can assume more responsibilities at home and at work. When feeling ready to face the real world, patients usually discharge themselves from outpatient therapy. Sometimes the staff need to set the discharge date if the patient continues to "hang around" instead of assuming reentry responsibilities after goals have been met. While physical, social, emotional, and intellectual abilities are less than before the injury, they are often good enough by now for the patient to function as a member of society.

CONCLUSION

The art therapist helps bridge the psychosocial aspects of head injury patients' rehabilitation. In art therapy, patients are given an opportunity to communicate nonverbally and verbally their overt and unconscious feelings. They express themselves about hospitalization, going home, and family and work issues; these feelings often include hostility, anger, confusion, and fear. They learn to accept and adapt to physical and mental disabilities and a new body image and self-concept. Through group pressure, they learn to limit inappropriate behaviors, and through group support, they are given encouragement and friendship.

Though greatly needed due to the large incidence of accidents, rehabilitation programs for head injury patients, particularly as outpatients, are unfortunately available on only a limited basis. Finding a position for an art therapist in one is even harder, due to lack of insurance reimbursement and understanding of our role in a medical model–oriented facility. It is hoped that this chapter has shown the contribution that art therapy can make to the general rehabilitation of a head injury patient.

REFERENCES

Bond, M. (1979). The stages of recovery from severe head injury with special reference to late outcome. *International Rehabilitation Medicine, 1,* 155–159.

Landgarten, H. (1981). *Clinical art therapy.* New York: Brunner/Mazel.

Leigh, D. (1979). Psychiatric aspects of head injury. *Psychiatry Digest, 40,* 21–33.

Silver, R. (1982). *Stimulus drawings and techniques in therapy, development and assessment.* New York: Trillium.

CHAPTER 11

Art Therapy for Patients with Alzheimer's Disease and Related Disorders

JUDITH WALD

Ten years ago, Alzheimer's disease was an ignored illness, unknown to the general public. Today it has gotten a great deal of attention in the media, yet *Alzheimer's* is still as misunderstood and misapplied a term as its popular predecessor, *senility*.

In proper medical usage, the term *senility* refers to the normal physical and mental changes that accompany aging, not "losing one's mind." Alzheimer's disease is one of the degenerative neurological disorders within the category of organic brain syndromes called *dementia*, which means "loss of mental faculties" (Blass, 1985, p. 37). An organic brain syndrome is the loss of cognitive functioning linked to an organic disease of the brain, with physical rather than psychological forces at play. Dementia specifically has a slow onset with insidious global loss of cognitive, intellectual, and memory functions, due to disease processes affecting the central nervous system.

Most state of the art nursing homes and day-care centers now have separate units for dementia patients. This arrangement permits the staff to focus on the strengths and deficits unique to this population. Working for 7 years in the Dementia Day Hospital Program at Burke Rehabilitation Center in White Plains, New York, I was able to develop an art therapy program specifically geared to the special needs of the dementia patient. In this chapter, the role of art therapy for patients with a dementing illness will be explored in the following areas: (1) evaluation and diagnosis—understanding of the disease for the treatment team, family, or caretaker; and (2) treatment and management—how to help the patient function at the highest level within the limits of the disease.

About two-thirds of older people with the dementia syndrome have Alzheimer's disease, and 10 to 40% of this group also have strokes (mixed dementia). Multi-infarct dementia (multiple small strokes), a cerebrovascular disease, is the second most common cause of dementia. Other degenerative diseases of the nervous system that can cause dementia are Parkinson's disease (in about one-half of its patients), Huntington's chorea, Pick's disease, infections such as Jakob-Kreutzfeldt disease and tertiary syphilis, and normal-pressure hydrocephalus.

Dementing illnesses account for half of the residents in nursing homes and are the fourth leading cause of death in the United States. Recognizing the scope of dementia has resulted in research efforts around the world to understand its biology and to develop drugs for its treatment. Support groups such as ADRDA, the Alzheimer's Disease and Related Disorders Association, have sprung up nationwide to help families and caretakers deal with a demented patient, as well as to lobby politically for improved insurance benefits and government research grants.

Just as dementia was until recently a shelved topic in medicine, the art therapy literature dealt with dementia under the general topic of geriatrics (See Crosson, 1976; Dewdney, 1975; Harrison, 1981; Landgarten, 1983; Weiss, 1984; Zeiger, 1976). Neurological changes that are a part of normal aging were addressed—changes in vision, hearing, and taste, reduced or distorted sensory input into the nervous system, and a slower rate of processing information. The main psychological issues addressed were overcoming depression and apathy, developing self-awareness and self-esteem, particularly through life review, sensory stimulation, positive reinforcement, and creative problem solving.

However, global cognitive impairments that characterize the dementia syndrome are not a normal process of aging. Alzheimer's disease, multi-infarct stroke, and Parkinson's disease are in fact illnesses, with chronic irreversible organic brain syndromes characterized by progressive loss of cognitive function. These impairments severely affect memory, intellect, language, and interpretation of sensory impressions. While long-term memory is better preserved, patients' short-term memory can be so severely affected that they forget from one minute to the next what they did or said, and keep repeating the same questions. As intellect fails, the patients lose ability to calculate, spell, and write. Patients' speech becomes confused, and train of thought is lost; they may talk in circumlocutions, confabulate, develop aphasia, and even become mute.

Nursing homes usually mix geriatric patients of different diagnoses. Patients come to art therapy groups at various functional levels, with a mixture of physical, psychological, and cognitive disabilities. It is therefore not surprising that the art therapy literature has for so long dealt with dementia under the general topic of geriatrics.

DIAGNOSIS AND EVALUATION

Patients in a dementia program have a variety of diagnoses determined after a battery of physical and psychological tests (definitive diagnosis of Alzheimer's disease and other degenerative diseases of the nervous system can only be confirmed by brain autopsy). Evaluation by psychologists and occupational therapists includes visual tasks that involve the copying and matching of shapes and patterns. Predominant signs of organicity are noted by perseverative patterns, incomplete shapes, fragmentation, misproportions, and concreteness. Such conventional graphic tests are useful and valid, but limited. One of the main characteristics of the Alzheimer's disease patient is difficulty in integrating and organizing information; the art therapist can use a variety of art tasks to ascertain more comprehensive information about the patient's visual perception and ability to process sensory input, translate it, and organize ideas into a graphic modality.

Art therapy can be used continually to evaluate the patient's deficits in orientation, memory, perception, and comprehension. Patients are asked to draw the following subjects: a self-portrait, the person sitting across the table, and a face, following the art therapist's step-by-step directions. Can the patient follow directions? Are the colors reality oriented? Does the drawing make sense to the patient and others? Are logical parts omitted? Does the patient notice misperceptions? A watercolor painting of a simple still-life arrangement such as a vase of flowers challenges the patient's perceptional, organizational, and manipulative skills. Can colors and shapes be named and identified? Can watercolor with its multiple steps so often taken for granted (wet the brush with water, choose a color, put the wet brush on the waterblock, move it on the paper, change the color by rinsing the brush, etc.) be coordinated and manipulated? Can the patient entitle the picture, sign his or her name? Does he or she remember what was drawn 5 minutes ago, or what was drawn in the last session? The House-Tree-Person Test can also be used for evaluation. Such art tasks reveal the strengths as well as the weaknesses of dementia patients and their emotional reaction to their situation. Artworks can help to determine the degree of deficits and the stage of dementia and evaluate what intellectual function is retained.

CHARACTERISTICS OF THE MOST PROMINENT DEMENTING ILLNESSES

The variety of diagnoses that comprise the dementia syndrome are characterized by different functional abilities and specific patterns. Alzheimer's disease has a gradual, insidious onset and progressive deterioration of cognitive functions such as language, perception, memory, and motor skills; the art therapist can note a gradual but progressive regression in the patient's artwork. With multi-infarct dementia (MID), the onset is sudden, and the clinical pattern is stepwise, with pockets of retained skills especially in memory and cognition; even some improvement can be noted between vascular insults of the multiple small strokes. The nature of the dysfunctions depends upon the locus of the strokes. Apraxia and difficulties in spatial tasks tend to characterize the MID patient; in art therapy, the patient has difficulty staying within the confines of the paper's borders and has problems coordinating the steps and spatial tasks involved in collages (choosing shapes, pasting shapes, arranging the picture space). The MID patient is more likely to remember what was done in art therapy sessions, while the Alzheimer's disease patient immediately forgets.

Parkinson's disease patients with dementia also have more clear pockets of retention of memory and intellect than Alzheimer's disease patients. However, upon closer examination, the Parkinson's patient tends to ramble from topic to topic both in conversation and in artwork, similar to stream of consciousness. For instance, the patient will start drawing the theme assigned in an art therapy session, gradually diverge from the theme with unclear forms and elements, which will in turn be reinterpreted with a new theme that has no connection to the original one. The Parkinson's patient with visual field cuts also tends to miss a large part of the picture surface, with the drawing resulting on the lower part of the paper and tablecloth. Drawing on one side of the paper points to strokes, and patients with large strokes may also portray the dementia syndrome with difficulties in cognition, particularly with language.

The art therapist encounters patients with other dementing illnesses on a less frequent basis. Huntington's chorea dementia can cause a patient to be impulsive in thought and actions. Drawings of lopsided figures reflect the patient's deteriorating physical gait. As the disease progresses, jerky, spastic movements restrict manipulative control of a crayon. The Huntington's dementia patient who develops expressive aphasia often responds well to nonverbal art expression, demonstrating some retained area of clearer cognition such as ability to interpret a theme (though in a concrete manner). One patient with a combination of Jakob-Kreutzfeldt disease and Guam Parkinson dementia was extremely ataxic, unable to connect a marker to a paper. Patients with tertiary syphilis dementia can be so manic that they can barely sit still long enough to draw. They are overly sensitive to any stimulus, auditory or visual, and even a line on a paper would be a starting point for an elaborate story. Attempts to refocus such manic confused patients often lead to further misperceptions and confabulations.

Depression can complicate a dementing illness such as Alzheimer's disease, and it is particularly common after strokes. The depression may be a psychological reaction to the dementia or a result of damage to the parts of the brain that mediate normal affective response. Pseudo-dementia is depression misdiagnosed as dementia, where the symptoms of depression are disguised as dementia (such as poor cognitive performance). Depression is represented in artworks by drawing at the bottom of the page, drawing objects disproportionately small in comparison to the picture space, dark or dull colors, isolated parts, or simplistic renditions. The patient may emphasize the aggressive components of depression by drawing such images as large clenched teeth. Behaviorally, the patient contributes minimally or totally refuses to participate.

Besides depression, psychosis may further complicate the dementia. Psychotic ideation surfaces in artworks in drawings of monsters, fused visual

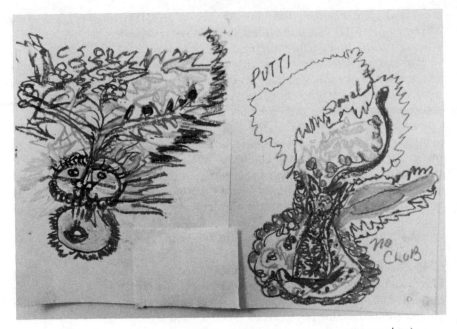

Figure 11.1. Vase of flowers transformed into a cat (on two separate occasions).

images such as a bird–person, house–face, or vase–cat (Wald, 1986b), bizarre drawings (two-headed people), x-ray-vision bodies (skeletal structure within a body), and bizarre descriptions of the product (''snakes and little people walking across a face''). In Figure 11.1, the patient began drawing the vase of flowers set up before her. However, psychotic ideation surfaced and the vases became transformed into cats (on two separate occasions.) The art therapist should present graphic renditions of depression or psychosis to the attending physician, who may prescribe medication to treat the depressive or psychotic elements of the dementing illness.

Keeping in mind these general distinctions between the major dementing illnesses and their manifestations in art therapy, one may follow the usual course of Alzheimer's disease, the most common of the dementias. Symptoms and course of illness do vary from case to case. Artworks, as well as the behaviors of the participant in art therapy sessions, help document the stage of illness.

COURSE OF ALZHEIMER'S DISEASE

In the early stages of Alzheimer's disease, the patient usually retains a proper outward appearance that masks the illness from the casual onlooker. A self-portrait can be well conceived, showing good organization in the face but increasing disorganization as the patient continues to draw (long neck, dis-

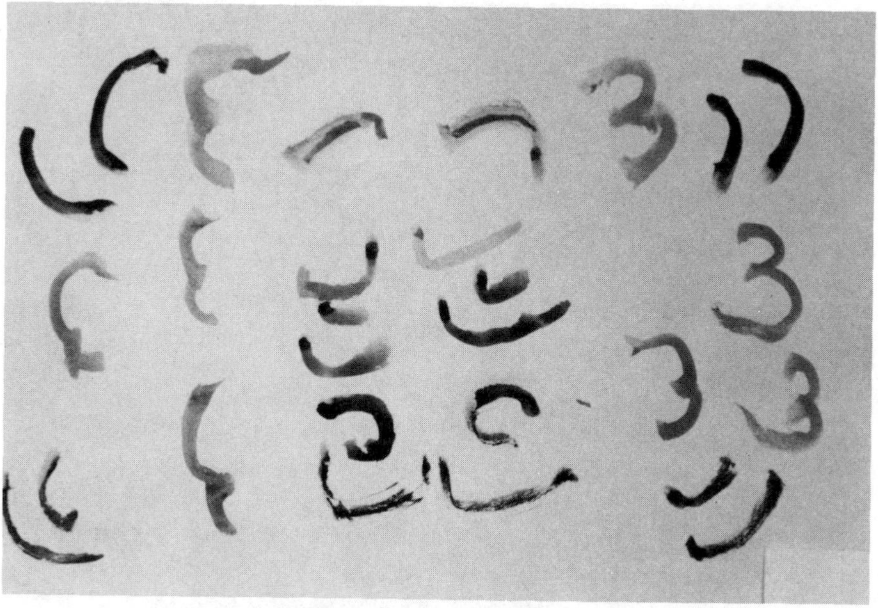

Figure 11.2. Perseveration with symmetry.

proportionate arms, confused hands, stick fingers, simplified body). Perseverative stereotypic behavior and inability to adapt to changing demands appear in perseveration in artwork—the patient goes over an outline many times, repeats the same drawing stroke endlessly, goes back and forth over an area until a hole forms through the paper, or is unable to stop a pattern. Perseveration is common to Alzheimer's disease. In Figure 11.2 the almost successful attempt at symmetry reveals an underlying obsessive–compulsive personality structure.

A patient may produce a good rendering, but repeat the same configuration from drawing to drawing (see Figs. 11.3, 11.4, 11.5, all drawn by the same patient). Note how the plant configuration was repeated yet gradually altered as the disease progressed. Intrusions are another mode of perseveration—when a subject or pattern lingers for weeks, no matter what instructions the art therapist gives or its relevance to the picture. At the early stage of the dementing illness, a high level of art skill is shown in well-developed detail of flowers with sturdy structure and grounding in a solid three-dimensional flowerpot on a table, much like the strong character of the patient. As her disease progressed, the flowers dropped lower, while the roots attempt to ground the plant in a circle, perhaps the remnant of the flowerpot. In a later stage, the patient still retained a three-dimensional concept in drawing a vase, but made a rectangle for a table. Roots still appeared, though not needed in a vase. Legs of the table become human feet with dainty shoes, showing percept contamination and psychotic ideation.

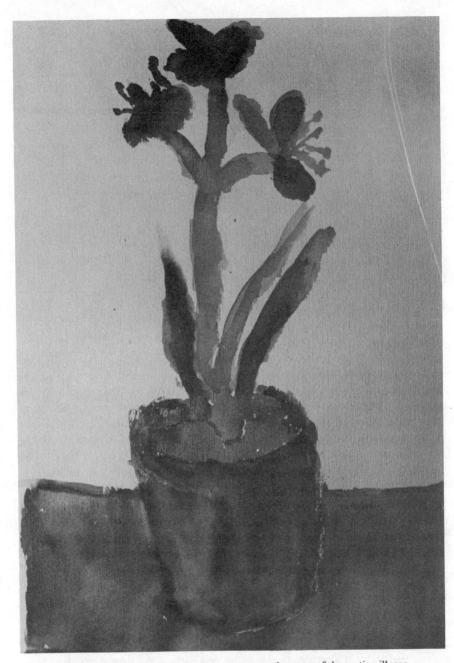

Figure 11.3. High level of skill seen at an early stage of dementing illness.

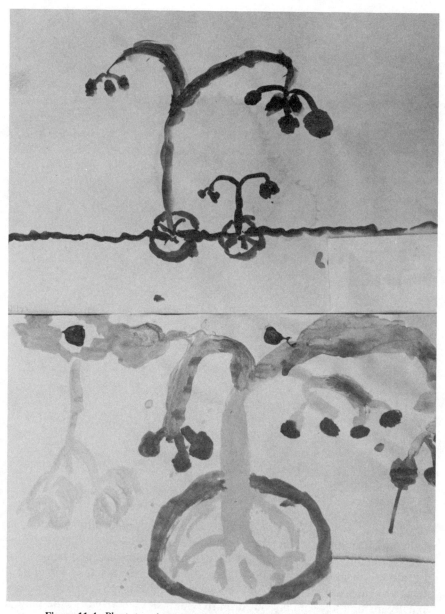

Figure 11.4. Plant–tree (on two separate occasions) as the disease progressed.

As language becomes confused and verbal output diminishes, the patient may omit the mouth in figure drawings. Short-term memory loss is seen in lack of retention of art therapy directions and inability to remember what was drawn after the session. At this early stage, the patient often recognizes deficiencies in the artwork, saying, "It doesn't look right," or "I used to

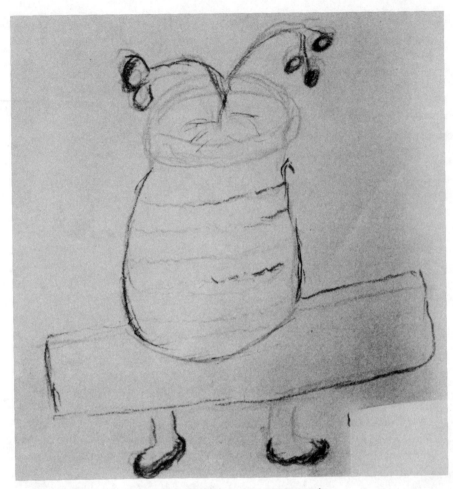

Figure 11.5. Vase on a table with human legs.

draw better.'' Unless denial is a strong element in personality makeup, he or she also admits to memory problems.

In the middle phase of Alzheimer's disease, as more learned behavior is lost and as adaptive mechanisms dependent upon memory fail, a decline is often noted in personal hygiene and social behavior. The patient may become sexually disinhibited and act out primitive fantasies. In artwork, the patient sometimes draws sexual parts, phallic shapes, bright lips. Sexual confusion may appear in the misidentification of the sex in a person drawing and even the sex of a real person. A patient who presents as socially appropriate may draw a navel on a clothed person, showing regression and dependency.

Personality changes can appear and exaggerate into psychotic ideation (Wald, 1984), and delusions can surface in artwork in bizarre drawings. Paranoid thinking may appear in out-of-context eyes, eyes looking sideways.

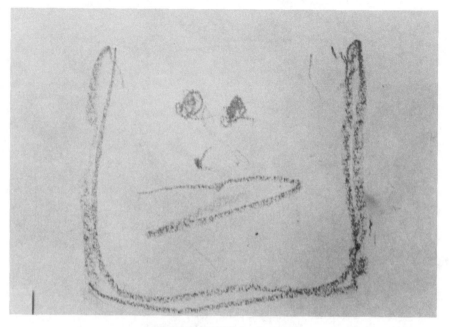

Figure 11.6. "Why, why me?"

Artwork becomes more chaotic, disorganized, and confused. For example, a collage done by a woman in early-stage Alzheimer's disease was full, well balanced, and clear; at the middle stage it showed impulsivity and confusion in its clutter.

In Figure 11.6, the patient drew a simplified version of a face. Incomplete rectangular-shaped face and open mouth show inability to complete a shape, a sign of organicity. Incompletions also point to specific areas of dysfunction: loss of cognitive abilities (lack of top of head), loss of speech skills (half-drawn mouth). This patient often cried out, "Why, why me?" showing insight into his disabilities.

As cognitive abilities decline, artwork is characterized by perceptual distortions, confusion in perspective, incorrect placement of parts, simplification (see Fig. 11.6), and disorganization. One patient demonstrated concrete thinking when instructed to paint the flowers in the vase—he literally painted colors on the flowers set before him! Asked to draw a nose to add to a face, a patient may write the word *nose* in the place of the nose. Perceptual loss, confusion, and agitation cause body and spatial disorientation. Loss of the body image appears in drawings where body parts are omitted or confused. Figures become distorted, regressed. The patient at this point rarely recognizes or shows concern about omissions or distortions. For the theme "Draw yourself and someone important to you," a patient drew herself, a large woman, and her thin husband (Fig. 11.7). Body concept

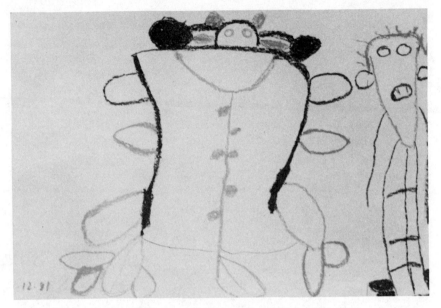

Figure 11.7. Drawing of self (center) and husband (right).

is confused, distorted, regressed. Some body parts are omitted, others re-peated in perseverative patterns until they became unrecognizable.

It should be noted that degenerative diseases of the nervous system typ-ically do not start symmetrically. Alzheimer's disease tends to affect one side of the cortex before the other, and deficits can be correlated with the part of the brain most heavily involved. In late stages, the disabilities become more global, and nearly all patients develop problems in speech, language, and comprehension. Motor skills deteriorate to the point where the caretaker must dress, feed, and toilet the patient. In art therapy, the patient also relies on others to get started and may draw over another patient's line. Artwork becomes incoherent, disconnected, and formless—primitive rhythms, frag-mented lines, and staccato dots. The patient no longer knows what to do with a crayon. Regressed and confused, patients may wash their hands in clay water, or eat or drink the art material, and not even notice their odd taste.

Diagnosis and evaluation serve the victim of a dementing illness from a clinical viewpoint. That is, the therapist or caretaker gains knowledge of what a patient can and cannot do, what the particular illness is, and what stage the illness is in. From this information, the therapist can move to establish treatment goals for working with the patient.

ART THERAPY GOALS

In establishing goals for an art therapy program, the therapist must keep in mind the terrible losses suffered by victims of a dementing illness—of intellect, memory, speech, and physical abilities. The primary goal is to help offset these losses by providing activities within a framework in which the patient can succeed. In art therapy, the patient is mentally, physically, and emotionally involved in making a visible, tangible product. The patient can take pride in this personal accomplishment, as long as the art therapist creates an environment geared for success by eliminating extraneous distractions, minimizing functional deficits, and giving encouragement and definition to attempts at artistic expression. Patients with previous art abilities have a special area where they can excel and get recognition and compliments from patients and staff, which boost their self-esteem.

Additional treatment goals are: to allow the release of pent-up emotions and the expression of underlying psychosis; to preserve a sense of pride and dignity as productive adults; to encourage reminiscence and life review; to provide a visual focus for reality orientation and memory retraining; to provide a nonverbal, visual means of communication for patients whose language skills are failing; and to bring patients out of personal isolation and despair by encouraging socialization and group support.

It should be noted that the focus of treatment goals for degenerative diseases such as Alzheimer's is by necessity supportive, not curative. Due to the regressive nature of dementing illnesses, art therapy is not used directly with the patient to break through such psychological defenses as denial, for this may be all that holds the patient together. The dementia syndrome is not treatable in the sense that physical problems such as high blood pressure, arthritis, vision or hearing loss, and psychiatric symptoms such as depression or psychosis may be alleviated. Once these "treatable symptoms" have been treated, one is left with the management of the dementia syndrome by the caretakers and by the patients themselves.

Art therapy provides an activity the patients can enjoy and cope with even as the dementia becomes severe. For patients who have never drawn or worked with their hands, the art therapy session is a pleasant, relaxing time to join others in a creative activity. Patients with a dementing illness need a focus; a piece of paper, a crayon, a topic, and seeing others draw provide this. While other populations can make choices and respond to the freedom of choosing media and topics, demented patients become more confused, agitated, and feel inadequate when left too much on their own. Art therapy gives patients a structured activity where they can release their emotions and focus their energy within safe boundaries.

PRECAUTIONS

The severe functional, visual, and perceptual deficits of dementing illnesses require the art therapist to present activities in an adapted manner. As patients may be unable to use scissors, the art therapist can supply precut shapes for collages. As patients have difficulty using water to moisten watercolor, the art therapist can place drops of water on the waterblocks before the session. To avoid the mixing of colors and brushes, a separate paint brush can be placed in each jar of tempera paint. Patients may paint beyond the picture edge, mistake clay for food and paints and glazes for drinks, forget how to use a brush, and be unable to sign their names. The art therapist must simplify tasks and instructions in order not to frustrate further, embarrass, or confuse the patients. When a patient paints off the picture edge or on the paint jar, or pastes on the wrong side of the paper, he or she should be quietly and gently redirected. As most art therapy sessions involve group work with patients at various stages and degrees of dementia, other staff personnel or volunteers must watch for confused primitive behavior such as attempts to eat or drink the art materials. Such a regressed patient may be kept aside at another table looking at art books. Considering all these practical constraints, group size should be limited to a very small number.

ART THERAPY ACTIVITIES

Painting with classical music in the background is a good way to provide an introduction to art therapy. Music that shows respect for the patients' mature tastes gives dignity to and creates interest in an activity they may avoid because they "have no talent" or think is childish. The art therapist may talk of how artists need some inspiration to get them started—an idea, a memory, a vision, a model, a scene, or music. In such a relaxed atmosphere patients often free-associate and recall experiences and emotions that are well suited to expression in watercolor. More "hyper," anxious patients often channel their energy in a painting, producing rippling designs with movement. The mandala form can be used to provide the structure of a circle wherein they can paint pleasing forms and colors. The art therapist may suggest to the patients that they simply move their brushes to the rhythm of the music to begin a pattern. For some lower-functioning patients the art therapist may need to place the brush in their hands and begin to move their hands to get them started. When patients get stuck and stop, the art therapist's expression of concern or a suggestion to change colors is usually enough to get them connected again. One is often amazed to see a group of such severely disabled people quietly painting away.

Bright poster paint is stimulating to the senses and helpful to the patient with failing eyesight. Applying poster paint with large brushes or sponge brushes is a good technique to use with the withdrawn, depressed, or highly controlled patient in order to encourage movement, freedom, and spontaneity. Holding up each completed painting, the patients are asked whether the picture reminds them of anything and to think of an interesting title. This gives definition to a patient's efforts, and is often fun for the group as well.

Sometimes the art therapist comes to the group with a specific theme or goal in mind, to find the patients already engaged in drawing or painting something on their own. Just seeing the art materials can stimulate ideas, and regular participation in art therapy sessions also creates a pattern of behavior and response. To help give the more recalcitrant patients a starting point, the therapist can draw a squiggle, a triangle, a square, or a circle, then tell the patients to exercise their imaginations and develop it into a design or picture. Comparing the results to those of great artists like Picasso, Chagall, and Klee elevates self-esteem and can bring up a discussion on modern art. Intellectually failing people appreciate and respond to a therapist's treating them like adults.

As memory loss is central to Alzheimer's disease and other dementing illnesses, themes that trigger reminiscence are especially valuable. So used to and demoralized by forgetting, the patients spark to life when they mentally connect with a past event. Topical themes that reinforce reality orientation can also stimulate old memories. For "School Days," patients can be encouraged to draw their elementary schools, an old schoolmate, think of how they got there, write anything they can remember from school such as a teacher's name, the name of the school, a favorite subject. "Holiday Memories," "Summer Vacation," and "A Special Outing" can lead to interesting artwork as well as stimulate discussion.

A life review project that continues for several sessions can be done on an 18-by-24-inch piece of paper divided into six sections. Above each section is a title to represent important phases of life—"Childhood," "School Days," "Special Occasion," "Adulthood," "Work," "The Present." The patients can concentrate on one section at a time, writing and drawing any pertinent memory. Other staff and volunteers can help focus the patients on reminiscence. Sharing the memories helps the patients to get to know each other better.

Another memory exercise is a series of collages, adding new shapes and textures at each session. However, collages can be confusing and frustrating because they involve too many materials and steps. Patients need help pasting. Some patients tend to paint with the white glue, mistaking it for white paint. Precut shapes are provided to avoid the misuse of scissors. Nevertheless, it is something almost everyone, with assistance in pasting can do without concern about drawing ability. The obsessive–compulsive patient thrives on creating a balanced collage, while a more creative patient can be playful in the placement of shapes. The resulting colorful designs are pleasing to everyone.

Memory retraining can also be implemented in art therapy by such sessions as a series on drawing people. The first session is run like an art class, with the art therapist drawing a face on an easel, asking the patients for suggestions as to the shape of the face, placement of parts, and recognition of missing parts. Step by step, with guidelines, patients attempt to follow on their paper. The results are usually quite good, and the patients are amazed at their art ability. In the next session, the patients are asked to try to remember the step-by-step directions of the last session. Subsequent sessions can include the themes: "Draw yourself," "Draw the person across from you," "Draw yourself and someone important to you" (see Fig. 11.7), "Draw your family," "Draw a model." Patients are reminded that it is for fun, to help memory retraining, and they should not be embarrassed with the results.

Clay can be too regressive for low-functioning patients, who often mistake it for food. However, it is excellent for higher-functioning individuals, giving them a three-dimensional, malleable material that can result in a concrete or functional object. A less impaired patient can follow the art therapist's directions step by step, and the resulting product gives a sense of productivity. More impaired patients enjoy banging the clay flat, often releasing pent-up anger in the process. Perseveration can result in a beautifully smoothed product, but the impulsive patient has difficulty controlling the medium. Patients have great difficulty following directions, so projects are designed to be simple; mobile shapes, tile pictures, a face or mask (using red clay for the slab face, and white clay for the features to minimize perceptual confusion).

To help patients interact with each other, patients can be paired together on a large piece of paper. When they are asked to work together on a picture or design that they both agree on, their actual dialogue may be nonsensical yet filled with warmth, humor, and mutual encouragement. A two-person collage also gets everyone involved, with leaders and followers assuming their roles. In a "round-robin" drawing, where one makes a mark and passes the crayon and the drawing to the next person, the group's attention is focused on a single task.

Another group project is filling in a full-size tracing of a man and woman. The art therapist can call on higher-functioning patients to draw the facial features, and others can draw patterns for the clothes or color in another's outline. This activity promotes social interaction and contributes to the patient's sense of body organization. Finally, the patients can give a name and profession to the full-size body tracings, even have them engage in a dialogue.

A clay project works well with a small group. Patients are asked to come up with an idea they can work on together. For a baseball game, one person rolled out the field, another the bases. Some patients made balls for the heads of the players, others rolled out cylinders for the bodies, legs, and arms. The more adept put the body parts together and later glazed the fired product. Other group clay projects include people on a bench, a plate of hors d'oeuvres, a main course of meatballs and spaghetti.

A smaller group is also conducive to a story picture. Beginning with "Once upon a time. . . ," the story develops from the group. The group discusses illustrations to add to the story line, and patients draw or add ideas to the story. In one story picture session, the group continued, with the assistance of the music therapist, to orchestrate rhythmic sounds to represent the monster, the men, the battle, and so on. Concluding with a dramatic musical reading heightened by sound effects was fun and creative for all.

In another example of a combination of music therapy and art therapy, art was brought into a music improvisation session. While most of the group played instruments, several patients were drawn aside and asked to listen to the mood, rhythms, and melody and respond graphically. One patient painted the rhythms, another a Mexican on a horse (as he felt the music had a Latin flavor), and another perseverated on a boat theme he had been stuck on since he had worked on a Columbus Day mural 4 months previously (however, the portholes had now become eyes). The fourth patient got totally confused by the combined stimulation of art and music and kept walking away, needing constant refocusing by the art therapist.

Murals give everyone a large, expansive surface on which to work together. Seated at a table, the patients may still stay isolated in their own space. Large brushes encourage freedom and spontaneity, and bright poster paint increases visual stimulation. Themes to encourage connection with other patients' space include a group abstract, water (waves, movement), and rhythms to music. Patients can be encouraged to work standing, or change seats in order to paint in another's area to elaborate on another's pattern. Thus they take interest in what the others have painted.

Mural paper on the wall is better for topics for reality orientation, for no one need work "upside down," which happens when sitting across from one another at a table. The patients can come up with a seasonal topic such as "Spring," "May Day," "Back to School," "Christmas and Chanukah." The topic is discussed, the patients reminisce about personal memories. Other topics could be carryovers from previous sessions where the patients drew trees or houses separately; the trees could be made into a forest, the houses into a village or city. As they come up with ideas, they or others can come forward to draw them with magic markers (which are bright and don't drip). The patients encourage each other. The art therapist can call on those patients he or she knows can draw a house or person to make these additions, so the mural has some stronger elements. When individual patients refuse to participate, they can be involved in some other way, such as suggesting ideas. Lower-functioning patients can fill in others' outlines, draw sky or grass, or follow the art therapist's finger to make a line. A good letterer can be asked to title the mural. For a theme such as "Happy Birthday" or "Happy New Year," some patients can draw large letters, the others add designs to create a confetti or festive effect. All the patients, having therefore interacted on some level with each other, feel good that they have participated and enjoy the end product. The more the art therapist intervenes with suggestions and encouragement, the more cohesive the resulting mural. Displaying the product on the wall provides a constant reminder of reality.

A Thanksgiving mural (Fig. 11.8) summarizes how one can work with a group of patients with dementing illnesses despite their severe deficits. The group discussed memories of Thanksgiving and plans for this year. Deciding to begin with a large dining table, a patient drew a rectangle without concern for perspective. Since there was no one with strong artistic skills, whoever

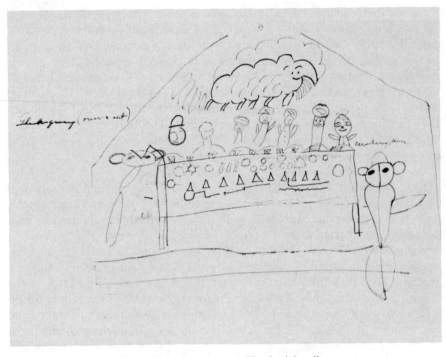

Figure 11.8. Group mural, Thanksgiving dinner.

was brave enough volunteered to draw a person. These "people" were simplified, regressed, distorted, some missing bodies, arms, noses, mouths. Other patients drew various shapes and lines to represent plates, glasses, food. One woman, when asked to draw cranberry sauce, wrote the word instead (concrete thinking). The therapist noted that the most important item, the turkey, was missing. A patient drew a whimsical turkey above the table, perseverating to make six feet, and adding a humanlike face. A patient who was proud of his ability to draw a house surrounded the scene with a house shape (note the disconnections). A humorous addition to this scene was the title "Thanksgiving (over and out)."

This Thanksgiving mural summarizes a variety of manifestations of organicity in artwork of patients with dementing illnesses: simplification, regression, perseveration, omissions, distortions, disconnections, incomplete shapes, concrete thinking, and lack of perspective.

CONCLUSION

In conclusion, art therapy serves important diagnostic, evaluative, management, and supportive functions in treating patients with dementing illnesses.

As a therapist working with a patient population that does not "improve" or "get better" in the traditional sense, I was often asked, "How do you hold onto yourself in the midst of the patient's increasing regression?" I kept in mind that at least these patients had led relatively full lives until their illness struck, at least their families or caretakers cared enough to give them the best medical treatment and day-care program. Feeling this support, the patients passed it on to other patients and expressed their appreciation to the therapist. I was also fortunate to work in a creative professional environment where the therapists supported one another and sensed when to relieve their colleagues. While the process of dementing illnesses is at this point irreversible, gains can nonetheless be seen in the therapists' and caretakers' abilities to manage the patients, and in the patients' adaptation to their declines. Demented patients kept as active and alert as possible in art therapy retain a sense of dignity while preserving their functions. The quality of life in its late stage is improved, which is indeed a major aim of geriatric care.

REFERENCES

Blass, J. P. (1985). Alzheimer's disease. *Disease a Month, 31*(4), 1–69.

Crosson, C. (1976). Geriatric patients: Problems of spontaneity. *American Journal of Art Therapy, 15*, 51–56.

Dewdney, I. (1975). An art therapy program for geriatric patients. In E. Ulman & P. Dachinger (Eds.), *Art therapy in theory and practice*. New York: Schocken.

Harrison, C. (1981). Therapeutic art programs around the world-XIII: Creative arts for older people in the community. *American Journal of Art Therapy, 19*, 99–101.

Landgarten, H. (1983). Art therapy for depressed elders. *Clinical Gerontologist, 2*(1), 45–53.

Wald, J. (1984). The graphic representation of regression in an Alzheimer's disease patient. *The Arts in Psychotherapy, 2*, 165–175.

Wald, J. (1986). Fusion of symbols, confusion of boundaries: Percept contamination in the art work of Alzheimer's disease patients. *Art Therapy, 3*, 74–80.

Weiss, J. C. (1984). *Expressive therapy with elders and the disabled: Touching the heart of life*. New York: Haworth.

Zeiger, B. (1976). Life reivew in art therapy with the aged. *American Journal of Art Therapy, 15*, 47–50.

CHAPTER 12

Art Therapy with the Unidentified Patient

ROBERT E. AULT

For many of us who entered the field of art therapy in the late fifties and early sixties, our work was primarily done in a variety of clinical institutions. Here clients identified as "patients" were deemed to be "sick" and carried a diagnostic label. A medical or special education model was most often used in conceptualizing clients, their needs, and their "treatment." At that time in history few of us were identified as art therapists; instead we were referred to by a variety of titles, including adjunctive therapists, activity therapists, special educators, art teachers, and so on. It was only later, with the creation of the American Art Therapy Association, that many of us scattered around the country began to identify ourselves as art therapists, although we had been using art in our work for years. Many of us, including myself, had entered the field without specific training in psychiatry or art therapy, but were artists with deeply felt humanitarian values and a semi-formed vision of how art could be helpful to people.

Conflict was a daily component of our practice and was experienced on many levels. Conflict resolution is a core component of the treatment process, and in work with patients support was available through supervision, education, and shared responsibility. The more difficult conflicts, then as now, have always been in our relationships with fellow workers and with ourselves. Professional boundaries were often strained or violated as we outgrew our old concepts and attempted to create a new profession. Concrete issues such as job descriptions, salaries, and so forth had to be renegotiated and often with much distress and little support. A deeper question also arose in regard to our own identity. What were we really: artists or therapists? What did we do with the chronic blessing or curse within ourselves, our need to create art? These were areas of major conflict and often guided or influenced decisions about our professional work. This chapter is about my own struggle with this conflict and how, through its resolution, I discovered a new arena of interaction outside of traditional institutional settings.

In November 1978, following 18 years of work as an activity/art therapist at the Menninger Foundation, primarily with adult inpatients, I decided I needed to make some type of professional move. I reduced my work at

Menninger's to half-time and opened a small art school. I also increased my time at Emporia State University, where I had been teaching in the graduate art therapy program since 1973.

The reasons for making such a move included a wish of long standing to reengage in the arena of art on a level that I'd enjoyed working on earlier but which had been eroded by clinical responsibilities. I'd always maintained my basic identity as an artist and was beginning to feel separated from that aspect of my life. Secondly, I had spent so many years with highly dysfunctional clients that I wanted contact with people on the other end of the scale, "normal" people from the community. Third, I wanted more economic rewards for my work. And finally, and probably of most importance, I felt a burning need to have autonomy over some aspect of my professional life, since I had worked for and within the structure of an institution for so long.

The school is basically a large studio located in a quiet but centrally located part of Topeka, Kansas. The main room, filled with easels, tables, still-life materials, plants, paintings, and even a canary, has a pleasant studio atmosphere. Here I conduct six classes per week. Three of the classes are for children ages 6 to 14, and three classes are for adults. The classes are kept to a limit of 8 students so they can be worked with individually. Instruction is primarily focused on drawing and painting. The classes have been full since the first week the school opened. Coupled with special time-limited summer classes, the enrollment averages between 50 and 60 students at any time. The students come primarily from middle-to upper-middle-class families throughout Topeka and are what I believe you would classify as "normal citizens." I have reserved a number of children's positions for below-cost services, and these are filled from lower-income families.

Early in this venture I observed that a percentage of clients came to the school seeking mental health services in the guise of art classes. Both children and adults exhibited symptoms that could be described, understood, and treated. These were not individuals who had been identified as patients or as suffering from mental illness, nor were they the sort of people who generally seek mental health care services from a therapist. They did not identify themselves as patients, yet they exhibited levels of personality and relationship dysfunction that often interfered with or inhibited their lives. By and large they were the nice but sometimes unhappy "neighbor types" who might occasionally seek out counsel from a minister during especially difficult times, but would not see themselves as patients. They came to art classes looking for help, though this was unacknowledged, and often experienced real changes taking place in their lives without any talk of therapy. I found that these unidentified patients could be served through what I considered rather minor changes of attitude and process, maximizing the "therapeutic" aspects of the art experience. I identify myself not as a therapist in that setting but rather as an art teacher. Granted, I have been a part of the psychiatric community for years and am known by some as having that background, but it is seldom mentioned. In fact, there are only three rules at the art school that I strictly enforce: First, there will be no coloring books; second, no number paintings; and third, no talk of Menninger's.

Before speaking of specific syndromes, it might be useful to define more clearly what I mean by unidentified patients. We all range up and down in our daily lives on a scale from healthy to pathological, yet the shifts remain in a generally acceptable norm. Illness, I believe, is characterized by a matter of degree of shifting into those areas of our personality that cause dysfuntion. Most people do retain some balance and continue to function in spite of internal conflicts and/or external realities that influence their lives. When these conflicts interfere with functioning, then we tend to identify these individuals as "ill" or if they seek help, as "patients." Clinically, we most often encounter those with severe degrees of pathology, but what happens to those who are moderately ill or have compensated somehow to cover, deny, or minimize these unresolved conflicted forces within their lives? Most go unrecognized, and untreated. In general, the health care system is not geared toward meeting their needs, although I believe they make up a high percentage of our population. Of those people who take art classes from me, about 25% fall into this category, and of these, only a handful have ever sought professional help. I often refer to this population that is crying for attention as "the great American wasteland."

As I interacted with these special art students I began to notice common patterns of history and behavior. These could be described and specific strategies of treatment developed to work with the problems they brought to the classes. I have divided these syndromes into those common to adults and those common to children. Each group will be described, and then I will present a description of how I have attempted to deal with these problems and the results of these interventions.

THE ADULTS

Adult Syndrome A

These adults can be described as functioning people in the community who exhibit some or all of the following characteristics:

1. They are chronically unhappy, and/or dissatisfied with some major aspect of their lives, such as their marriage, their role in life, or something more vague and undefined.
2. They are mostly females, from 25 to 65 years of age. Although I've observed some males with the same syndrome, most of my students are female.
3. They exhibit mild to moderate depression. Most are well off financially and are not overly concerned with the basic issues of survival such as food and shelter.

4. Most of the clients have somatic complaints such as headaches, backaches, weight control problems, and sleep disturbances.

5. They are often out of touch with their own feelings, especially those of aggression and/or anger.

6. They often describe a general feeling of being unfulfilled and searching for something to satisfy this hunger, such as classes. Often they have a history of movement through many types of classes such as cooking, music, dance, great books, and so on.

7. They often have multiple involvements in social clubs or organizations, or the reverse; they often face social isolation, especially after their children leave home.

8. Many drink too much but are not really alcoholics, or they take a variety of prescribed medications but never use illegal drugs.

9. Often they are oriented toward traditional sex role models that are stereotyped. These are the "in-betweeners," having some awareness of the repression and dependency of these roles yet being unable to move on into more responsible and/or independent roles.

10. Often they are very right brain oriented, resulting in poor self-esteem as they have failed at left brain functioning in their daily lives. These are often bright women who can't keep a checkbook straight.

11. Many speak of marriages that have become arrangements lacking any real warmth or intimacy. Often they report multiple marriages over a period of years.

12. There is nothing they can really claim as their own, separate from their children's or husband's accomplishments. They often identify themselves as Mrs. John Doe.

In general these are bright, decent, successful middle-to upper-middle-class nonworking females, who go through life feeling shortchanged, concluding that happiness or good feelings are not a part of their lives. They are friends and neighbors who keep their troubles mostly to themselves. Most have a circle of friends and are able to raise families successfully, yet they suffer a great deal.

Adult Syndrome B

The second group I wish to describe displays many of the characteristics of the first group but to greater degrees. Added to this list are more disturbances in interpersonal relations.

1. They are often seen or experienced as rather insensitive people who struggle with their own aggression. Often their hostility is expressed in subtle but effective verbalizations and/or acts, such as making messes, misuse of time, and so on.

2. They are often characterized by a sense of drifting in their lives and are angry at the world.

3. Often there is a rather high degree of suppression of their feelings resulting in extreme rigidity, or problems with expressing their anger too much.

4. There is often more severe dependence, yet rejection of the care and attention they demand.

5. They generally have a smaller group of friends and often complain of loneliness.

6. These are people who more often use the professional services of a minister or a counselor. They do not identify themselves as patients, however. Usually these contacts are initiated by school counselors they contact because of their children's problems.

7. Finally, these are often people that are overinvolved in their children's lives and seek self-esteem from the children's accomplishments.

Adult Syndrome C

1. These are often patients or former patients who exhibit more severe degrees of personality dysfunction.

2. Chronic difficulty in interpersonal relationships is common.

3. They often act out anger or hostility in not so subtle ways, creating a sense of tension in the group.

4. They often attempt to misuse the relationship with the teacher, expecting to be taken care of and picked up after, and/or they talk about their personal lives, demanding the teacher to be their therapist.

5. There is a general sense of their not being a part of any group. They are usually loners who are isolated and isolating.

All adult groups I have tried to describe have the capacity to get involved and use the experience of interacting with both the activity of art and the interpersonal relationship with the instructor and others in the class. I have observed real growth and change in these people. The three groups differ only in the degree of intensity of symptoms. They respond to similar handling. The methods of working are similar to basic activity or art therapy as we've practiced it in the context of a hospital for years.

Therapeutic Interactions

The following is a list of elements in the process that I feel are helpful in fostering change toward better functioning. They involve not only specific treatment strategies but also characteristics of the mileu itself.

1. One should provide an interested, caring, and stimulating environment in which to work. A relaxed studio atmosphere including music, coffee, a lot of plants, art equipment, the smell of turpentine, and a canary seems to work best for me. The place itself becomes very important as people begin to identify with it. The location is also of critical importance. A safe, middle-income, residential location that is convenient to get to seems to have been very important. Low-rent Bohemia is definitely out.

2. One should teach skills in art while at the same time maximizing decision making by the student. As students gain more skills, they often report a good feeling of having control over something and the satisfaction of mastery. It is important that the work go beyond the norm and avoid stereotyping of imagery and/or technique, yet at the same time be something the students can claim as theirs. Often this is a first-time experience for them.

3. One should encourage discussions of feelings related to art; how it feels as well as what one thinks. I often use feeling language in working with these people. Aesthetics is a process of relating both intellectually and emotionally and both should be considered and used.

4. One should encourage group formation and the development of a support system. For example, cards are always sent when someone is ill.

5. One should encourage participation in art groups in the community to enlarge the circle of involvements.

6. It has been helpful to have occasional student art shows where the students show off as "artists" to friends and family.

7. I often talk about the art and lives of people recognized as "real" artists who have suffered some form of mental illness: Audubon and his bouts with severe depression, Monet and his difficulties during the time his eyesight became bad, Utrillo and his problems with alcohol, and, of course, Van Gogh and Winston Churchill.

8. I actively share a lot about my own professional and personal life. This can certainly be done with discretion so as not to burden people with another's problems, but it also allows them to get more involved. I listen to them, provide an empathic ear, sometimes advise or counsel, or share experiences. I maintain the willingness to be open with people while at the same time carefully retaining a sense of structure and purpose to our meeting. Touching is also a part of the work that has to be carefully understood and used. A hand on the shoulder, a pat on the back, or an occasional hug can sometimes communicate better than words and is used when comfortable and appropriate for both the student and myself.

The results of this work can be both dramatic and satisfying. Many of the students seem to blossom and report they are feeling and doing better than they have in years. There is a reduction in symptoms previously described, and generally they seem more engaged in life, have improvements in self-esteem, and experience more control over themselves and their families. Many become active in amateur art groups and begin to refer to themselves as artists, often with the support of spouses. With many former patients, the studio has at times been utilized as a way of weathering difficulties and avoiding hospitalization. We've been able to set schedules, structure time, offer support either directly or through the group, and help the person make it through difficult times. Of course, it does not always work, and in spite of such efforts, difficulties sometimes are too great to be dealt with through this environment alone. Generally our experience has been positive, however.

What I have attempted to describe is a particular treatment process that is most often "unidentified" so as to be more palatable. Many of those served would actively reject an open treatment model and would resist identifying themselves as patients, yet they come, they get involved, and many seem to make major changes in their personal lives. Some of these changes include decisions to reenter college at middle age, to complete projects that had been put aside, to review friendships, or to improve relationships with spouses and families.

THE CHILDREN

During the course of a week I have contact with between 20 and 30 children. They range in ages from 6 to 13 and are divided among three classes. About half the students are boys and half are girls; their average age is 9. The students often stay in class for a period of time ranging from several weeks to 3 years. Most of the children are referred to me through school personnel or parents, because of their interest or skills in art. They are, by and large, from families where art, creativity, and education are held as values. Occasionally I have students from more isolated rural areas, but most have had some elementary school art and have shown enough interest to alert a teacher. Many teachers report a marked change in the student's behavior during "art times" in the classroom and want to expand or capitalize on this method of self-regulation. The majority of these kids are well behaved, bright, serious students and are a pleasure to work with. There is a percentage, though, who are brought to class for other reasons, which I will try to describe.

The Westboro Syndrome

Westboro is an upper-class neighborhood in Topeka that is characterized as the old-money, high-prestige section of town. The homes are large, rambling, stone houses, with well-groomed lawns, exuding a sense of order and social and economic well-being. The men are the basic income producers, and most are professionals such as doctors and lawyers or successful businessmen. These people are often the ones that middle-class Americans idealize. On the surface all appears well, yet many of the children suffer from a particular complex of symptoms or characteristics that I've grouped together and call the Westboro syndrome simply because so many I see of this sort come from this neighborhood. These are the bright, gifted children whom teachers often find very disruptive and to be low achievers in public school despite their advantages of high intelligence.

Children's Symptoms

The following is a list of behaviors and/or symptoms that are common to many of these children. They may not exhibit all these characteristics but generally fit into a profile of this nature.

1. These children are often hyperactive, tense, and intense.
2. They are very achievement oriented to the point where they feel compelled to produce a product in a very short time (30 minutes).
3. They have very low tolerance for frustration or failure.
4. They often misuse materials, or there seems to be no respect or value placed on materials.
5. There is often high value placed in the home on the child's uniqueness. While many of the children strive to be different and draw attention to themselves under the guise of being creative, their work is often highly stereotypical.
6. Often these children have multiple involvements in self-development classes such as music lessons, sports, scouts, chess club, and drama groups.
7. Many of these kids have difficulty in school. They are characterized by teachers as having a short attention span, are discipline problems in class, and, although bright, work below their abilities. Parents often deny there is anything wrong with the child but rather believe that the problem is with the school and the teachers.
8. Many are narcissistic, overly indulged children who later experience problems of acting out as they reach adolescence.
9. Often these are hyperstimulated kids with little internal resources to turn to when external stimulation is removed. They are often, as Edith Kramer describes (Ulman & Dachinger, 1975), empty and suffer depression and the real pain of boredom.

Common Patterns of Parenting

As I began working with these children I noticed a very specific pattern to the parenting of many of the kids. First, and of great importance, is the lack of good fathering. Many of the fathers are away from the home a great deal or are erratic in their relationships with their children. It isn't that they don't love their kids, it's just that they have chosen to place priorities of time and energy in other areas and leave the parenting mostly to the mothers. There is a tendency to substitute material goods for emotional goods. These fathers, generally, are hard-working high achievers who often sacrifice family needs to those of their professions and businesses.

The mothers of these children also seem to exhibit common characteristics. Generally they are self-sacrificing, somewhat infantile women who suffer from loneliness and dependency. They often have difficulty differentiating themselves from their children. The children are often seen as extensions of the mothers and are used through their achievements and activities to counter the emptiness, low self-esteem, and depression of these women. Again, denial is very much a part of the relationship, not only with themselves and their families but with the rest of society. There is a high value placed on appearances, and prestige choices are often made in favor of human choices. They are loving mothers who are extremely interested in their kids, are sincere in their attempts to do what is best for the family, yet are at times blind to the imposition of their will on the child and the price that it extracts.

Therapeutic Goals

The therapeutic goals of the art experience for these children along with the art instruction goals include the following:

1. To allow children to differentiate from their parents more clearly by establishing a separate arena of interaction
2. To help establish some area they can claim as theirs alone
3. To channel energy into more constructive and creative uses
4. To delay gratification by investing more in what they do
5. To develop an identity with a skill, which is very important in changing the self-concept
6. To provide a consistent relationship with an adult male

Techniques

1. Provide a milieu that is structured yet relaxed and respectful of individuals.
2. Maximize participation by the student in decision making, such as choosing what he or she wants to paint. I assist by teaching how to produce it but they decide what they want to do.
3. Insist—absolutely—on proper and respectful use of materials.
4. Allow challenging and testing of authority. Permit humor, joking, teasing, by the children and vice versa.

5. Allow openness of expression of feelings within boundaries of respecting each other's rights.
6. Counsel mothers to allow their children more space. I do not allow parents in the studio while the class is in session.
7. Capitalize on competitiveness. Have contests with enough categories so everyone wins a ribbon.
8. Adjust materials to those demanding more time and investment. At times make adjustments in material use toward more structured activities.
9. Sometimes separate students from the children's class and put one or two into adult classes.
10. Use a lot of appropriate touching.

Results

After the children attend the classes for approximately 2 months I begin to note changes in their behavior. Common observations of both the children and the parents are as follows:

1. Overall, the children tend to slow down their hyperactivity. They seem to relax and are able to invest more into their work.
2. There usually develops a rather intense investment in the relationship with the teacher. They often begin to bring in work they have done outside of class for me to see. They also bring in objects they have found, special things they have received, and so on. It seems very important that they share these with me.
3. Parents and teachers begin to report that students have made marked improvement in their schoolwork and their ability to concentrate and follow the structure of the school program.
4. Children often assume the identity as the "artist" in their school classes.
5. There usually develops a greater openness on the part of the parents to discuss the child more realistically. The parents are often quite relieved and appreciative of the changes that have taken place.

Overall, I believe the children make significant changes in the areas of cognitive functioning, self-concept and self-confidence, independence, and coping with the tension that had been such a big part of their lives. Their artwork also changes, not only in terms of the skill with which it is made but also in terms of becoming more personal. Other students often make comments such as, "That picture looks like Mary's work."

Children with Special Problems

There is one other group of children who use the services of the school, but with whom I have not had as much success. These students are often very responsive to the structure and process, but the changes they make alarm the parents, and they are frequently not allowed to remain in the class. Following is a list of characteristics of this group and a discussion of the results of the art experience for them.

Symptoms and/or Characteristics

1. They are often very bright, sensitive young children, ages 5 or 6, preschool or in their first year of school. They are identified by the parent as "special," "the next Leonardo," "young geniuses," and so forth. Parents often pursue me to get them into class at an early age. They also check me out first by calling other parents or asking for a vita.
2. The children are socially isolated, have few peer friendships, and tend to be a part of the adult world rather than the children's world. They often have difficulty with peers as they see themselves as different.
3. They suffer from depression.
4. There is often a high degree of suppression of their own feelings.
5. High skill levels in drawing and painting are common although these are often stereotyped productions such as cartoon drawing. Some of these children are doing oil painting at age 6.
6. Their art products are highly prized by the parents, and everything is framed and hung in the home.
7. They are very protected by parents.
8. I have frequently observed at times a retardation in physical growth. These are often small, delicate children.
9. The children often have overly involved mothers who want to stay in class and question me extensively after class. They are often tense women suffering from low self-esteem seeking their own identity or place in history through the child.

Results

As you can gather, these children have experienced patterns of parenting similar to those described in the first group, yet they are different. They are generally younger, and the intensity of the relationship with the mother is stronger.

Very quickly these children start looking better, with the expression of more affect. They begin to interact more with the others in the class, and hang on to me physically. As they begin to shift in the imagery toward that which is more age appropriate, the parents often experience great anxiety at the "loss of skill." The parents then remove the child from the class and search for a more understanding teacher. It is sad not to be able to counter more effectively the forces at work that control these children's and parents' lives at this early stage. Intervention usually occurs later as the children enter the school system and experience great difficulty, and/or failure.

EXAMPLES

The following vignettes are about three people, two adults and a child, who have used the services of the academy. I am reluctant to refer to them as case studies as I do not identify them, nor do they identify themselves, as psychiatric cases. They are normal people dealing with negative circumstances in their lives and they come for and receive art instruction. As the stories illustrate, there is creative power in the art process itself, and when that power is combined with an understanding and supportive relationship and milieu, major changes can occur. The changes evolve without "psychiatric" intervention such as that which characterizes psychotherapy or counseling.

RAMON

A 56-year-old physician, Ramon began his work at the academy with a profusion of apologies. He was sure he had no talent nor skill and would not be able to learn or perform as I might expect him to. He was brought by his wife Catherine, a former student of some years ago, who had both enjoyed the experience and achieved a rather high measure of success. She was concerned about her husband, a gifted pathologist, who because of a physical handicap was limited in the range of activities he could do. She felt he needed to make better use of his leisure time, which he most often spent watching T.V. or "withdrawing more into his books." Retirement without meaningful activity loomed as a problem rather than an opportunity.

Ramon was also concerned that as he reached the age of retirement he would have nothing to occupy him in a meaningful way, as his medical practice did. He had tried a variety of hobbies including music but had been unable to stick with any of them. With the strict discipline he imposed on himself to practice the piano, it finally became an intolerable source of anger and frustration and was dropped after a year.

The couple joined an adult class of eight students that meets once a week for a 2-hour session. They each do their own thing and seem to enjoy the time together. Catherine usually works across the studio on her more realistic painting while Ramon has chosen a different path.

Figure 12.1 is an acrylic painting titled "Reaching for What You Want." Ramon explains it as follows: "You should reach up for what you want, or you dream of. The chains represent your negative thoughts that hold you back from obtaining your golden dream."

In Figure 12.1 Ramon has chosen to minimize the drawing aspect of the imagery, concentrating more on a variety of symbolic and technical effects such as color relationships, pointillism, and hard-edge designing. These are done in a relaxed atmosphere that is both instructive and supportive.

The first paintings were accompanied with apologies and declarations of how valueless they were. In spite of these comments, though, he ventured to hang several in his office at the hospital. To his amazement and pleasure he found his colleagues and friends were both interested and delighted.

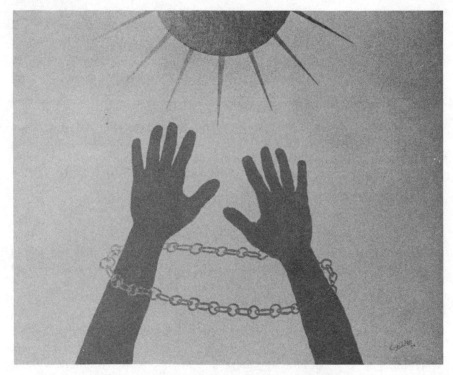

Figure 12.1. Ramon: a hard-edge design.

People began coming to his office to see his most recent work. He gave several away to friends who admired the artwork. As he related these stories he appeared puzzled over these positive responses but showed pleasure as well. The making of artworks has clearly opened a new experience to both Ramon and Catherine. It is something that each can do, find pleasure in, and share, thus lessening the stress imposed by his retirement.

He continues to create, has now bought an easel and paints to use at home, is framing his work, and, hopefully, will continue with it indefinitely. He was never identified as a patient although I believe he responded therapeutically to both the therapist/teacher and the art process.

J.C.

A rather thin, bespectacled 11-year-old boy who speaks with a distinct nasal twang, J.C. has had some hard knocks in his life. He was brought to the academy by his "folks" following urging by their friends at a local donut shop. His "folks" would often spend their evenings there drinking coffee and socializing while the boy sat and occupied himself by drawing fanciful pictures of underground caves filled with military activity. These were usually done with pencil and markers on the backs of used sheets of paper. Figures 12.2 and 12.3 are drawings done at the donut shop and illustrate the creativeness, control, and violent themes that have been typical of his work.

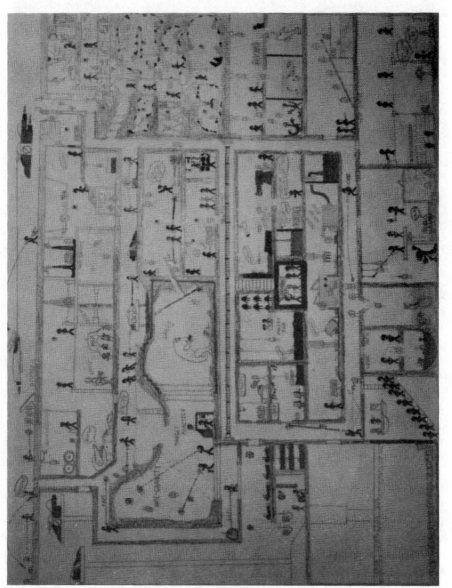

Figure 12.2. J.C.: mechanical imagery.

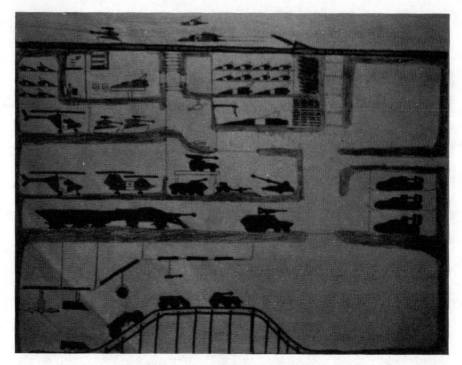

Figure 12.3. J.C.: mechanical imagery, detail.

He was enrolled at the academy in a children's class of eight students aged 7 to 13, which met once a week for 1½ hours. There he initially isolated himself again, relating more easily to me as an adult than to his peers. The first intervention was with the materials and size of the drawings. While allowing his social isolation, I gradually moved him to larger painting projects and jokingly made him my "main man." He seemed to enjoy the specialness of our relationship and felt supported as he explored less controllable materials and imagery.

After several weeks of class the boy's "dad," as he was called, came to pick up J.C. and stayed and talked about the boy and his background. The "folks" turned out to be his grandparents who had raised him after his mother, their daughter, had divorced and threatened to give him to the state for care, declaring herself unwilling or unable to provide a home and parenting. There was also a suggestion the boy had been mistreated, as he was plagued with a variety of phobias and fears. The grandfather also suffers phobic symptoms and is on medical leave from his job.

Many months later J.C. continued to take art from me but had acquired a therapist. He is much more sociable, seems more comfortable, and his speech has improved. He still likes to work with mechanical subjects such as cars, planes, and architectural structures, but his behavior and imagery seem more age appropriate (see Fig. 12.4). Throughout our work together I

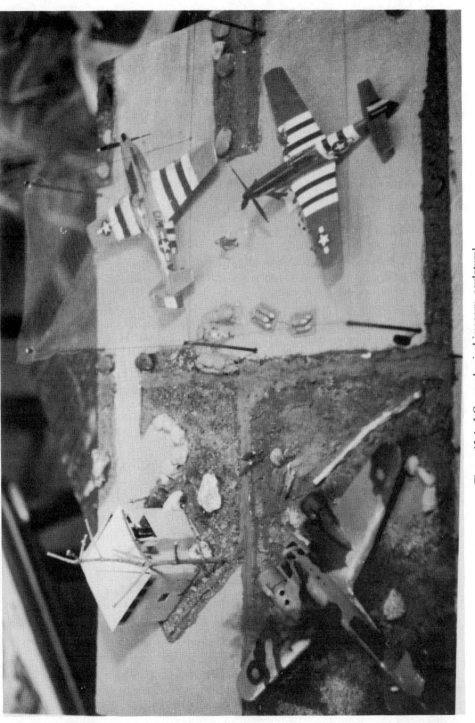

Figure 12.4. J.C.: mechanical imagery, sculptural.

have never identified him or his family as patients, but have worked in as therapeutic a manner as possible. It seemed important that the boy have a good art teacher and friend rather than another mental health worker.

DOROTHY

A woman in her sixties, Dorothy has now attended classes at the Academy for 5 years. Before enrolling she had been to other classes in the community, and I had been warned not to accept her as a student because she'd "take too much of my time." I ignored these comments and enrolled her in an adult class consisting mostly of middle-aged women. To my surprise and relief, instead of experiencing her in a negative way, I found her to be delightful. She worked hard, was responsive to instruction, and was a very nice and decent person. We seemed to hit it off and have both enjoyed our relationship over these years.

A year after she began art classes, her husband, a retired businessman, died very suddenly and unexpectedly. Dorothy plunged into the emotional task of mourning the loss, made more difficult because she was of a generation where women typically maintained a strong dependency on their mates. For the first time in her life she was indeed on her own. To compound matters, within months after his death she was diagnosed as having a cancerous tumor, which was removed surgically.

Throughout these difficult times of her life, though, she maintained contact with her "art class." She continued to paint and talk as she grieved and put her life back in order. This process continues as she has discovered she not only can survive but can thrive.

Figure 12.5 was started just before her husband's death. It was a pleasant landscape that she planned to hang in a prominent place in their home. With his loss the strong emotional associations were simply too much for her to continue and it was set aside for more than a year. The day finally arrived, though, when with encouragement she was able to get it out and bring the project to completion. I supported her through this process and felt the painting had an excellent cathartic impact on her. Today she continues to grow and try out new experiences. Her life instead of closing up has opened. She has expanded the use of the academy during the years to be a place of support, acceptance, and care, all elements of a therapeutic experience.

IMPLICATIONS FOR ART THERAPISTS

What I have attempted to describe in this chapter is another arena for the services of art therapists outside of traditional clinical institutions. What was initially conceptualized as an art school quickly included adaptations of clinical understanding and technique as I attempted to respond to the special needs of students. It is an area of great need, it is financially feasible, and it offers an expanded view of the field of art therapy.

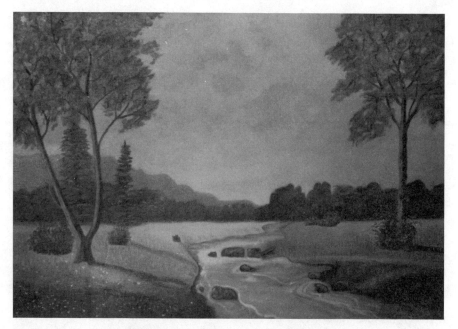

Figure 12.5. Dorothy: a pleasant landscape.

I believe this mainstreaming of clinical-based processes with the "normal" population can and should be a major focus of the art therapy profession in the future. As this occurs, I believe we will see a further acceptance on all levels of society of the "therapeutic" dimension of art. There is evidence that this is occurring already, and the implications are very exciting. Hopefully art will then move out of the commercial vise it is in now, and into a position more oriented toward the needs of a larger population. It is a sad fact that for years those receiving the best education and treatment have been those who have been taken out of the mainstream and put into special education or institutions.

For myself, I have found the use of art therapy with the unidentified patient to be a new direction that is revitalizing important personal and professional needs. It is an area calling for the creative, sensitive understanding and participation of future art therapists.

REFERENCES

Ulman, E., & Dachinger, P. (1975). *Art therapy in theory and practice*. New York: Schocken.

CHAPTER 13

Artistic Giftedness in the Multiply Handicapped

DAVID HENLEY

Entering the art studio, the slightly built boy of 10 strides briskly over to the paper closet and, after much rummaging, selects a large sheet of heavy rag paper. While setting up his drawing materials, Jason pauses to gaze up into the sunlight that filters through the room. He begins to rock his head slowly back and forth as the rays are refracted through his prismlike corrective glasses. When he tires of playing within this kaleidoscope of light and color, he turns his full attention to the oil crayons that will similarly stimulate his visual senses. He giggles, issues a birdlike trill, then begins to draw, alternating between large sweeping arcs and rapid back-and-forth strokes. His eyeglasses remain just inches off the paper as he follows each of his lines around the composition, many of which spill off the paper. The composition evolves swiftly, with large blocks of geometric forms springing up in a flurry of scribbling that appears to be just barely controlled. As the images become articulated one can sense his mounting excitement—he becomes wildly animated with displays of almost euphoric emotion. Buildings, trees, power lines, two people posed in bed outside emerge, as he adds layer after layer of built-up surface. Some images gradually fade from view or are obliterated under his constant reworking. He has been coloring with his right hand, but Jason suddenly switches to his left as he crosses the midline of the pictorial field. Then he ceases drawing and signs to no one in particular, "finish color." He offers the piece one quick glance, then turns to the next piece of paper with equal exuberance and tenacity. Four of these works will be completed within the 40-minute studio session.

This vignette describes the art process of a 10-year-old child who is at once hearing impaired, legally blind, and autistic. It is an unusual case in that the child is developmentally disabled to a degree that would typically inhibit an individual from developing such fine concentration and artistic expression. The peers in this child's classes are mired in developmentally arrested artistic stages of random and semicontrolled scribbling or the rudimentary schematic stages of representation. They demonstrate little of the intense concentration, compositional awareness, deft use of medium, nor have they evolved such an individual style of imagery making. What makes this child different from his similarly retarded peers? With what frequency do the multiply-handicapped populations harbor individuals with such potential?

This chapter will explore the incidence of artistic giftedness in multiply handicapped children. It will concentrate upon visual artists who have developed the capacity to draw, paint, or sculpt with uncommon ability. For the purposes of this Chapter, two case examples will be discussed with the emphasis placed upon aesthetic, therapeutic, and ethical considerations. The children who were identified during the study suffered in varying degrees from sensory impairments, mental retardation, and emotional handicaps. Despite the profundity of their disorders, they were able to compensate for and surmount these obstacles by mobilizing their inner resources and innate aptitudes. The resulting artworks do, however, reflect the stages of symptomatology of each individual as was demonstrated in the first case vignette. Yet, as we shall observe, the pathology inherent in this form of artistic capability is an integral, almost vital part of their distinctive and unique artistic vision.

LITERATURE REVIEW

In 1977, Lorna Selfe published her seminal case history that awakened the fields of art education, psychology, and art criticism to an alien form of artistic giftedness. Not since Itard's account of the *Wild Boy of Aveyron* had a single subject stirred such interdisciplinary debate and study (1962). Selfe's case was that of Nadia, an autistic, functionally retarded girl of 5 years of age, who was able to draw realistically with a facility and verve usually associated with only the most mature artists. So great was this child's virtuosity that the artwork was subsequently compared to that of artists such as Hockney and Daumier (Pariser, 1981) and astoundingly to that of such masters as Delacroix and Rembrandt (Arnheim, 1980) and Leonardo (Winner, 1986).

This instance of artistic giftedness prompted a great deal of commentary by a wide range of art critics, educators, and psychologists. (Contributions by art therapists are noticeably absent from the literature.) Most investigators concluded that it was not really a gift at all, but a highly idiosyncratic aberration that was symptomatic of Nadia's incapacity to communicate through language, cope with interpersonal relations (outside of the child's family), or conceptualize her very surroundings. Regardless of whether Nadia's drawing ability constituted an elaborate symptom or highly refined skill, her pictures remain sensational examples of art created by the multiply handicapped child. Nadia's horse drawings bear out the sense that a confident and exceedingly sensitive draftswoman was at work (Fig. 13.1). In these works, the exuberance and vitality of the line reveal the hot-blooded beast in motion,

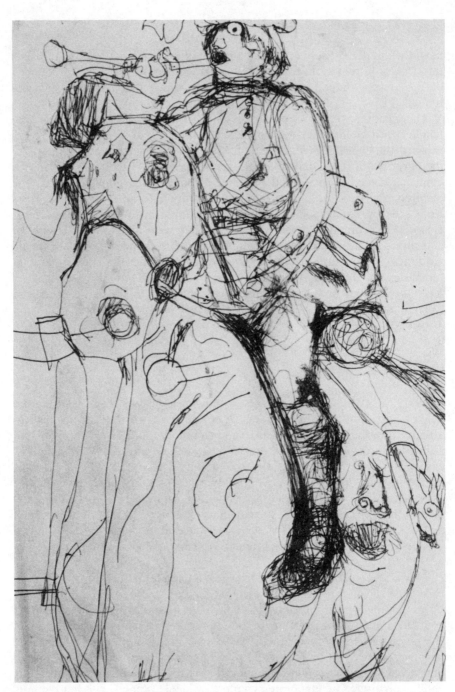

Figure 13.1. Nadia's celebrated "Horse and Rider," which was completed at 5 years of age, was drawn from memory. The rendering displays extraordinary precosity in draftsmanship, yet retains an autistic edge. (From Selfe, 1977. Reprinted with permission of the author and Academic Press.)

its nostrils snorting, its muscular legs thundering against the turf. The line work conveys the animal's form and movement with a spectacular economy of means. As with most seasoned artists, Nadia would focus intensely upon one idiosyncratic apsect of her composition—in this case the leg of the rider is worked and reworked with the same perseveration and compulsion evident in the work of Jason, the deaf and blind child.

Consistent with much of the art produced by the multiply handicapped, aspects of the child's symptomatology surface throughout the imagery. In contrast to the vitality depicted in the horse, the rider is rendered as a puppet-like figure, sitting rigid and bug-eyed as he toots his tiny horn. Draped from the saddle, like so much baggage, are a grotesque human head and the body of a rabbit. These are disturbing images that constitute the autistic artist's statement of who she is and about her mode of being in the world. Whether the autistic content of these works constitutes such a pathological element that it negates the artistic viability remains a question that will be addressed later in the discussion.

Another instance of artistic exceptionality is the case of Richard Wawro, who gained notoriety in Laurence Becker's documentary film entitled *With Eyes Wide Open* (1982). This young man from Scotland is visually impaired, cognitively and communication handicapped, with behavioral mannerisms suggestive of secondary autism. Without formal instruction, Wawro has completed thousands of oil pastels, mostly of landscapes of domestic and exotic settings (Fig. 13.2). The work bears the indelible mark of a multiply handicapped (MH) gifted artist in his eccentric handling of the oil pastel medium. Countless layers are built upon each other, resulting in unusual color gradations, perspective, and atmospheric effects. The draftsmanship is not sophisticated as in the Nadia drawings, but possesses a naive charm in its crisp and airy images of rural life.

In 1978 Rawley Silver brought forth a case study of a severely commu-nication handicapped 14-year-old boy who displayed a wide range of self-stimulatory mannerisms. His work reveals another instance in which a pre-cise and sensitive use of line and form combines with an array of sensory and affective deficits to produce works of uncommon quality. His wooded landscapes drawn from imagination are hauntingly beautiful (Fig. 13.3). The trees are depicted in an endless cycle of growth, maturity, and decay. The compositional sense is fantastic, as some areas are left untouched, or, rather, left with an aching sense of void, while others are teeming with densely interconnected saplings, underbrush, stately trunks, and fallen branches. In the later works the imagery takes on an hallucinatory astuteness, where each twig, bud, and bark crease is depicted with almost frightening acuity.

In each of these cases we find a certain consistency of common pictorial elements. These elements may be utilized to aid in the identification and characterization of the gifted, multiply handicapped artist, so that working criteria can be established. By utilizing such criteria, the author sought to avoid stereotyping the art of the multiply handicapped on a presupposed or

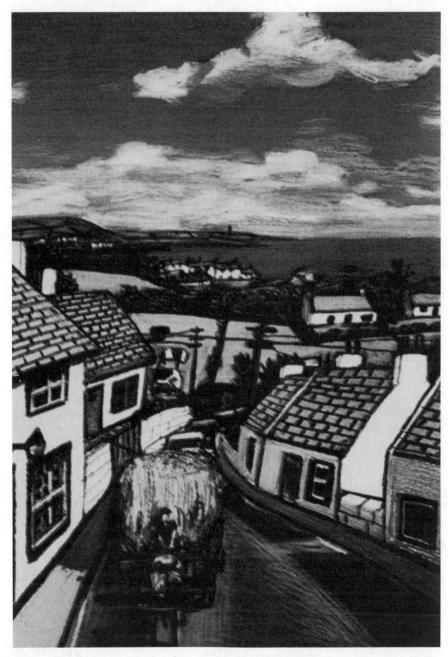

Figure 13.2. Richard Wawro's landscapes depend upon obsessive layering of oil crayon, which creates unusual depth and a strangeness of color. (Reprinted with permission of Laurence A. Becker.)

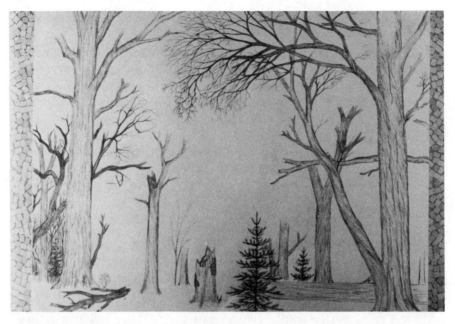

Figure 13.3. Charlie's pencil work sensitively captures the ebb and flow of nature's cycle of birth, growth, death, and rebirth. Its visual intensity and detailing speak of compelling affective issues that were worked through during the art process. (From Silver, 1978. Reprinted with permission of the author.)

judgmental basis. The thrust of this chapter is an attempt to recognize a school of art that is at once unique and worthy of serious appreciation and art criticism.

CLIENT ASSESSMENT

The study was undertaken between 1982 and 1987 at two educational facilities that provide service for clients with multiple handicaps. These included various combinations of mental retardation, communication disorders, sensory impairments such as blindness or deafness, and behavioral disturbances. A large percentage of the behavioral disturbances were aligned with congenital etiologies, particularly autism, rather than environmental, cultural, or social deprivation. The clients ranged from 9 to 21 years old, and all were participating in therapeutic, education, or recreational art programs at the time of screening.

The clients were assessed for artistic giftedness according to criteria that differ appreciably from those that are employed to assess giftedness within the normal population. The criteria were developed to reflect the clients' potential against the inhibiting factors posed by the severity of the handicapping condition. The criteria are:

1. Artworks that show a highly developed style or theme maintaining a degree of consistency and individuality.

2. Artworks whose content and style display a virtual absence of cultural, commercial media, or peer influence. This implies a high degree of individual originality and even eccentricity.

3. Artworks that display a precocious use of perspective(s) or drafting skill.

4. Artworks that are of the abstract mode, that are reminiscent of historically or critically accepted norms of art. These artworks should be highly developed stylistically and demonstrate sophisticated use of design elements.

5. Artworks in which objects or figures are rendered in an extraordinarily realistic way, with the inclusion of many details that elaborate the ideas.

Methodology

The criteria were applied to each of the individuals initially referred to the study and rated by the author and his assistants. These included several practicing artists, critics, and art therapists from the United States and Great Britain. It was established that three out of the five criteria would qualify the artist for gifted status. Criteria 1 and 2 were considered essential for qualification. At least one out of criteria 3, 4, and 5 were deemed necessary in order to qualify the artist as gifted. However, these three criteria were at times expanded or reworked in order to accommodate the more eccentric forms of artistic expression.

The criteria were applied in concert with a questionnaire that attempted to characterize the nature of the client's creative process. This creative process profile was adapted from a notation system authored by Laurie Wilson and used in New York University's art therapy program. The focus of this questionnaire centered upon the client's response to the medium, to the therapist, and to the group dynamics in his or her peer group. It recorded the preferences of medium, subject matter, manner of application, and use of materials. It characterized the client's affect during and after the work was completed, behavior during the art process with special emphasis upon self-stimulatory mannerisms, perseveration and obsessive or ritualized behavior. However the greatest focus is upon the art productions: the quality of line, form, and color. While actual diagnosis of pathology was avoided during this assessment, the fact that imagery displayed symptomatic elements was considered pertinent information, and this was meticulously recorded. Because most of these clients were nonverbal or communication disordered, little emphasis was placed upon verbal elaboration, except in instances where this material was volunteered.

TABLE 13.1. Clients Identified as Possessing Artistic Abilities at Institution A

Client	Age	IQ	Etiology	Criteria	Studio Focus
Male	16	34	Down's syndrome, hearing imparied	1,2,4	Figurative drawing, mono-chromatic, reminiscent of African totemic art
Male	21	30	Down's syndrome	1,2,4	Figurative works incorporating unarticulated geometric forms
Male	16	28	Down's Syndrome, congenital birth defects	1,3,4	Figurative works in drawings and paintings that are strongly reminiscent of abstract expressionism
Male	19	22	Anoxia, behaviorally disturbed	1,5	Draws weed pods, microscopic objects through a microscope, dandelion seeds with expert realism

Results

Institution A supplied a total of 87 clients, with 52 males and 35 females being screened for the criteria according to the research procedure. Of these numbers, 4 clients were identified as possessing artistic abilities (see Table 13.1), with another 3 being regarded as having the potential. The clients in this survey represented the lower end of the cognitive–behavioral functioning scale, with severe mental retardation being the predominant disability.

Institution B supplied a total of 36 multiply disabled clients with 12 males and 24 females. Each of these clients was hearing impaired and had two or more additionally complicating conditions. Of these clients, 4 were identified as being gifted (see Table 13.2), with 1 regarded as having potential. Once the population was identified, attention was turned to the aspects of exceptionality regarding the multiply handicapped artists' art productions and creative process. After the author had observed 20 to 60 studio sessions and

TABLE 13.2. Clients Identified as Gifted at Institution B

Client	Age	IQ	Etiology	Criteria	Studio Focus
Male	21	49	Hearing impaired, autistic	1,2,3,4	Draws mechanical objects from memory of imagination (see case example)
Male	21	53	Deaf, legally blind	1,3,5	Draws urban landscapes with multiperspectives (see case example)
Male	20	70	Hearing impaired, cerebral palsy	1,3,5	Draws realistically from life and imagination;
Male	10	40	Deaf, legally blind, autistic	1,2,3	Draws buildings in landscape settings

studied scores of artworks, the research was utilized to notate the client's behavior, affect, medium, thematic preferences, and interpersonal relations during the art-making sequences. After reviewing the art process notes, the 8 individuals outlined earlier were observed to possess striking similarities in their creative processes.

With a single exception, the mentally retarded and sensory impaired individuals displayed a highly focused, idiosyncratic quality with regard to their art techniques, styles, contents of the artwork, and behavior while engaged in the art process. As will be elucidated in the case examples, repetition and preservation emerged as a predominant element in both the imagery evoked and the choice or manner of use of the art medium. Perseveration of this kind remains a common behavioral trait among these populations. It should be noted, however, that the perseveration described in these instances constituted a highly evolved, aesthetically integral form of graphic expression based upon repetitive use of design elements.

Accompanying the perseverative aspects of the art process and artwork was a pronounced resistance to change, whether it be in response to psychotherapeutic intervention, art technique instruction, or attempts at expanding social interactions. Five of the 8 clients displayed a compelling need to maintain different degrees of ritualized behavior, routines, or environmental constancy during the studio session. Spontaneous interpersonal interactions were notably lacking in 3 of the 8 clients while engaged in the art process. These individuals displayed withdrawn or socially indifferent reactions to peers and only passively endured the interventions of staff. Of the 5 that related, 3 communicated through sign language, another was limited to friendly affect and gesture, with only 1 of the 8 being verbally articulate.

In effect, 6 of the 8 clients displayed the symptomatology associated with autism. This incidence of secondary autism surfaced both in the overt behaviors of the clients during their art making, in their interpersonal relations with staff and peers and in the artwork itself, as the following case presentations illustrate.

CASE EXAMPLES

Marcus

One can usually anticipate Marcus as he approaches the art studio. Out in the hallways he is making strange grunting sounds while tracing the outlines of the doorway and running his hand along the underside of the railings. He will also smell each of the objects touched, bringing each scent to his nose and lips in a ritual that virtually announces his arrival to the weekly art therapy sessions. Finally through the door, he pauses to check a loose toggle switch on the drill press, then rushes to the tool chest for an adjustable wrench to tighten down its locknut. I finally extricate him from his compulsive mechanical work and point him toward his flat file, where his sketch books and matted drawings are stored. He thumbs through the pencil drawings of transistors, halogen tubes, and other esoteric objects, as if to greet his friends after a long week's absence. Once acclimated, Marcus is ready to draw.

Marcus is 18 years old, hearing impaired, with a long history of psychiatric problems. It is hard to imagine his formative years on the wards, growing up in a psychiatric institution, not being able to hear, speak, or otherwise convey personal needs and concerns so basic to daily life. Marcus endured those years but in the process developed the highly ritualized and aggressive behaviors that provide a modicum of physical protection and emotional peace in the unfathomable world around him. His pugnacious temper did not serve him as well once he was transferred to a residential school for deaf children. Despite the caring and empathic ministrations of his teachers and counselors, Marcus remained an aggressive autisticlike child who had great difficulty adjusting to mainstream life outside of the psychiatric setting.

Marcus soon found sanctuary within the art studio where he was referred to individual art therapy sessions given his low verbal abilities and aversion to peers or groups of any kind. The time spent in art therapy allowed Marcus to relax his defenses within a sheltered yet stimulating art environment. Initially he remained suspicious and withdrawn, yet he eventually was lured from his shell by the tantalizing array of interesting props, tools, and media that were available for his exclusive use. Shelves of anatomical castings, crystals, minerals, pieces of driftwood, and a turtle skeleton were arranged for study on one sunlit shelf. Discarded clockworks, television debris, and gutted electrical motors were also around for tinkering and still-life sketching. Stacks of drawing paper, media, construction equipment, and solitary work enclaves were set up to encourage participation. Marcus became especially intrigued by the electrical junk and soon began to study and render these objects in pencil with increasingly intense concentration. While engaged in the drawing process he often let loose without warning a startling array of sound effects and hand mannerisms. These episodes seemed to act as a kind of safety valve, in which the buildup of tension or anxiety was dissipated in one wildly animated instant. In other instances, he appeared to be celebrating his artistic prowess with an exuberant display of affective expression. Regardless of its context, Marcus utilized the art process as a vital avenue of energy release, in a manner that was at once productive and appropriate in his school setting.

The initial drawings that emerged involved a bizarre series of cartoonlike depictions of stick figures being catapulted or somersaulted off various chutes, ladders, and rooftops (Fig. 13.4). These pictographs soon gave way to increasingly realistic depictions of film projectors and conveyer belt assemblies, with the stick figures rendered as unarticulated objects or disposable accessories to be manipulated or controlled by the machines. In later works, these schematic figures were omitted altogether as the electronic gadgetry emerged as the all-pervasive subject matter. Marcus was to perseverate upon

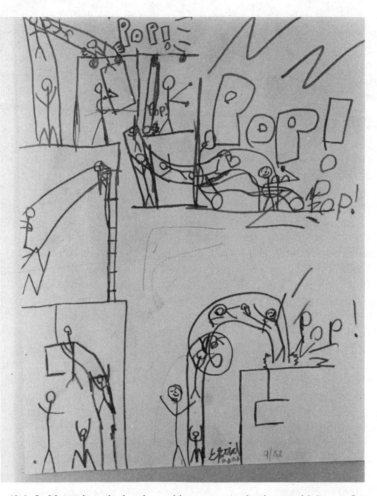

Figure 13.4. In Marcus's early drawings, objects were predominant, with human figures being relegated to incidental schemas who seem to be activated by the ubiquitous machinery.

mechanical objects drawn from imagination, memory, or life for the next 2 years of art involvement. He would not deviate from using his own personal #2 pencil, which he mercilessly ground to a nub in search of an acceptable point. Usually he would sit motionless for up to 10 minutes, then begin to sketch his ideas in the air above the paper, then gradually make contact with the paper ever so slightly. Finally, his line work would be heavily drawn in thick black pencil lines that overpowered the preliminary sketching.

As Marcus developed in his eccentric style of drawing, it became apparent that his work was moving beyond mere expressions of autistic symptomatology toward a viable, albeit idiosyncratic, kind of artistic giftedness. Meticulously rendered images of machine components, wiring schematics, and

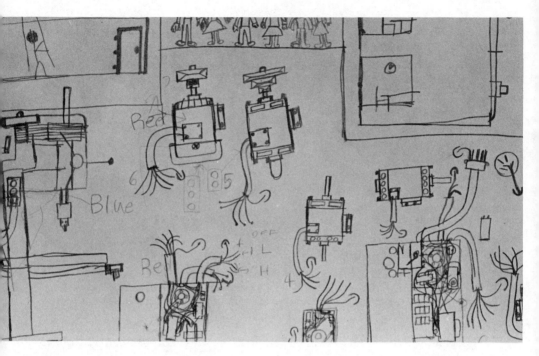

Figure 13.5. Marcus's mature machine-oriented drawings were drawn from imagination, memory, and life in a rigid, compartmentalized format.

household appliances soon overflowed from his sketchbooks. He arranged his pictorial fields in strange gridlike compostions, with certain forms remaining compartmentalized while others spilled off the page with total abandon (Fig. 13.5).

For an entire year, Marcus was allowed to pursue his art without being subjected to any art instruction, psychotherapeutic intervention, or any other form of staff expectation beyond maintaining appropriate studio conduct. Once Marcus displayed an adjustment to the studio regimen and became comfortable with my meddling, cautious interventions were implemented in order to promote both aesthetic and mental growth.

These interventions sought to address both psychodynamic, art educational, and developmental issues, in ways that were minimally provocative and anxiety producing. Issues such as the young man's preoccupation with inanimate machinery, his aversion to persons at school or at home, and his incessant ritualization and self-stimulations emerged as the salient problems to be addressed.

The main intervention sought to incorporate more animate, living imagery into the art productions. Since Marcus participated in a school horticulture program, I decided this would be an appropriate point from which to depart. Starting with seed propagation, we prepared topsoil, germinated bean seeds,

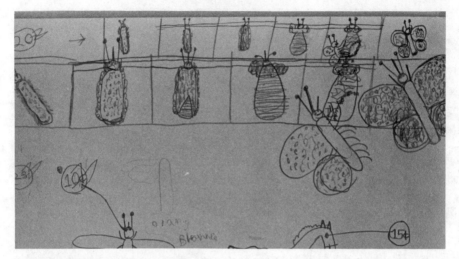

Figure 13.6. One of Marcus's breakthrough pieces was the metamorphosis of the butterfly. In this piece, inanimate machines gave way to living beings who are in the midst of profound change—a fitting metaphor for the intrapsychic changes occurring in the child during the course of the art therapy.

planted, watered, and over the weeks to come observed together the wonder of growing life.

While Marcus participated enthusiastically in this horticultural activity, the author made little effort to integrate it into his art process. It remained a purely adjunct activity, until the child demonstrated the capacity to assimilate this new theme into the image making. One did not have to wait long for Marcus to make use of this motivational intervention. Without prompting, he spontaneously cut and sectioned off a 4-by-12-inch piece of paper and began to depict the plant's entire growth sequence with stunning detail. Only several months after the initial horticultural project, Marcus was creating new and increasingly varied growth sequences. One depicted the metamorphosis of a caterpillar evolving through stages until a butterfly emerged from a cocoon (Fig. 13.6).

Eventually, Marcus would draw both animate and inanimate forms spontaneously, yet he never portrayed the human figure on an equally articulated level. His life drawings retain a mechanical, robotic quality, or they regress completely to faceless ciphers and stick figures. In his final studio sessions, Marcus astounded me by suggesting that he draw a self-portrait posed in a graduation cap and gown. This marked the only instance in 3 years where Marcus rendered the human figure without some level of prompting or suggestion. He was provided with a mirror, yet it was discarded in favor of utilizing a haptic approach to studying his body. Marcus literally *felt* each of his limbs, trunk, and face as he painstakingly concentrated upon each facet of his figure. The finished portrait is a fully articulated study that powerfully and graphically reflects the artist's struggle as he recorded the unfamiliar features of his own body (Fig. 13.7). It successfully terminated

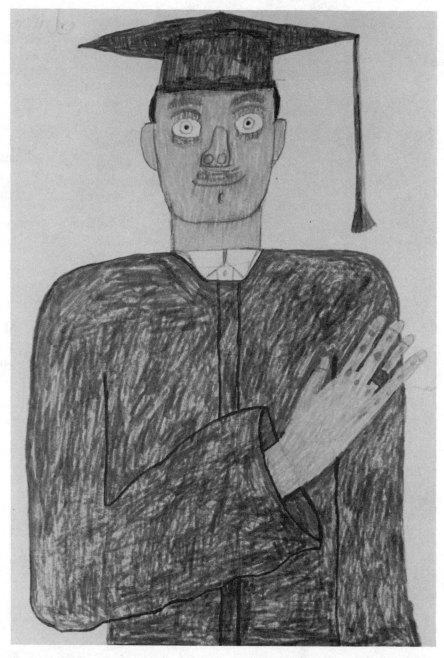

Figure 13.7. This culminating self-portrait was created as part of the termination process. Marcus literally carried the picture with him during his graduation ceremony as a kind of "diploma."

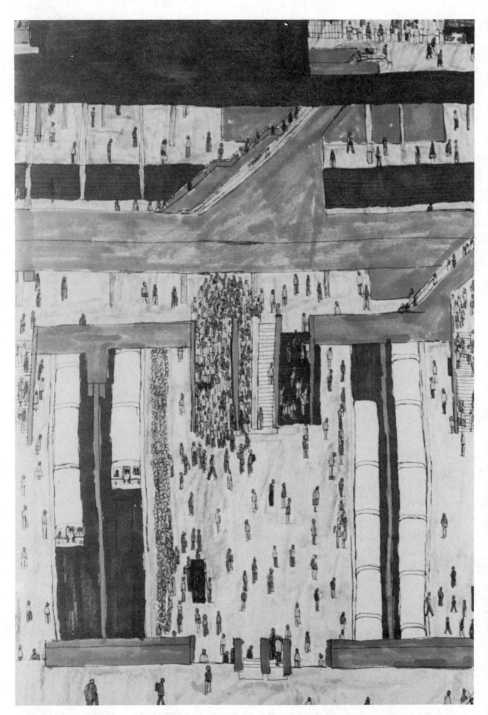

Figure 13.8. Sean's vistas were created with little planning or sketching. They emerged during a frantic spontaneous process that was punctuated by intensive self-stimulation and gesturing.

the 3-year journey from bizarre pictographic images, through the drafts-manship of the mechanical stages, toward the final phase where the growth processes assumed vital importance in the art and life of this multiply hand-icapped young artist.

SEAN

Figure 13.8 depicts a view from some distant observation point, high up in New York City's Port Authority Bus Terminal. This cavernous crossroads of the metropolitan area is rendered with dramatic perspective and an almost awe-inspiring sense of scale. On the uppermost level commuters are seen emerging from escalators, some of which disappear through turnstiles that lead to the bus gates. Mid-level, pedestrians climb the stairs, mill about in waiting rooms, or stand strangely alone as if lost or disoriented. Under the maze of walls, corridors, and utility tunnels, the subway trains arrive at their platforms that are packed with waiting strangers. Hundreds of other people walk about briskly as New Yorkers or travelers are apt to do, toting their shopping bundles and other baggage toward Times Square and beyond. In one far corner, an isolated silhouette leans against a girder reading the paper, dwarfed by the massive forms of concrete and steel.

The creator of this urban panorama is a 19-year-old man who is congen-itally deaf and legally blind. His functional vision is difficult to gauge since he has only one eye (the other being a porcelain prosthesis) and needs the magnification of a thick corrective lens. Despite the severity of his sensory handicaps and moderate mental retardation, Sean is somehow able to in-corporate visually the vast landscapes that appear in Figures 13.8, 13.9, and 13.10.

Working from memory and life, Sean displays near photographic retention as he renders the visual images with uncanny accuracy. Besides retracing his mental image of the scene, Sean will freely improvise, adding objects of his imagination to the composition that contribute to a highly individualized view of inner-city life. Sean's manner of working is no less eccentric. He begins by choosing a variety of wide-point and fine-point felt markers, which he alternates depending upon the scale of the scene. Then without observable planning or deliberation, he boldly draws a flourish of horizontal, diagonal, or vertical lines intermixed with details that seem completely out of context. The expected method of laying out the major forms and the gradual buildup of detail within an organized framework are not seen. Lines, forms, and minute figures spread diagonally across the paper, giving little indication of what the artist has in mind. Eventually, the viewer can begin to make out the enormous shapes that comprise office buildings or housing projects that are drawn without the benefit of either straight-edge or T-square. Sean's robust, kinesthetic style of drawing offers a striking contrast to the persev-erative qualities of the artwork.

Sean's element of perseveration is carried through in the limited themes

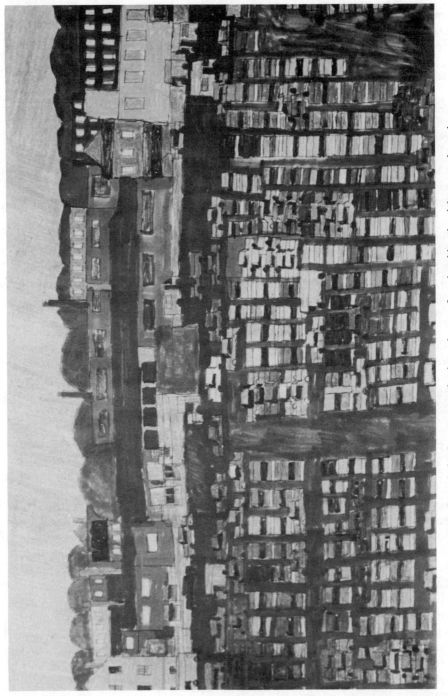

Figure 13.9. Sean derived enormous vicarious pleasure from invoking the sights, sounds, and actions of the inner city.

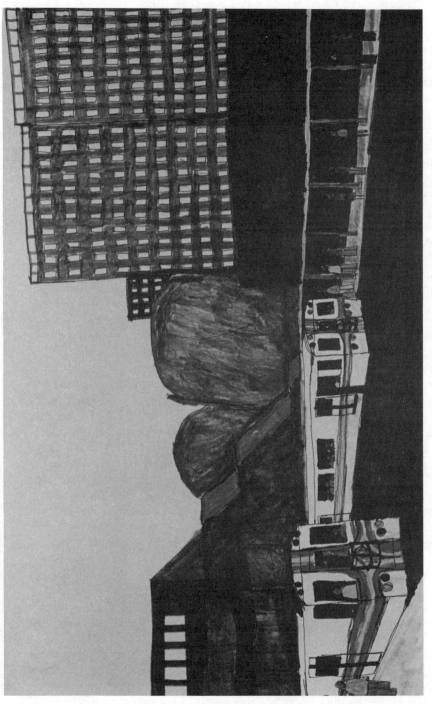

Figure 13.10. Sean did countless studies of housing projects. The hundreds of windows were drawn without the use of a T-square or straight-edge and impart an obsessive and abstract quality that breaks up the enormous mass of the buildings.

257

and medium usage that characterize his work. Yet the stereotypical trains, buses, crowds, and street scenes are animated in exciting concert. Sean condenses this vision of urban life without resorting to hyperrealistic detail. Instead, the myriad of color, form, and rhythm is orchestrated so that the essence of the scene emerges. The result is a rich and varied tapestry of considerable complexity, which retains the naïveté indicative of a self-taught, multiply handicapped artist.

One of Sean's preferred themes is the housing projects, where hundreds of windows are depicted without the use of a ruler. Sometimes 15 to 20 across, these windows act as a fascinating design element that provides the viewer with glimpses of the worlds behind the buildings walls. In some instances an arm can be made out watering a plant, or a torn curtain waves in a breeze. One depicts a portion of a policeman at his desk; in another, one can identify an IV bottle at the bed of a hospital patient, all rendered within an area less than 1/4 of an inch square.

After one views a series of these works, the elements of design begin to take on an abstract quality. They are effective in this stylistic sense, because Sean naturally breaks up the pieces with intersecting and rhythmic lines and forms. Wide expanses of color traverse the field while pockets of detail play out a range of fascinating vignettes. Colors playfully interact with bands and blocks of solid hues that create rich contrasts to the intricacies of the figure's clothing, minute advertisements, and other fine details. The rendering of space does not adhere to the conventional rules of perspective; its multi-dimensional views constitute a viable design device that shares a long tradition in eastern and post-modernist circles. In all, the art productions work not only because of their unusual compositional treatment, but also because of the freshness of the artistic vision and a personal sense of wit and charm.

Sean's creative process is accompanied by self-stimulatory mannerisms that include a range of sound effects and bizarre head movements. As in the case of Jason, one can observe these behaviors becoming more frequent and intensifying as the piece progresses and takes on shape. In these instances, this behavior appears as a celebratory display of the intense pleasure provided by the art experience.

Because these mannerisms remained benign displays that were not associated with other more seriously disturbed behaviors, I did not address them as issues that warranted therapeutic intervention. But Sean did encounter some problems initially that inhibited him from exploiting his full potential. In the first studio sessions, Sean insisted on completing each piece in one sitting and would resist storing a work in progress until the following week. The result was an increase in careless drawing that bordered upon scribbling and the advent of agitated behavior as the 1-hour sessions drew to a close. This situation had an adverse effect upon both the outcome of the artwork and the emotional well-being of the client. Thus I implemented what was to be the only major intervention in the art therapy treatment of this individual.

It was thought that Sean was responding adversely to a defective sense of object constancy. Once the cherished artwork was removed from his supervision, he assumed, as many visually impaired and multiply handicapped individuals do, that the piece was given over to unknown forces. Once the work in progress was surrendered, he essentially had lost control over its destiny, allowing for potential damage, theft, or other forms of object annihilation to occur. He therefore guarded each piece when finished, carefully supervising its matting or display.

To address this issue, I sought to provide Sean with a secure facility to store his artwork where he could maintain unfinished works with a sense of preservation. Sean also was provided with a designer set of markers that were contained within this flat file, assuring him that he would find his yellows unsoiled and the tips uncrushed from careless student use. Over a period of several months, these arrangements were assimilated into Sean's routines and became part of the highly structured regimen that allowed him to work with less stress and anxiety.

With the decrease of agitation and anxiety Sean was better able to concentrate upon developing his artistic style. He soon began to experiment with large-scale drawing, often working on murals that incorporated whole city blocks. He also began to use paint when appropriate with his drawings. Expansive areas of sky, water, and open land were better rendered with acrylic or tempera than the omnipresent markers, which posed both logistic and aesthetic limitations.

Additionally, the vista format of incorporating vast pictorial fields eventually gave way to a zoom lens effect. Subjects were being investigated at closer range, as in Figure 13.11, where pedestrians and commuters are seen descending stairwells and passing by newsstands.

Observing this young man as he pores over the work, his intact eye only an inch away from the paper, one realizes that an extraordinary process is taking place. The fact that he is able to give such intricate form to his artistic vision in light of the severity of his sensory and cognitive deficits is truly remarkable. The perseveration and naïveté invested in the artwork in no way detract from its richness and aesthetic value, but, on the contrary, endow it with an endearing eccentricity that many established artists would be hard pressed to approximate.

DISCUSSION

The artwork that has emerged in this study provides us with a highly vivid, thought-provoking profile of gifted multiply handicapped artists. We have seen that, despite their extensive sensory impairments, cognitive deficits, and behavioral idiosyncrasies, these individuals share many of the attributes that characterize seasoned, practicing artists. They are endowed with the single-minded intensity that allows for complete concentration and high pro-

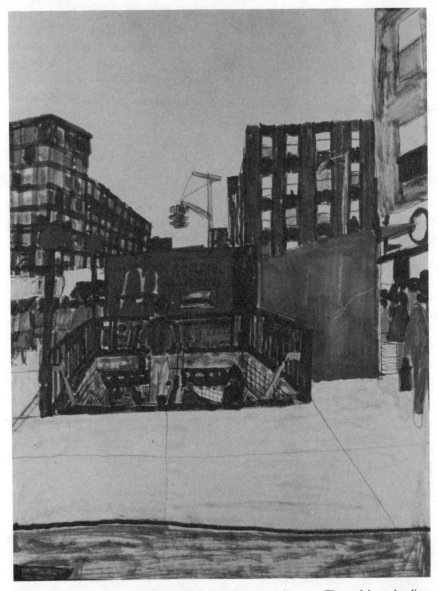

Figure 13.11. Sean's later works tended to focus upon street vignettes. They celebrated ordinary occurrences that were caught and transformed by the astute observations of a special artist.

ductivity. They utilize a complex system of design devices that contribute to the originality of their artistic vision. They are astute observers and somehow retain visual information with remarkable accuracy. Lastly, they are endowed with a colorful and innocent eccentricity that remains uncontaminated by the cult and the sensational that are so pervasive in the modern art scene. The nature of this eccentricity is a result of the complex interplay between their congenital handicaps and the environment in which they attempt to function. With these issues in mind, we can begin to expand and contrast these attributes with the art and art process of the normally functioning artist.

It was evident that virtually all of our gifted multiply handicapped artists displayed intensive, self-directed motivation that bordered upon an all-consuming obsession to create their art. They worked oblivious to academic performance or social protocol and dispensed with most other obligations that are ordinarily imposed upon a student in the process of making art. In several cases, their compulsion to create suggested almost pathological levels of impulsivity, perseveration, and an autisticlike withdrawal while engaged in their art process. From a developmental viewpoint, all of these artists demonstrated an intense thirst for sensory stimulation and an unusual degree of identification or incorporation with their subject matter. Edith Kramer has commented that their very impulsivity and perseveration seemed to lend an enormous energy to their artwork, enough that their sense of self and their art were virtually indistinguishable (1975).

Indeed, these were not the art processes of casual participants, but the urgent workings of self-absorbed, high-powered artists whose investments of emotion and energy suggest there was more at stake than creating a mere picture. In their spontaneous, deft handling of the medium and their unconcern for rational deliberation or extensive planning, they remind me of the calligraphic artists of medieval Japan. These monks and literati approached their silk and rice paper with absolute decisiveness and an astute intuitive approach to their medium. Little emphasis was placed upon premediation or societal norms by these Zen painters; rather their goal, after years of self-discipline and training, was to free up their hand and eye, to work their dazzling feats unencumbered by the limitations posed by overintellectualization.

While it may seem ludicrous to compare the incapacitated and retarded multiply handicapped individual with the artisitically revered, spiritually advanced Zen monk, commonalities nevertheless exist. The spiritual and artistic training undergone by the Zen painters of sixteenth century Japan aimed to approximate the same state of thoughtless innocence that is the hallmark of our multiply handicapped gifted artists. After years of rigorous study they forced themselves to renounce such teachings, suppressing the expectation to follow the conventions of Oriental design, in favor of painting in the same kinesthetic, furiously robust manner found in our MH artists. In their emphasis upon creating in meditative, reclusive environments they can be similarly compared to both MH artists and modern artists. What we may clinically denote as being withdrawn, obsessive, or autisticlike, parallels the self-imposed isolation and sense of preoccupation that are so predominant in many normal-functioning artists during their creative process.

Another inference that we can draw concerns the manner in which the MH artists' work evolves as compared to that of the normal artist. In 5 of our 8 cases, the MH indivdiual's growth in regard to stylistic sophistication was predicated upon producing work in series. These distinctly different but interrelated groups of works employed similar media, thematic content, scale, and technique. Each element was repeated for as long as the artist deemed necessary, until it slowly evolved into a new experimental design. The artist may have created works in series in order to solve a personal design problem, work through an impulse, or develop an area of interest to its fullest conclusion.

Regardless of context, our 5 MH artisits reconvened their motifs until they focused upon one element within these works, then utilized this element as a point of departure for developing new works and subsequently new series. This is a sophisticated and effective manner of prompting artistic growth, and not, as some clinicians may suggest, an extension of purely perseverative behavior. For within the works of these 5 individuals is an upwardly spiraling movement, where works are developed, resolved, reach a point of saturation, then splinter off into related but discernibly novel directions. For example, our Down's syndrome young man created scores of geometric figures by utilizing simple squares, cones, circles, and rectangles as graphic building blocks to form schemas. Each figure contained a slightly new and varied combination of forms and emphasis. In one set of drawings the predominant composition would be circular and cone like; in the next it would be multiples of rectangles; in another just squares would be utilized.

While none of these robotic figures ever portrayed movement, there was a fascinating internal rhythmic movement that pervaded each deceptively simple figure.

Our MH artists additionally displayed extraordinary sensorial acuity in spite of the sensory deficits in evidence. This sense of spatial ability has been studied in both normal and retarded artistic populations, most notably by Gardner (1983). Gardner has designated spatial ability as a type of intelligence whereby the individual is somehow endowed with the capacity to incorporate visually and internalize imagery deemed pertinent in his or her environment. In this category would be visual stimuli that for some reason are interesting, attractive, useful, or even compelling to the individual. These images are selected from among other elements in the environment and committed to visual memory, then subsequently put to graphic use.

Spatial acuity has been documented anecdotally in writings or interviews with mature artists such as Picasso, Van Gogh, Rodin, and countless others, who report powerful and vivid experiences of visualization. This faculty seems to be equally or extraordinarily shared by 4 of our 8 MH artists, as they drew their highly elaborated and realistically correct images from memory (and to a lesser extent, imagination). Writers such as Rayala (1981) have explored the possibility that such remarkable visual memory employs the phenomenon of eidetic imagery, whereby certain mental images remain projected in the mind's eye for extended periods, thereby remaining accessible for the artist to draw upon. This theory is certainly an attractive one, but it cannot explain satisfactorily how each of our MH individuals adds, subtracts, and otherwise improvises upon his or her themes. One example concerns the case of Sean, who was commissioned to draw the skyline of Trenton, New Jersey. Sean was driven past the city's skyline several times, and was then taken back to the studio to begin work. The result was a realistically correct record of his impressions, with each building, landscape, and object rendered faithfully in realistic terms. Yet, eventually, to everyone's delight, he began to improvise, adding a group of joggers in one corner, a child on a skateboard, and a fishing boat making its way down the Delaware River.

The theory of eidetic imagery requires that the omnipresent mental image be transcribed in the most literal fashion, as if tracing an overhead projection of the image onto the paper. Not in any of the eight cases did this transcription occur—there were substantial elements of interpretation and spontaneity in each of these productions.

It has been well documented among deaf, blind, autistic, and mentally retarded individuals that incoming audiovisual stimuli may be processed with decided hypersensitivity. In other words, due to distortions or other aberrations of the sensory apparatus, the individual may experience the ticking of a clock as an insufferable din or the changing of a traffic light as a hallucinogenic light show. These distortions inevitably lead to the self-stimulatory mechanisms we witnessed in the opening passage—Jason pausing to rock his head to catch the reflections of sunlight. These phenomena are almost certainly in evidence with our MH artists during their art process and in response to their finished art products. In the case of Sean, it is reasonable to assume that he derives uncommon stimulation from such overpowering images of skyscrapers and the atriums of large buildings. For a relatively sheltered, almost blind individual, one can only speculate what effects the roar of a subway train or the view from the World Trade Center has on his distorted or hypersensitive perceptions. In his attempts to process these overwhelming stimuli, Sean may have been compelled to depict incessantly the salient features of other inner-city scenes; the monumental forms, the bustling movements, the montage of color, form, and texture. For such an immobile individual, this process may have constituted a vicarious experiencing of the freedoms that come with movement—freedoms that are ordinarily denied him by his disability and the protectiveness of his school and home environment. His art then becomes invested with a powerful element of wish fulfillment that was symbolically conveyed each time Sean reconvened the images in his art productions. Thus the creative process becomes an act of liberation, whereupon physical limitations are symbolically surmounted, and the concomitant feelings of isolation and powerlessness can yield to those of mastery and control. The issues of mastery and control emerged in symbolic terms throughout the art processes of MH individuals. Sean's preoccupation with inner-city life may have been as terrifying as it was tantalizing. Managing the onslaught of sensations and exercising a degree of control over the chaos of the urban street may have given rise to the gridlike, highly structured format evoked in his art. Marcus may have been similarly awed by the mysterious electrical forces that pervaded his art. The machines that harness such omnipotent power may have prompted an equally compelling need to invoke and symbolize such concerns as a means of managing such terrifying force. The case of Jason bears this out in a most graphic way. In keeping with his autistic symptomatology, Jason resisted drawing figures in his architectonic-dominated work. However, after 3 years of art-therapeutic intervention Jason began to render the figure in a most cautious and idiosyncratic manner. His figures strangely appear not as animate beings that freely interact with each other and the environment but as frozen pictures mounted to the wall or as faces whose images appear on the television set. By imprisoning these figures and by robbing them of their animation, Jason was able to effect a measure of control over those who populated his real-life and imaginary environments. He devised this most ingenious design so as to communicate his own vulnerability and reticence in the face of the perceived danger in an otherwise uncontrollable world.

All through the history of art, artists have been compelled to express highly personal symbolic images. They never cease to utilize design devices that graphically convey the breadth of their own concerns, those of their culture, and indeed, the existential predicament of the human condition. Thus the iconography that has emerged in these artworks remains a testament to the power of art, which has been conveyed with a special poignancy by our MH artists.

A final question regarding the art of this population: Does it fulfill the requirements of aesthetic integrity and should it therefore be awarded consideration as a truly viable form of high art? Despite the fact that our subjects dutifully met the author's criteria and for this chapter's purposes were given the distinction of being artistically gifted, there is no inference that their work will gain acceptance in the communities of art criticism and appreciation.

The reasons underlie a constant source of interdisciplinary debate among the mental health professions, educators, and artists themselves. It is the issue of symptomatology that seems to trouble the art criticism community most when attempting to assign such art its place in the aesthetic hierarchy. Does the presence of pathology within a given work of art or artist detract from its aesthetic value? Why is it acceptable for an artist such as Francis Bacon to depict dismembered, eviscerated, and otherwise distorted images as "high art" while an equally facile autistic artist is invalidated?

In recent years a group of artists, critics, and authors have argued for parity between the art of intact artists and the art of outsiders, those who are mentally ill, eccentric, primitive, or otherwise outside the cultural norm. Jean Dubuffet describes art brut as:

works executed by people untouched by artistic culture, works in which im-
itation—contrary to what occurs among intellectuals—has little or no part, so
that their makers derive everything (subjects, choice of materials used, means
of transposition, rhythms, ways of patterning, etc.) from their own resources
and not from the conventions of classic art or the art that happens to be
fashionable. Here we find art at its purest and crudest; we see it being wholly
reinvented at every stage of the operation by its maker, acting entirely on his
own. This, then, is art springing solely from its makers's knack of invention.
(1967, p.8)

Michel Thevoz writes of the aesthetic viability (1976, pp. 198–201) of the
art of the autistic as a sense of liberation from constraint, an upsurge of
innovation and resourcefulness, a breakthrough into unsuspected worlds that
make one think twice about the so-called "primitive" character of these
works, as the pontiffs of the constituted art forms would have us regard it.
Roger Cardinal (1979) has emerged as one of the few art critics who view
the artwork of Nadia and other outsider savants as being worthy of serious
aesthetic study and appreciation, despite the presence of mental retardation
and emotional disturbance.

In Cardinal's (1979) review of Selfe's (1977) book he writes of his aston-
ishment at Nadia's gifts: her superb draftsmanship, her dark humor, her
splendid composition. He sees the elements that convey agitation, flamboy-
ance, and grotesqueness not as deficits but as declarations of the fantastic.
Cardinal prizes Nadia's unkempt, unsupervised, and improvisatory qualities.
Like Dubuffet, Cardinal takes issue with terms like *beautiful* when describing
a work of art, preferring instead adjectives such as *intense* and *interesting*.

All of these writers would agree with Licht (1987) when he states that the
creators of art brut do not ask to be understood, nor do they beckon us to
follow them on their explorations. It is at our own risk that we look at these
works and ponder their importance. What we stand to gain is an extended
vision of the boundaries of art and greater freedom from convention (p. 28).

Yet other writers express reservations concerning the aesthetic merit of
autistic art or art brut. In recent conversations with Edith Kramer (personal
communication, 1987), she has maintained that culture remains a vital in-
gredient in order to "cook" the art product properly. Kramer has described
the art process as being essentially integrated with the influence of culture
combining with cognition, dexterity, and affective expression to create viable
art successfully. While Kramer appreciates the work of our multiply handicapped artists, she resolutely opposes Dubuffet's rejection of culture and
art historical influences, especially when applied to normally functioning
artists who embrace art brut. Kramer sees a need for suffusing art with social
meaning, so as to enrich and heal society's cultural ills. Thus it becomes an
almost moral responsibility for the artist to master his or her cultural alienation and to present a human's individuality as it persists within or in spite
of the modern environment. Those artists who choose to feign cultural naïveté or maintain a hostile stance toward their culture, Kramer asserts, are

in fact acquiescing to and feeding the very institutions they denounce. Kramer sees this as an eerie process whereby protestors are absorbed and digested by commercial galleries—their protests are thus transformed into marketable commodities (personal communication, 1986).

Other writers attack art brut and particularly the appreciation of the art of the retarded as succumbing to a naive romanticism. Pariser (1981) warns the viewer not to assume that "aesthetic effects always proceed from the aesthetic causes" (p. 27). In dismissing the work of Nadia as pseudo-art, Pariser points out that without a conceptual understanding of her subject matter, or without the capacity to internalize her representations, her renderings remain purely mechanical or perceptual–optical manifestations. Rayala (1981) counters by reminding Pariser that the fact that the individual has somehow suspended cognitive and conceptual modes of thought in favor of aesthetic pursuits does not demonstrate that the aesthetic involvement is a low-order human activity.

This is where the crux of the argument may lie. Despite the meticulousness of Lorna Selfe's investigation of Nadia's cognitive and perceptual abilities, little insight emerged concerning Nadia's internal world. If he or she remains incommunicado, the cognitive investigator is at a loss to appraise an individual's potential accurately. The nonverbal world of elective or congenital mutes cuts us off from sharing their thoughts, concerns, and perceptions.

CONCLUSIONS

Over the course of 2 years of researching and preparing this chapter, it became apparent that more questions would arise than answers would be found. The provocative nature of this subject extends beyond the practice of art therapy and enters the realms of aesthetics, art criticism, and art advocacy. In conclusion I hope to sort out these interrelationships while also exploring the issues of practical concern to the art therapist who endeavors to meet the complex needs of the MH artist.

One of the original questions posed in this research was where the art of exceptionally gifted autistic, retarded, and MH artists should rightly be placed, whether it be within the realm of fine art or even that of Dubuffet's art brut.

I feel that there is sufficient support for the argument that this art is a form of art brut and is indeed worthy of serious study and critical appreciation. The qualifying criteria established during the study's tenure (against which the MH individuals were rated) certainly conform to the model set forth by Dubuffet. In my view, the MH artists exemplify Dubuffet's required condition of autistic withdrawal and isolation, in which a state of near egolessness pervades both the artists and their art. These artists also share the outsider's obsession with using bizarre and incongruous design elements. These include the rendering of distorted, primitivistic figures, gridlike or rigid compositions, the use of words, symbols, or other pictographic elements. One distinction that can be raised is that the MH population comprised children and young adults, whose etiologies were primarily severe and complex congenital conditions. In contrast the art brut artists are a heterogeneous group of peasants, eccentrics, mystics, and psychiatric patients who possess limited awareness of culture or aesthetics. Because of the fundamental difference between the two populations, the MH group seems as yet unable to achieve the peculiar sophistication that is reached by the outsider adults. It is reasonable to suggest that the art of autistic savants and gifted retardates can be considered a precursor or immature form of art brut, with the factors of age, functioning level, and etiology inhibiting their full designation.

The question next arises as to whether awarding this designation does in fact create an association between the art of the MH and established fine art. Indeed placing this art under the rubric of art brut may prove to be a dubious distinction since many critics remain skeptical of its aesthetic worth. One can counter by reasserting that there are distinct similarities between the art processes of mature, intact artists and those of the MH artists. Throughout this chapter I drew close parallels between their powers of visualization, their intense concentration, and the nature of their artistic evolution. In regard to their art products, we find that there is a growing movement of international art connoisseurs that are exhibiting MH artwork beyond the hospital walls, in mainstream galleries in the art community. What is significant about these exhibits is that the curatorial emphasis has been upon the aesthetic merit, without the yoke of pathology such work usually wears. In Europe especially, there is increasing interest in handling the work of autistic and retarded artists. Several established galleries, such as the Kunstler Aus Stetten in Germany and the Art En Marge in Belgium, have successfully introduced this art to the public by mounting professional-quality exhibits and by publishing catalogs and portfolios of the exhibited works. Respected critics in Britain and France have also responded by writing catalog essays and media presentations that accompany the visual art displays (see MaClagen, 1987).

With this increase of exposure and public awareness have come improved opportunities for MH artists to work with quality media and techniques in proper studio environments. There are now efforts to remove the more adaptable artists from institutions and place them in ateliers, under sheltered conditions conducive to creating serious work.

Yet despite these heartening developments in art advocacy, the issue of aesthetics still remains unsettled. Although the promotion and orientation of the art-viewing public are crucial steps in fostering art appreciation, they can also serve to skirt the issue of aesthetic viability. For the public is continuously presented with shrewdly conceived and provocative art sensations that retain little staying power. Thus I become uneasy at the thought of using the acceptance and consumption habits of a fickle public to resolve so vital an issue.

To face this question squarely, we must first purge the notion of sympathy or advocacy when criticizing the handicapped or mentally ill artist. We must then return to the argument set forth by Kramer, who maintains that much outsider art is lacking in sufficient integration and evocative power to be considered true art. Kramer (1975) views artistic expression that is reliant upon stereotypic or pictographic representation as representing constricting mechanisms that are used in the service of defense (i.e., repression, identification with the aggressor). Therefore, work that remains oblivious to or resists the conventional bonds of communication cannot serve as an analogue for a broad range of human experiences. It is not until the artist succeeds in producing symbolic images that serve both *self-expression* and *communication* that fully formed art emerges.

One can argue still that this is a rather narrow definition of art, one that dismisses not only autistic art and art brut but much of post-modern neoexpressionism as well. However, I have found this line of thinking to have a direct bearing upon the argument at hand.

In studying MH art, I have found that most of the works had difficulty standing alone without the benefit of some reference to the artist and his or her history. Regardless of the graphic intensity achieved or the freshness of artistic vision, the works seem strangely incomplete, as if they were still in gestation. In some cases it is the artist's naive approach to technique that detracts from its aesthetic impact. (One only has to compare the primitivistic figures of an art brut or MH artist with the highly sophisticated primitivism of a Dubuffet to appreciate this point.) More often, there is a sense that the artist lacks the resources to grow or the freedom to change and expand through his or her art. For instance, if I were to respond to the cityscapes created by our deaf and blind artist without reference to his background, I could find his work interesting in its idiosyncratic charm and its freshness of vision. However, there is pronounced stereotypy and obsession—there is little relaxed movement, and because of its rigidity it generates little excitement for the eye. The same holds true for Marcus, whose rigidly compartmentalized images are more like bizarre, internal blueprints or a form of graphic discourse with the self. This is graphically evident in Nadia's case; her extraordinary drawing gifts are weakened by the absence of a context or concept within the work. Her renderings of horses and roosters are exquisite indeed, especially when viewed in the original, yet they fall short of being art since the figures seem to languish in a blank void or emerge out of a confused scribble.

These impressions can be revised, however, once the work is put into proper perspective. Viewed in the context of their maker they do "provide a glimpse into a world beyond our logic and our physical experience and thus allow us to commune briefly with those forces that are astir in all of us but to which we dare not respond" (Licht, 1987, p. 28). This is especially true in Nadia's case, due to the mysterious transient nature of her gifts, which makes such a glimpse all the more precious. Yet as exciting as this glimpse is, I feel strongly that our enlightenment and appreciation of these works are predicated upon comprehending the circumstances that brought the work into being. Perhaps I am suggesting that they work best as a kind of "conceptual art," narrative elements combined with the visual art, ideally, with videotapes that allow us a full experience of the artist's process. On the other hand, art therapists must guard against becoming preoccupied with the "amazing story" beind the artwork. By allowing the sensational elements to take hold of our thinking, we may end up embellishing a case history only to compensate for empty or meager artistic quality.

It is reasonable then to conclude that the truly gifted MH artist will strike a firm balance in which the sensational aspects of the case history and the extraordinary art products exert an equally compelling influence. With the integration of both case history and art comes a broadened viewing, one that begins to comply with Kramer's requirements for fully "formed" aesthetic experience.

The last points that I wish to take up are directed toward the problem of ethics and the practice of art therapy as applied to this population.

In his review of *Nadia,* Nigel Dennis (1977) attacked Lorna Selfe and the other staff psychologists as having victimized rather than helped her. Since the child rarely again spontaneously drew in her grand style after the age of 6, he charged that their testing and training program interfered with Nadia's creative development. Dennis argues that the cognitively oriented attempts at teaching the child to relate, verbalize, and function at a more "trainable" level hindered the preservation of her one admirable characteristic. This, Dennis maintained, irreparably destroyed her "priceless gift in order to create an average state of subnormality" (p. 15). Pariser defends Selfe by maintaining that Nadia's treatment was in her best interests and that we must approach all autistic children by assuming that they are unhappy in their isolation, even if it means sacrificing their extraordinary artistic gifts. We can agree with Pariser to the extent that Selfe's intentions were nothing less than professionally ethical and her investigation exhaustively thorough. It would be naive to subscribe to the romantic notion that the multiply handicapped or autistic individual should be left to his or her own devices in a world of sensory deprivation and distortion. As therapists and educators, it is our responsibility to counteract the effects of developmental arrest and attempt to advance autonomous functioning to the furthest degree possible. Yet Dennis raises a significant and disturbing point for the research and practicing art therapist to ponder.

I feel that the problem is soluble, however, if we look to the child and his or her emotional and cognitive needs for guidance; for each individual case will dictate special interventions. For instance, in my work with Sean, there was little reason to interfere with his behavior and the nature of his art productions, since they functioned adaptively for a deaf and blind individual. His self-stimulations were not autistic in the sense that he was shutting out stimuli, but rather, they were due to hypersensory stimulation and distortion. His need for routine was an understandable requirement for him as a visually impaired person, and his adherence to a limited subject matter constituted a legitimate interest that was not solely a matter of neurotic perseveration. Therefore very few interventions aimed to modify either his behavior or his artistic style. However, in Marcus's case, his compulsiveness to render purely inanimate objects was a symptom of autistic withdrawal. Thus therapeutic interventions were implemented that encouraged him to explore and cautiously confront those issues that arose in his day-to-day interactions and in his art. In this case, art-therapeutic interventions had a positive impact upon his emotional life without compromising his skill and joy at rendering his favored mechanical objects.

In Nadia's case it is still a matter of speculation as to what circumstances led to her loss of drawing prowess. Several reviewers pointed to the increased emphasis upon speech therapy that caused Nadia to shift her attention away from drawing. Others felt that Nadia drew solely for those special people in her life, and with their loss her desire to create diminished. In any case, we are certain that Nadia was never worked with by an art therapist who given the opportunity, could have fostered her artistic ability while also promoting social, cognitive, and communication development. Without the benefit of art-therapeutic interventions, little emphasis was placed upon developing pictorial organization or conceptualization in her work. No one intervened to give Nadia a context for her drawings such as a Lowenfeld Motivation would serve to accomplish, nor were there attempts to expand her visual vocabulary over a sustained period of time. More importantly, Nadia was not supported by an art therapist during the gradual but dramatic artistic regression that marked such a turning point in her artistic career—for this was not Lorna Selfe's profession or mission.

In our work with these clients, art therapists begin by fostering any strength in evidence by cautious and sensitive interventions that cause minimum client anxiety or stress. Although art therapy and the art experience should be a growth process, these interventions must respect the client's resistance to change, for it is an indication of vulnerability and confusion over expectations that the client may not fully comprehend.

We may next concentrate upon providing a stable yet sensorially stimulating environment where the timid client is encouraged to explore, solve problems, and take creative risks without resorting to stultifying defenses (Kramer, 1971). The art therapist can assist in this process by providing a model with which the MH client can identify, incorporating appropriate behaviors and artistic skills into his or her own creative and behavioral repertoire. By remaining calm, firm, and consistent in the face of bizarre or other acting-out behaviors, we communicate our commitment to assist the multiply handicapped individual to make positive and productive changes in the art studio. The art process can then be promoted as a serious educational and therapeutic activity that engages and challenges the multifaceted faculties of the MH individual. Ultimately, the goal is to open channels for the sublimation of the client's ideas, concerns, and issues that may otherwise remain indefinitely inaccessible.

Finally, the growing interest in the art of the multiply handicapped and other outsider artists has given rise to the concern for protecting the vulnerable client amidst increased public exposure. Because this is extraordinary, even sensational, material, there are inherent dangers in regard to promotion and research in accordance with our ethical obligations.

From a promotional standpoint, it is true that the art therapist is in an ideal position to recognize and introduce this art to the art-viewing public. While in some cases this exposure can foster a positive and welcome boost to the client's self-esteem, I think it wise that the art therapist extricate himself or herself from an advocacy role. In working with several of these clients I have found myself in the uneasy role of promoter, and sometimes even "agent," making it ethically problematic to maintain a conflict-free sphere as a therapist.

Because of the sheer diversity of promotional and advocacy issues, the situation demands that there be appointed trustees who can relieve the art therapist of these extended duties by administering affairs that remain outside the therapeutic sphere. For instance, an autistic child artist in Great Britain received more than 700 requests for original drawings after he was featured in a BBC documentary. To cope with this tidal wave of public acclaim, a management team was appointed that included a publisher to satisfy the demand for art prints, an attorney for copyright and other legal concerns, a financial advisor who worked out a trust foundation, and an agent to handle the exhibition and sale of the artwork, all of whom volunteered their services on a strictly noncommission basis. While a staff of this sort seems cumbersome and almost ludicrous in light of the fact that the child remains oblivious to all the commotion, he and his family were effectively shielded and spared from exploitation. The art therapist also benefits in that he or she can remain concerned solely with the client's creative and emotional well-being.

However, the art therapist who researches this or any population may still be ethically at risk, in that we may inadvertently exploit the client by reducing him or her to a clinical subject or object of our professional attention. In keeping with the art therapist's humanistic ideals, I feel that our research must not be based solely upon satisfying professional curiosity, but should also attempt to contribute something to the client's welfare. For instance, the 3 days that I spent making art with Nadia could have been construed as a self-serving intrusion unless there was demonstrated a genuine concern for her well-being. In this case, I attempted to compensate Nadia and her family for my visit by devising strategies that helped the family cope with inappropriate behaviors and helping structure leisure time by reawakening her drive to make art. By maintaining a balance between conducting empirical research and offering therapeutic support, the art therapist can gain insights into this extraordinary population in a way that is beneficial for all.

REFERENCES

Arnheim, R. (1980). The puzzle of Nadia's drawings. *Arts and Psychotherapy, 7,* 75-85.

Becker, L. (1982). *With eyes wide open.* Documentary film.

Cardinal, R. (1972). *Outsider art.* New York: Praeger.

Cardinal, R. (1979). Drawing without words. *Comparison, 10,* 3–21.

Dennis, N. (1978). Portrait of the artist. *New York Review of Books, 25,* 8–15.

Dubuffet, J. (1967). *L'art brut.* Paris: Gallimard.

Gardner, H. (1983). *Frames of mind.* New York: Basic.

Itard, M. (1962). *Wild boy of Aveyron.* New York: Century.

Kramer, E. (1971). *Art as therapy with children.* New York: Schocken.

Kramer, E. (1975). Art and Emptiness. In E. Ulman (Ed.), *Art Therapy—Theory and Practice.* New York: Schocken.

Licht, F. (1987). *Beyond the reach of critics?* From Jean Debuffet and Art Brut, Catalog Essay of Peggy Guggenheim Collection. New York: Guggenheim Foundation.

MaClagan, D. (1987). *From the outside in.* Catalog Essay "In Another World." London: Art House, South Bank Centre.

Pariser, D. (1981). Nadia's drawings. *Studies in Art Education, 22*(2), 20–29.

Rayala, M. (1981). On Nadia's drawings. *Studies in Art Education, 22*(2), 70–71.

Selfe, L. (1977). *Nadia.* New York: Academic.

Silver, R. (1978). *Developing cognitive and creative skills through art.* Baltimore: University Park Press.

Thevoz, M. (1976). *Art brut.* New York: Rizzoli.

Winner, E. (1986, August). How kids draw. *Psychology Today,* pp. 20–29.

PART 2

New Methods

HARRIET WADESON

The essence of art is creativity. Less obviously, the essence of psycho-therapy also entails creativity as therapists help individuals to develop more satisfying ways of living. Therefore, it follows that art therapists are likely to be very creative people working in a most creative modality.

This creativity is applied to art and work with individual clients, and in addition, to innovative ways art making can be applied to the enterprise of enhancing human functioning. As a creative modality in and of itself, tra-ditional art therapy offers a foundation for seemingly endless creativity in ways that can be built upon, modified, combined, refined, and applied.

This section of the book provides examples of some of art therapy's innovative methods. It is important to bear in mind, however, that the ac-tivities of art therapy are not a mere bag of tricks nor a dazzling array of gimmicks. New methods grow out of new needs and possibilities. They are never an end in themselves, but always a means to achieve a larger end in the realm of human functioning.

The new methods described in the following chapters are of two kinds: those in which art expression is combined with other modalities, such as computer animation, photography, or psychodrama, and those in which art therapy techniques are delineated or developed for specific purposes, such as initial engagement with children or cutting through superficial expression among depressed patients. Undergirding most of this work are new ways of thinking about art therapy.

Although art therapy's roots reach back to prehistoric cave paintings, we reach forward as well, embracing the high-tech possibilities of the late twen-tieth century. Jerry L. Fryrear and Irene E. Corbit have utilized electronic high technology to create new possibilities of self-confrontation by combin-ing Polaroid® portrait making and video with art and movement. In their chapter "Visual Transitions: Metaphor for Change" they detail how they have adapted procedures for work with children, groups, and families and have applied them to many problem-solving areas.

As it has in so many areas of our lives, the computer has entered art therapy as well. Devorah Samet Canter describes her work with youngsters in creating computer animation to expand expression of fantasy in her chapter "Art Therapy and Computers."

Another combination is described by Jean Peterson with Leigh Files in a view of group therapy possibilities from a psychodramatic perspective that unites the ancient uses of art and drama for healing rituals in the chapter "The Marriage of Art Therapy and Psychodrama." The authors not only suggest a variety of techniques for encouraging spontaneity, reflection, and group connectedness, but also provide a framework for the conceptualization of the healing processes of art and enactment.

Lenore Steinhardt also offers us a new perspective in her chapter "Six Starting Points in Art Therapy with Children." Although the techniques she describes in working with children are not new, she focuses on the crucial task of initial engagement with the child. After noting the child's approach to the art therapy session and his or her internal organization, Steinhardt selects an art engagement activity best suited to the particular child. The six techniques fall along a continuum of children's responses, from enthusiastic engagement with independence and responsibility to detachment and resistance.

In her work with depressed patients, Susan Buchalter-Katz found that her patients responded to art in a pleasant stereotypic manner, avoiding their more painful feelings. In order to enable them to move toward positive change, she developed a more directive approach and found "barrier" drawings a useful vehicle for self-confrontation and sharing among depressed patients. Her chapter, "'Barrier' Drawings for Depressed Patients" describes the evolution of this technique and a comparison of spontaneous drawings and "barrier" drawings.

These chapters describe new ways of working and new techniques that other art therapists may wish to try. But even more, they give us a view of each author's thinking about the work that stimulates this sort of creativity in approach. Such exposure is contagious; this kind of sharing can stimulate the creativity of other art therapists to develop new methods and thereby expand the repertoire of the entire profession. Hopefully, this section will provide encouragement for further development of art therapists' professional creativity as they assess the needs of their clients and experiment with creative ways of using art to meet those challenges.

CHAPTER 14

Visual Transitions

Metaphor for Change

JERRY L. FRYREAR AND IRENE E. CORBIT

The *visual transitions* procedure features a blending of visual arts, photography, movement, video, and verbal psychotherapy or group process. It focuses on providing group members or individual clients with experiential exercises that allow them to observe, through photographs of themselves, their present state (indicating some type of rigidity or constriction) and also a more preferred state (indicating a new level of coping or openness). The still photography and the artwork are combined to reveal new relationships between these two facets of self. The participants utilize body movement as a means of characterizing and sensitizing the feelings and emotions of these states. The movement and the discussion of the artwork are shared with the other group members or the therapist, who imitate these same poses to achieve a psychodramatic mirroring effect. Video provides group members with a graphic medium to facilitate the transition between the two states and also acts as a reinforcement tool. Visual transitions therapy attempts to label artistically and verbally two points on a continuum—a constricted behavior on one end and a more relaxed, confident behavior on the other. The artworks, including the still photos, the movement, and the video, become metaphors for the change needed to help the individuals move in a more positive direction on this continuum.

Visual transitions therapy offers three distinct advantages: It is primarily a visual art therapy method; it is multimodal; and it provides a metaphor for change in the therapy program.

Regarding the first advantage, that the method is primarily a visual art therapy technique, Wadeson (1980) has discussed the advantages of art therapy: the primacy of imagery in early personality formation; its centrality in unconscious phenomena, including dreams; objectification in the tangible art product; permanence of the art object; and art's spatial matrix rather

The authors are indebted to Ms. Barbara Butler for her tact, patience, and word-processing wizardry.

than linear feature, permitting it more readily to represent certain experience. Wadeson states further that art therapy also fosters creative and physical energy stimulated by art making.

We agree with McNiff (1987) in his position that the psyche is expressing itself in a variety of forms. By providing a multimodal arts approach, we allow the individual client to experience multiple avenues for change and personal growth. One client may respond more to the movement aspects of the therapy, another client may resonate with the photography, a third may find the visual artwork to be the significant portion of the therapy. Still another may be surprised and positively confronted by the video playback. All clients seem to benefit from the sense of universality provided by the verbal sharing part of the therapy.

We believe that the metaphor for change aspect of visual transitions therapy is important and significant. As we all know, therapeutic change is extremely difficult. Furthermore, therapy is only successful if, sooner or later, a client makes some changes in her or his life. Visual transitions therapy provides for metaphorical change within the therapy session. Change is illustrated metaphorically by two poses, by the two photographs resulting from the poses, by the integration of the poses and the artwork, and by the movement that the client demonstrates and experiences when making the transition from one pose to the other. Furthermore, in the video playback portion of the therapy, a client is confronted with the reality that change, at least the metaphorical change in the therapy session, is certainly possible.

Using the expressive means of visual transitions, the client gains awareness, experiences the constriction kinesthetically, and uses discussion and sometimes psychodramatic techniques to move beyond the constriction. Once the impasse is dislodged, the client is able to experience alternatives in being. Change becomes a choice. Visual records of possible new behavior choices are available through the still photos and videotaping. How then can the client deny the possibility of change?

Watzlawick, Weakland, and Fisch (1974) suggest implementing small changes in behavior patterns to upset perfectionistic needs in order to enable one to work toward greater behavior changes. They say that "the target of change is the attempted solution, and the tactic chosen has to be translated into the person's own language" (p. 113). In visual transitions we are presenting a method in which the client is creating his or her own solution to the problem. The art and body language are unique to that person.

Rosen, speaking of Milton Erickson, discusses change also: "If a pattern can be changed even in some small way there is a possibility for further change. As we have seen many times this is one of Erickson's basic approaches to therapy—to initiate a small change" (1982, p. 126).

Houston uses body movement to facilitate change in workshop participants. Using imagery, she has group members visualize their bodies achieving greater flexibility and mobility. She then asks them to follow through the visualized movements with body movement. She says:

To change the modality we must change the metaphor. In our research we have found the metaphors which provide for the personalizing of body parts and states can often give us the charged imagery that then creates those channels of communication for dialogue with our innate body image. (1982, p. 12)

Visual transitions therapy then has three major advantages and, in that respect, represents an advance in art therapy. First, it is a visual art therapy approach, and has the advantages well documented for art therapy. A second advantage is its multimodal format, featuring a blending of art, photography, movement, video, and group or individual psychotherapy processes. The third advantage is its built-in provision for metaphoric change.

THE BASIC MODEL

The basic model is a group model, but with small adaptations it can be applied to individual or family therapy. No particular size of group is more desirable than any other, although obviously, size will be restricted by the room available. Time also creates obvious restrictions. We have found that the ideal time allotment for the program with a group of between 14 and 18 participants is approximately 3 hours. With less time, or more people, the pace is not as leisurely and there is less time spent upon the members individually.

The sessions begin with nonverbal introductions. This technique acquaints group members with alternative, visual–kinesthetic means of expressing themselves. Group members sit on the floor in a circle. One by one, they introduce themselves to the group nonverbally either from their sitting positions or by moving into the circle and relating to group members in their own unique ways. As a rule, this exercise is begun by the group leaders who model their own methods of nonverbal introductions. A few enthusiastic participants have introduced themselves by way of a dance or somersault. This beginning exercise helps to loosen the group and begins to get members more closely in touch with their bodies and accustomed to relying on the visual sense.

Videotaping can occur throughout the entire session or during any predetermined significant portion. Release forms are, of course, a necessity in videotaping any therapeutic group activity. If any participants request that they not be videotaped or that any portion of the tape involving them be erased, these requests are honored. The videotaping, if need be, can be eliminated altogether if equipment is not available.

In the next segment of the session, participants form into pairs to photograph one another. They use instant cameras and take two photographs of each other. One pose depicts "as I was." This pose reflects the participant "as I was" before therapy, "as I was" during a time of emotional conflict, or "as I was" when I became entrapped by personal constrictions.

The second pose portrays "as I would like to be." This pose reflects how the participant would like to be or feel ideally. Many participants take a great deal of time discussing and deciding on these poses. Background props and improvised costumes are frequently used.

The poses or postures are often overstated. Someone who had experienced or is experiencing a bout with depression might curl into a fetal position to express this condition nonverbally. Another who was or is fearful might assume a cringing position.

In the second pose, the participant explores and models a body posture that often exaggerates a sense of well-being or change.

After the still photos are made, the participants are provided with art materials including, but not necessarily limited to, poster board, craypas (oil pastels), chalks, scissors, glue, and colored marking pens.

Each group member then cuts out and mounts the two photographs on poster board in whatever way he or she wishes, somehow relating the two images to each other with the art materials. When the art projects are completed, members form pairs or small groups to discuss their work with one another.

After the small groups have processed their work, they form a large circle. Each member shows his or her artwork and explains how the two images are related in the art. Immediately after each member's sharing turn, he or she demonstrates the first pose with his or her body, then the second. The member is encouraged to repeat the two poses, choosing one word or phrase to describe each pose. The group member concentrates upon the feeling aspect of each pose and the movement necessary to get from one pose to the other. The entire group then joins the presenter in duplicating his or her movements. Much as in the psychodrama technique of mirroring, empathy is developed in assuming the body poses of another person.

The presenter is asked to be aware of personal feelings and body sensations in moving from one pose to the other. Is the pose strained or awkward? Does the presenter feel trapped or joyous? The transition is enacted like a group choreography, with members not only becoming aware of their empathic feelings with the presenter, but also attending to personal body sensations and feelings during the reenactment. Each member, therefore, experiences directly the movements described and enacted by himself or herself and every other group member.

If time permits, the group members might, during this phase, explore their transitions even further by following the transitional action in meditation. One private client who had drawn a rainbow around herself in the "after" pose took that image into meditation. She visualized herself being surrounded by the rainbow and later described the elated feelings of a natural high that influenced her life in the following weeks.

The videotape of this phase of the therapy program can be replayed directly after each member's presentation, or at the end of the workshop. Each member can then see himself or herself going through the transition from "as I was" to "as I would like to be." Both the artwork and the movement become metaphors for change, as do the images captured by the still film and the moving tape.

During one workshop presentation of visual transitions, a woman informed us at the end of the workshop that she was angry because we hadn't given her the same opportunity to present her artwork and movements that we had given the other members. We argued that, yes, she had presented.

"No," she said, "you passed me by in the group."

When the videotape of her was replayed showing 3 or 4 minutes of her presenting her work, she was amazed. "I wouldn't have believed it," she said. The denial aspect of her personal defense system was far more powerful than she had previously suspected.

The last phase of the program is the general sharing of the experience, relating the experience to more elaborate possible change in the outside world, and sharing common experiences and feelings. It is not unusual for several individuals in a group to demonstrate very similar poses and transitional movements. This similarity is helpful in convincing the group members of the universality of their concerns—a common experience in verbal group therapies also. This also is a time for closure, a time in which members may deal with any unspoken issues or feelings.

CASE EXAMPLE: ELIZABETH

A 34-year-old divorced woman who works as an administrative assistant in a large corporation, Elizabeth took part in a 7-week visual transitions group in which she produced the following art based on her two photographs. The "as I am" pose for Elizabeth is labeled "I can't" (standing slump shouldered, arms crossed, head down), and her "as I want to be" pose is labeled "I can" (illustrated by jumping into the air with heels clicking: Fig. 14.1). Her comments about the artwork follow:

ELIZABETH: In my first pose, I'm pressing on my right leg and chewing on my lip—and my arms are crossed as a way of holding myself together.

THERAPIST (demonstrating the same pose): I'm feeling having been aggressed upon—a lot of hurt.

ELIZABETH: I was the middle of five children—the scapegoat. I was moody and temperamental, and I would stand like this a lot [indicating first pose] . . . a feeling like "I don't need anybody." I wouldn't let them know I was hurting, and I wouldn't let anyone in.

ELIZABETH (illustrating second pose): I've noticed that when I feel really good about something, or I'm happy about something, I'll give a hop, skip and jump [similar to pose], and it feels so good.

THERAPIST: One thing for sure, you can't jump while you're holding your arms crossed and biting your lip.

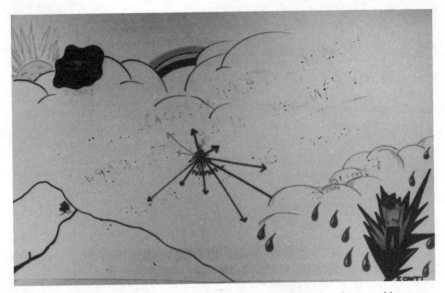

Figure 14.1. Visual transition photographs and artwork by Elizabeth, a 34-year-old woman.

ELIZABETH: Right. I wasn't aware that body posture could actually make you feel a certain way.

ELIZABETH (about her decision to grow): It was a decision to either give up, or go on. I asked myself, "Are you, or aren't you?" When I made that decision [to go on], I decided not to go on, filled with torment. I felt like if I had a sense of hope, I could try. Ever since then, I'm not

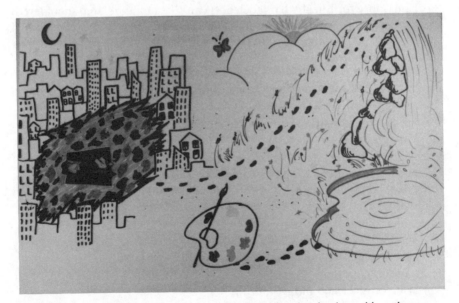

Figure 14.2. A tranquil piece of art done by Elizabeth after the visual transitions therapy.

at a loss of control over my life. If I lose it tomorrow, it'll be all right—but I know I won't be the one that does it—and I feel peaceful about that. But for a long time, I didn't. Because I knew I could always do that if I couldn't take it anymore. But now, I know I don't want to.

A subsequent art object was created by Elizabeth in which she pictures herself at peace within the elements of the city, in juxtaposition to the tranquility of her worlds of art and nature (Fig. 14.2).

VARIATIONS ON VISUAL TRANSITIONS

Variations on the theme of visual transitions can be as numerous and creative as the imagination of the facilitator allows. We have developed variations of our concept to include group work, family therapy work, sandtray work with children, humor, conflict resolution, and more.

Sandtray Uses With Children

The sandtray is a therapeutic tool developed from a Jungian concept by Kalff of Zurich, Switzerland (1980). In her work with children who are experiencing conflict due to divorce, abuse, loss, or family strife, Corbit offers the sandtray as a means of resolving these conflicts. The sandtray is a tray 19½ by 28½ by 3 inches in size, filled with sterilized play sand. The child develops a scene in the sandtray, choosing from hundreds of toys and symbolic objects. The child's inner conflict is reflected in his or her production in the sand.

Included among the children's favorites are monsters and dinosaurs, soldiers, little dolls and action figures, cars and airplanes, houses, fences, and trees. A child in therapy will often select the same or similar objects each week, but create a slightly different scene.

As the child begins to gain control over the events in the sandtray, this control generalizes inwardly. Around this time, the therapist begins to receive reports from the parents or teacher that the child's behavior has begun to improve.

A visual transitions technique for the sandtray was developed by Corbit when she saw the applicability of using a photo paper doll of the child in the sandtray. Using this technique, the child begins to plan his or her sandtray, then poses for an instant action picture. The child's image is cut out and mounted on a piece of poster board. A "stand" is cut out of the poster board and glued to the back of the figure—such as with old paper dolls or stand-up Valentines. The child then places his or her own figure into the sandtray, interacting with the other figures in the tray. In this way, the child actually becomes a part of his or her scene in the sand.

CASE EXAMPLE: HOLLY

Holly, a 6-year-old girl, was brought into therapy with Corbit because of her profound fears. She refused to leave her mother's side at home or out shopping. She panicked when she had to go up in an elevator, so they usually took the stairs. In discussing the child's history, the mother said that Holly had accidentally locked herself into a bathroom at preschool when she was 3 years old. The mother felt that this incident precipitated Holly's fears.

Holly was asked if she would like to work on her fears using art therapy. She liked to draw, and readily agreed. Corbit asked her to draw a picture of an elevator. Next, she was asked to pose for an instant photograph as if she were about to step onto the elevator. This was fun for Holly. She enjoyed cutting out her image and gluing it onto her picture. In the completed product, she could see herself smiling as she was about to step onto the elevator.

In the next phase of the therapy, Corbit asked Holly to close her eyes and relax. Holly was asked to go, in her imagination, into a building with an elevator. She could take as many friends and protectors with her as she cared to, so that she would feel safe. Next, in her imagination, she was to press the elevator button going to the second floor. When they arrived at the second floor, everyone was to get off the elevator. Corbit asked her, "Did everyone get off?" Holly nodded her head. "Who do you want to come down with you?" Corbit asked. "Just my Mommy," Holly replied. "Do you feel safe?" Corbit asked. Again Holly nodded her head. In a later session, Holly's mother reported that Holly had gone to the dentist's office and ridden the elevator without any qualms.

In a recent session, Holly began a sandtray. Corbit asked her if she would like to put herself into the sandtray. "How can I do that?" Holly asked. "We'll take a 'brave' picture of you, and put the picture into the tray," Corbit answered. Holly posed for the instant picture in which she was to feel brave. The photograph was cut out, mounted, and a stand was then glued onto the back of the figure. The sandtray contained many frightening figures, but "brave" Holly stood up to them. We then took an instant photograph of the sandtray so that Holly could have her own copy of the scene (Fig. 14.3).

The mother's next report to Corbit was that Holly had gone shopping with her, but this time she was able to be separated from mother without becoming panicked.

Family Therapy Applications

The visual transitions method can be used with enmeshed families or families in distress. During the sessions, the therapist looks for clues to the problem or problems, just like any other family therapist: Who is the identified patient in the family? Where are the subgroups in the family? What does each family member perceive to be the problem? Who needs what and from whom?

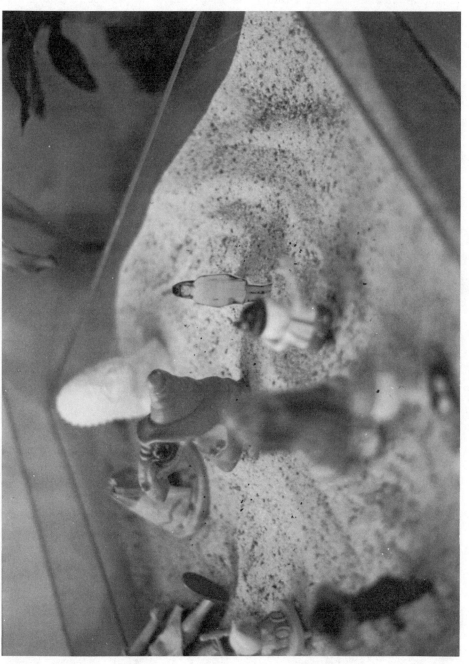

Figure 14.3. Fearless Holly in the sandtray.

The application of visual transitions helps the family to recreate their problem visually, and then create a visual solution. In this process, family members are asked to pose for full-body instant photographs that symbolize the role each member plays in the family. The interpretation of this directive is left entirely to the family member posing for his or her photograph. When all photographs are completed, family members are given scissors, glue, marking pens, craypas, and a piece of 22-by-28-inch poster board. This large poster board allows the family members the space and flexibility to create their own world.

Next, family members cut out their images from the photographs, and as a family unit decide how the photographs should be placed onto the poster board. There is usually a great deal of discussion in deciding how and where these images should be placed. When all family members agree as to the placement of the figures, the images are then glued to the poster board. Family members next create a background for their picture. This aspect of the exercise, too, calls for cooperation of family members. This is the time for the therapist to observe such factors as: Who begins the artwork? Who directs the group? Who withholds? Who sabotages the work of others? All of this information is vital to the family therapist.

In the next segment of the exercise, family members are asked to pose individually for photographs depicting themselves in their ideal family. There

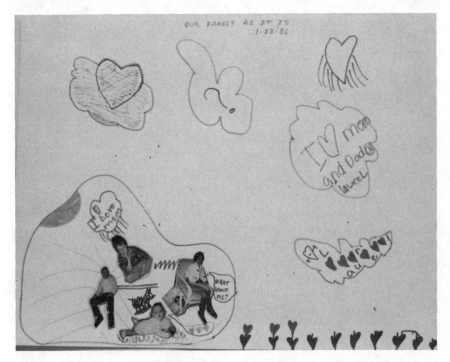

Figure 14.4. A family at odds.

is usually less acting out in this part of the process because family members can say nonverbally things that they couldn't communicate in the past. Maybe they would like to see Dad become more involved in the family. Possibly they are beginning to individuate from the family and ask nonverbally for more freedom.

In one family therapy session, Corbit was working with a family that consisted of mother, father, 6-month-old baby, and a 7-year-old son from father's first marriage. The family struggled with the first picture. The baby (Laurel) was placed close to mother, father and mother were separated by the children, and the 7-year-old contended for his position in the family (Fig. 14.4).

At mother's suggestion, the second picture, the ideal family picture, showed all family members in a circular or mandala shape so that everyone could have access to everyone else. This gave the family some valuable visual information of where they have been in the family system, and ultimately where they could be (Fig. 14.5).

Humor

One element that seems to be missing from psychiatric wards and therapy sessions is humor. Doctors are serious, the staff are serious, patients are serious. O'Connell, an advocate for humor in psychotherapy (Hirsch & O'Connell, 1984), sees "the sense of humor (or lack of it) as the essential criterion of the actualization process" (p. 554). O'Connell says that "a sense

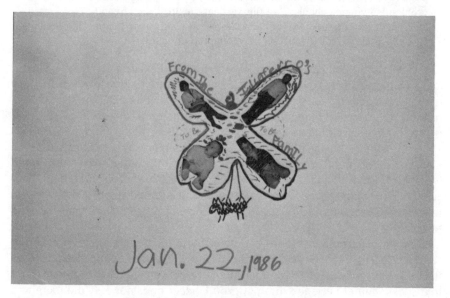

Figure 14.5. The same family in harmony.

of humor is the end result of self-training for the expansion of one's sense of worth and feelings of universal belonging, plus the development of an appreciation for the basic paradoxes of the human condition" (p. 554).

Visual transitions can be a powerful force in eliciting humorous responses from patients and clients. In her work as consultant on an alcohol and chemical abuse unit of a hospital, Corbit initiated the use of visual transitions within patient groups. Depressed and withdrawn patients were able to bring themselves out of their depressed mood states when asked to photograph one another in humorous poses. The patients were asked to select a photography partner and to help one another create a humorous pose, then to photograph the pose. Other patients in the group were encouraged to give support and advice to the photography subject.

After the photographs were shot and discussed within the group, and sometimes second photographs taken, group members were asked to cut out their images and to glue them onto pieces of poster board (usually 14 by 20 inches or half a piece of poster board). Next, they provided the background for their humorous poses using colored marking pens and craypas. The spirit within the group by the end of the session was always high. Sometimes chronically depressed patients stated that they hadn't laughed so hard in ages.

In an article on humor in psychotherapy, Salameh (1983) writes:

> One of the important goals of psychotherapy with regard to creativity factors is to help patients surpass their constrictions and develop a greater awareness of creative alternatives. Furthermore, an effective therapeutic intervention prepares clients to deal with life resourcefully by providing them with a creative problem-solving mechanism. In this respect, healthy humor can be considered as a creatively therapeutic problem-solving modality representing the human capacity for survival, continuity, and adaptation. (p. 81).

At a "Humor in Health Care" workshop in Houston, co-led by Corbit and O'Connell, participants were asked to identify a constriction in their lives. Constrictions consist of such ego identity elements as the use of control, boundary building, active or passive competition, distancing, self-guilt, perfectionism, invidious comparisons, resistance, and so on (O'Connell, 1981). Working in teams of four, workshop participants were asked to assume a pose symbolizing their constriction. Then, with the aid of their fellow team members, the participants were asked to create a humorous pose that transcended their constriction. In this exercise, it seemed important for group members to receive the advice, support, and encouragement from others on the team.

Workshop participants then cut out and mounted their images representing "constriction" and "moving past constriction." After creating a background for both pictures with colored marking pens and/or craypas, the teams met to discuss their experience. In their group discussions not only did members explain their work to others, but through the act of verbalizing they came to a new level of understanding of their own process.

While working at a school for emotionally disturbed children, Corbit asked students to pose as staff members and other students. This activity generated a new sense of intimacy for staff and students alike as the principal, teachers, and students attempted to outdo one another with their silly poses. The principal assumed a relaxed pose with his feet up on the desk, which delighted the students. The students cut out the pictures, mounted and labeled them, then had an exhibit of their projects in the entry hall.

Jung's Concept of the Shadow

Jung writes of his concept of shadow that "if we are able to see our own shadow and can bear knowing about it, then a small part of the problem has already been solved: we have at least brought up the personal unconscious" (1971, p. 20). We have developed a visual transitions variation to recognize and encounter one's shadow qualities. Shadow, we feel, can be more palatable to group members when encountered in this manner rather than in some more damning or condemning way.

Shadow workshops begin with a slide presentation of images that might depict shadow qualities of one's personality, or aspects of the personality that are unconscious to the person, either positive or negative. These slides include the Warlock, the Witch, the Gossip, the Harlot, the Shrew, the Fool, the Hero, the Heroine, the Priest, and the Naive Woman. Participants are asked to acknowledge any feeling reaction they might encounter while viewing the slides. They then take a few minutes to search inwardly for aspects of their personal shadows. These shadow clues might also come from dreams or from projections upon others.

The participants are then asked to translate their shadow qualities into a pose. Working in pairs, the group members photograph one another. Their second pose is their "ego" pose, a pose that indicates how they see themselves, or how they project themselves to the outer world. In their work of integrating shadow, the workshop members concentrate on befriending their shadow qualities as they compose a picture using both aspects of themselves: ego and shadow. Sometimes a third photograph is required to achieve the integration of these qualities. The images are cut out, arranged, and mounted onto a piece of poster board. Creating the picture takes considerable reflective time for sorting out ego and shadow, and for the integration of these aspects.

We are certainly cognizant that working with shadow elements of oneself entails risk, and many potential participants are simply not ready for such a confrontational procedure. To date, we have only used this variation with mental health professionals who are attending the workshop for training rather than therapy. We ask these participants early in the session to take responsibility for themselves, and to gauge their self-disclosures. We must urge caution in using this particular variation with therapy clients early in the therapeutic process.

We have also found that more in-depth work is accomplished if the group

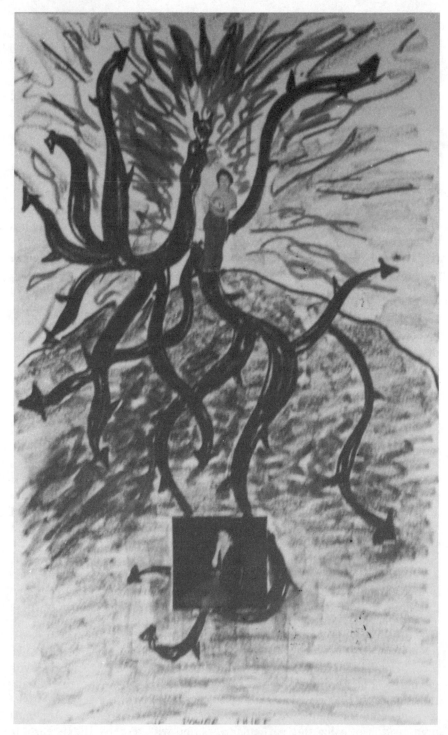

Figure 14.6. The Power Thief.

members meet in small teams, usually two photography pairs. After meeting in teams, the group then meets as a whole to share any part of the exercise that the participants feel comfortable relating to the larger group.

One woman in a recent shadow workshop identified her personal shadow as the Power Thief. Her artwork represented the power thief as a snakelike, multitendriled creature (Fig. 14.6).

Conflict Resolution

Yet another variation on the basic model is the use of visual transitions to help with the resolution of intrapsychic conflicts. Clients are instructed to pose, not for before and after constrictions, but in a way that represents both sides of a conflict. Common conflicts include safety versus risk taking, dependence versus independence, and the desire to be dominant in inter-personal relationships as opposed to deferential. Conflicts among psycho-logical needs are also very common. The need to nurture versus the need for succor, the need for change versus the need for order, the need for achievement versus maternal needs—these are common psychological con-flicts that are experienced to some degree by most of us.

The visual transitions therapy is used in much the same way as the basic model outlined earlier. Clients pose for both sides of the conflict, then in-tegrate the photographs into artwork using craypas and other materials. Rather than act out the two poses with movement, however, the group leader or therapist helps the client to resolve the conflict using psychodramatic or gestalt techniques. In order to illustrate the conflict resolution variation, we will present a case of a man, a workshop participant, who was struggling with a career change decision (Fig. 14.7). His comments follow.

As I explained in my little group I've got a bit of a problem, a dilemma. I have a graphic design business that I started 3 years ago, and then about a year ago I decided I wanted to pursue a doctorate in psychology. Anyway, I launched my program in psychology. I'm 6 months into it and I know that I want to graduate in 2 years. It will be organizational psychology, and stress management is my specialty.

So I've got these great designs about my future for the next 20 or 30 years or whatever where I really want to do something in that arena. And graphic design and printing and all of that has been my last 25 years of my life. This new little business called Brochures Unlimited, I'm not making a whole lot of money but it surprised me; I've hung in there, I'm paying the bills, paying for my schooling. It's my little child. I don't want to give it up and turn it over and tell it good-bye and so I'm still going to own it. I'm a one-person operation but here lately and for some time to come I'm sure I'm wondering what I'm going to do about hiring someone to come in and manage that business and then the pains of trying to separate myself from it.

So that's kind of what my picture indicates. This is my company that I built and started out with a few hundred dollars and hope and questions of uncertainty, risk. As a businessman I risk everything every day. Anyway

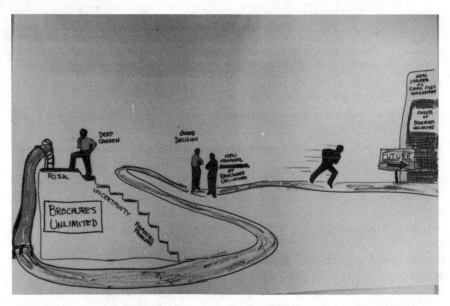

Figure 14.7. A man in career transition.

this picture represents deep concern. It's not worry. I'm not really worried about anything. I don't *have* to go into stress management, but I want to. I think I'm just not worried but I'm really concerned about what I'm going to do.

Anyway, so this is the place that I'm at now [pointing to his image at top of slide] and this is a slide. I thought about doing stair steps, but when I do this it's going to be kind of quick. Soon, in the next year or so I'll get on this sliding board and this is kind of the road. This is me right here where I feel pretty confident that I made a good decision. [pointing to image in center of poster] This little alter ego right here that came off the back side of the photo is the person who is going to take my business over and manage it. For some reason I was really playing with where I would position that person. Notice I've positioned him slightly below me. [laughter from group, discussion of gender of manager] Well, I could have drawn a skirt on it. I'm more concerned with the quality of the individual.

Once this is resolved right here, then this is me. [running figure] No stops or reservations. This is my future out here. [right side of poster] I consciously made the decision these are the two things I am working with. My new career is the biggest and it's on top, but within that my Brochures Unlimited that I am still going to hold onto. That is my whole scenario that I am concerned with right now. It's certainly not as deep as some I've heard and I think that once I find this person [manager] and after I've finally decided what to do I want to let them manage it. They might hire some production workers to do the work. By the way, I do my own writing, my own production work, I do my own photography, and I'm my own printer by trade. I don't think anybody is going to do all that. I've been thinking this person is going to be just like me. But there's not going to be one just like me! They'll be doing a little differently from me. That will be a tough time but I can handle it.

RESEARCH PROGRAM

To date, we have carried out one formal, extended research program to assess the effectiveness of visual transitions. We also have many informal comments from participants and our own observations of its effectiveness with diverse clients.

In order to test the effectiveness of visual transitions in a formal program, we (Corbit, Fryrear, & Evans) asked for volunteers to participate in a 7-week group experience. Eleven people agreed to the program. Each participant filled out the Personal Orientation Inventory (Shostrom, 1974) and the Adjective Check List (Heilbrun & Gough, 1965) prior to and at the end of the 7 weeks, and each filled out an extensive questionnaire about the experience after the 7 weeks. The Personal Orientation Inventory is a paper-and-pencil measure of self-actualization and includes subscales of Spontaneity, Self-Regard, Self-Acceptance, as well as nine others. The Adjective Check List has 24 standard subscales. We were interested only in three— Number of Favorable Adjectives Checked, Number of Unfavorable Adjectives Checked, and Personal Adjustment.

The results of the Personal Orientation Inventory and the Adjective Check List indicated overall positive growth among the participants. Two of the Personal Orientation Inventory subscales showed positive changes (before therapy to after therapy) at the .07 level of confidence, and two of the three Adjective Check List subscales showed changes in the positive direction.

The questionnaire contained many positive comments and overall high ratings. Responses to the questionnaire showed that the workshop participants experienced personal growth from the visual transitions experience and also felt that the therapy approach shows promise as an advance in art therapy. Our informal observations and feedback from participants all over the world have been in a similar vein, and have enabled us to refine and expand the procedure as we learn more about it. We anticipate that further refinement and expansion will be an ongoing process.

IMPRESSIONS OF CROSS-CULTURAL DIFFERENCES

During the past few years, as we have developed and expanded visual transitions, we have had occasion to present the model in far-flung areas of the world. In the United States, we have carried out workshops in Houston, Washington, D.C., Miami, Chicago, and Los Angeles. Outside the United States, we have led workshops or presented the model in Toronto, Cardiff,

Frankfurt, and Zagreb. Although we have not studied cultural differences systematically, several impressions stand out in our memories.

North Americans, particularly U.S. citizens, are in a hurry. We hurry through the poses, we dash off the artwork, we move quickly. There are exceptions, of course, and art therapists represent one exception. Art therapists seem to spend more time on the poses and artwork than do other participants.

Europeans, conversely, take time with the art. They spend more time meditating and conceptualizing before actually snapping the shutter or applying the pen. We had that impression in both West Germany and Yugoslavia.

We carried out a workshop with the staff of a state psychiatric hospital in West Germany. They took more time with the art, and we also were impressed with the formality of the participants. The participants were careful to show their posters to each of the other group members and seemed determined to express individuality. We were also intrigued that, compared with both North Americans and Yugoslavians, the West German participants seemed to use more abstract symbols. We carry with us a memory of posters full of triangles, circles, geometric shapes of all kinds.

In Yugoslavia, we worked with a number of mental health workers from different parts of Eastern Europe. We were impressed with the relaxed, "laid-back" atmosphere in the group. People laughed and joked, took a leisurely approach. We also have a memory of nature scenes. The Yugoslavian participants seemed to use nature scenes in the backgrounds of the "after" photos more than people in other parts of the world. The "natural life" seems to be part of the ideal mentally healthy existence there. We also have the impression that the Yugoslavian participants used black and white backgrounds for the "before" pictures and color for the "after" photo backgrounds, more than has been our experience other places.

There is always the danger of stereotyping, of overgeneralizing from limited data and experience. We wish to emphasize that these few comments are impressions only, and we certainly have no hard data to back up these assertions. One thing we can say for certain, however, is that the nonverbal nature of visual transitions has allowed us to share the experience with people of widely differing backgrounds and languages. The art, the photographs, need little in the way of verbal interpretation or even verbal description. The poses speak for themselves, and the video and movement components need no verbal explanations.

SUMMARY AND CONCLUSIONS

Visual transitions seems to be a powerful tool for change, incorporating art, still photography, movement, video playback, and verbal psychotherapy in a single program. It has three noticeable advantages: It is primarily visual, with the well-known advantages visual media bring to therapy; it is multi-

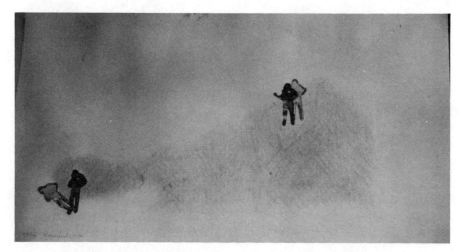

Figure 14.8. "She saw where she was, and she saw where she wanted to be."

modal, enabling clients to use a choice or a combination of modalities to achieve therapeutic change and personal growth; it provides for metaphoric change within the therapeutic session, rather than relying on the client's resources outside of therapy to initiate the small changes that lead to larger ones.

As a therapy method, it can be used with adults, with children, with families, with groups or individuals. Corbit has used the method successfully with children and families and both authors have used it with adults individually and in groups.

We have developed several variations on the basic model, including sand-tray uses, family therapy, conflict resolution, and humor, and we continue to refine and enlarge the approach. Research data and personal testimonials lead us to be optimistic about the effectiveness of the basic model, and we will continue to evaluate and use the method with diverse groups of people.

Shortly after presenting a workshop on visual transitions at the 1983 annual conference of the American Art Therapy Association in Chicago, we received copies of a poem written by a group participant, Helga Schafarczyk, who had come to the meeting from Germany. She said that she had written a poem on the airplane on her return trip. Figure 14.8 expresses graphically a line from the poem. Printed with her permission, the poem reads:

> *She had been walking for so many years:*
> *There were so many ways to try.*
> *There were so many rooms to discover.*
> *There were so many things to do.*
> *There were so many people to know.*
> *There were so many emotions to feel.*

>*She stopped:*
> *Where am I?*
> *Where do I want to be?*
>*And a friendly voice told her:*
> *Define where you are.*
> *Define where you want to be.*
>*And she made two pictures of herself, expressing*
>*Now and then:*
>*She took the scissors and cut herself out*
>   *carefully,*
>   *Not to get hurt.*
>*She picked up her shadow gently,*
>   *Not to get lost.*
>*She let them move around slowly,*
>   *Not to get exhausted.*
>*She fixed them all in the right position*
>   *quickly,*
>   *Not to get indecisive.*
>*And she saw where she was.*
>*And she saw where she wanted to be:*
>   *Now and then.*
>   *Contemplation—realization.*
>   *Stay or move?*
>*And she looked up and the gentle voice told her:*
>   *Realize! You've already found the answer.*
>*And she knew that it was so easy to stay.*
>*And she knew that it was so easy to go.*
>*And she arose.*

REFERENCES

Heilbrun, A. B., & Gough, H. (1965). *The Adjective Checklist*. Palo Alto: Consulting Psychologists Press.

Hirsch, V., & O'Connell, W. (1984). No laughing matter: The lack of humor in current psychotherapies. In J. Harriman (Ed.), *Does psychotherapy really help people?* Springfield, IL: Charles C. Thomas.

Houston, J. (1982). *The possible human*. Los Angeles: J. P. Tarcher.

Jung, C. G. (1971). *The archetypes and the collective unconscious* (Vol. 9, Part 1, of the *Collected Works of C. G. Jung*). Princeton: Princeton University Press.

Kalff, D. M. (1980). *Sandplay*. Santa Monica: Sigo.

McNiff, S. (1987). Pantheon of creative arts therapies: An integrative image of the profession. *Journal of Integrative & Eclectic Therapy, 6*(3), 259–281.

O'Connell, W. (1981). Natural high therapy. In R. Corsini (Ed.), *Innovative psychotherapies*. New York: Wiley.

Rosen, S. (1982). *My voice will go with you: The teaching tales of Milton Erickson.* New York: Norton.

Salameh, W. (1983). Humor in psychotherapy: Past outlooks, present status, and future frontiers. In P. McGhee & J. Goldstein (Eds.), *Handbook of humor research.* New York: Springer-Verlag.

Shostrom, E. (1974). *Personal orientation inventory.* San Diego: Edits.

Wadeson, H. (1980). *Art psychotherapy.* New York: Wiley.

Watzlawick, P., Weakland, J., & Fisch, R. (1974). *Change: Principles of problem formation and problem resolution.* New York: Norton.

CHAPTER 15

Art Therapy and Computers

DEVORAH SAMET CANTER

If there's one thing we can be sure of, it's the fact that we can look forward to an accelerating future of technological advances. The arts will not be immune to these changes, as they have already been greatly affected by computer technology. Computers are currently in use as electronic palettes, animation stands, music generators, and 3D sculpting devices. And with the usage of computers for storage of patient records, it's obvious that these technological advances will have a major impact in every aspect of art therapy.

Computers, with their animation, music, and drawing software, can be an integral part of the client–therapist relationship. By combining powerful user-friendly hardware and software in treatment programs, psychological and psychiatric institutions, hospitals, schools, and nursing homes, art therapists can develop innovative art therapy techniques.

Joe Nathan, computer education specialist, has written and lectured on the creative and educational applications for computers. He believes that the most advanced and effective use of computers requires rethinking attidues, which will provide opportunities for creative experimentation, thus changing traditional patterns and practices. He writes: "Computers can do much more, but they cannot do these tasks for us—we must be open, thoughtful and brave enough to do them ourselves (1985, p. 231).

Whether computers can advance art therapy techniques depends entirely on our innate curiosity as artists to explore and investigate this new medium. The possibilities are endless and the results can prove to be greater than we ever expected.

As an art therapist and art teacher I have used the Apple® Macintosh™ computer and "creativity software" as tools for therapy and education. In art therapy sessions I primarily use the Macintosh and animation software called VideoWorks II™. Instead of just drawing static pictures on paper to portray their thoughts and feelings, emotionally disturbed children and adolescents use VideoWorks II to illustrate and animate their fantasies. In this case the computer is used as a story-telling device, or electronic puppet stage in which clients can easily move pictures around the computer screen to tell a story about their personal problems. This technique has proven to be an effective tool in a therapeutic milieu and will be further discussed later through case studies in this chapter.

PURPOSE

This chapter will address the potential of applying computers and creativity software (art-related software) in art therapy sessions. These new tools will give art therapists better insight into their clients' worlds and further their technological advancement. Also presented will be case studies illustrating how the Macintosh computer and specially designed creativity software can both bring out creative talents and reduce behavioral problems for clients with learning disabilities. These youngsters have difficulties expressing themselves through the use of common art materials because of problems with fine motor coordination and/or impulsive or destructive personalities. Using computers allows these clients to express themselves in new ways, while at the same time keeping their hands clean. There has also been a noticeable increase of self-esteem on the part of clients who have interacted with the computer over a short period of time.

Computers and computer-based therapy are constructive and beneficial tools for clients with learning disabilities because they provide calming effects and creative and intellectual skills, are versatile, and allow immediate feedback.

Exploring the possibilities of combining traditional art therapy tools such as clay, plaster, and so on with computers, animation, and music programs will advance art therapy into the future. While this technology may not be fully integrated into the lives of our generation, it surely will be for our child and adolescent clients.

BACKGROUND

In our educational and psychiatric institutions today we find a myriad of computer systems used for administrative purposes and psychological testing. What many art therapists may not be aware of, however, is the capability to transform these hardware systems into tools that can be used in the creation of both music and art. Not all computer systems are equipped to run art, music, and animation software, although in some cases specially designed hardware peripherals may be added on to equip them to do so. Hardware peripherals are the extra hardware that enhance the functionality of a computer.

The Apple Macintosh's increased capability to produce graphics, sound, and animation and its revolutionary easy-to-use approach to computing have helped me implement these new approaches to art therapy using computers.

In the future computers will become even more friendly and easy to use. Interactive programming languages are now designed so that the user can interact with the computer to learn just about anything. In Hamburg, Germany, at the Centre for Research into Sign Language and Communication of the Deaf, Rolf Schulmeister has developed a sign language dictionary on the Macintosh that will be able to produce visual sign language in the form of animated pictures or movies. The Macintosh provides an easy way to represent signs by pictures and to simulate movements by animation. A dictionary of sign language could be a useful learning tool for those people who live or work with the deaf: hearing parents, teachers, nurses, doctors, and child care personnel. Computers can grant quick random access into an existing animation.

In Chicago, Illinois, at Schwab Rehabilitation Center, computers are used with the severely handicapped to help them control their environments. Computers allow patients access to control electrical equipment in their homes such as televisions, lights, radios, and telephones. In the occupational department at Schwab, computers are also used for daily living skills with stroke patients. Therapists use software programs that tell stories pertaining to actual daily problems, and clients interact with therapists by discussing how they would solve these problems. Themes pertaining to spending money and other daily living skills are included. Ismene Munch (personal communication), director of the Occupational Therapy and Therapeutic Recreation Department, believes that computers are important tools to use in rehabilitation because they can adjust to different levels of difficulty, unlike paper and pencil.

LITERATURE REVIEW

Computers: Educational and Therapeutic Opinions

In his chapter titled "Toys with Minds of Their Own," Howard Gardner (1982) envisions a time when computer toys will allow students in a classroom to locate their mental metier, to advance at their own speed and in their own way, aided by the very best "minds" (p. 233). Computers are ideal instruments for play, says Robert Taylor, professor at Columbia University's Teachers College. He believes educational programs should not just be instruments to help children learn reading, writing, and arithmetic. Instead, they should encourage the key developmental components of play, including the strengthening of children's creativity, their gift for fantasy and imagination, their ability to play roles and build models of the real world, their curiosity, and their hunger for exploration, discovery, and experimentation (D'Ignazio, 1984).

Computers can also change the way people think about themselves, asserts Sherry Turkle (1984). She believes that mirrors, literal and metaphorical, play an important role in human development. In literature, music, visual arts, or computer programming, they allow us to see ourselves from the outside, and objectify aspects of ourselves we had perceived only from within. In her studies with children and computers she found that some children are able to see computers as a "mirror of their mind." These children made explicit use of computational metaphors to think about themselves. Turkle states, "looking at the detail of how they [computers] provide a vantage point for understanding something helps us understand how computer metaphors can turn into a new popular psychology for the culture at large" (p. 155).

Computer journalist Sharon Zardetto Aker (1986) has found that animation software for the Macintosh enhances prereading skills, letter and name recognition, letter sounds, rhymes, premath skills, rote counting, numeral recognition, one-to-one correspondence, quantity, conservation of number, ordinal numbers, simple operations, and other skills such as shape discrimination, spatial relationships, object classification, and pattern recognition (pp. 83–88).

Art therapists who wish to begin implementing computers and creativity software in their sessions must first understand how difficult it is for some users to overcome the immediate challenges of just "using" the computer. Once these initial investigations (and fears) have been overcome, tremendous breakthroughs in learning, creativity, and self-esteem will occur. A basic understanding of the computer's capabilities is very important for art therapists to have if they are going to employ computers in their clinical work with clients.

HARDWARE

We are bombarded everyday by advertisements that claim theirs is the best or most powerful computer. The choices to be made as to what kind of computer hardware to purchase may be confusing and overwhelming.

IBM®, Atari®, Amiga®, and Apple® all produce computers that create graphics and sound. The key questions are what kind of graphic resolution the computer produces, how difficult is it to get up and running on your computer, and what other kinds of software it will allow you to use. For instance, some computers are primarily used for producing text. Word processing may be their only function. Other computers may be able to run color graphics, animation, and sound, but the user interface (how you use the computer) may be poor, and traveling with your computer or transporting it from work to home may not be convenient.

I have found that the Apple Macintosh to be the ideal computer system to use in art therapy, because it is a pixel-based (bit-mapped) graphic computer. While using a Macintosh, the user doesn't have to remember obscure commands like DIR or A:*/B:*/.

The Macintosh is a portable computer, meaning it can be packed up in a carrying case and transported from home to work. It can even be stored underneath a chair in an airplane, and it weighs approximately 20 pounds.

The "mouse" of the Macintosh ("Mac") is a moveable cursor or pointer. As you move the mouse around on a flat surface it moves the cursor on the screen. The user clicks the button on the mouse to control the computer.

On the top of the screen is a row of words called the menu bar. Each word is the name of a menu, under which is seen another set of words that represents the choices that are available to the user. Each menu is accessed by placing the mouse cursor on the menu name itself and holding the mouse button down. When the menu is opened, the user pulls the mouse cursor down the menu to select the particular command desired; thus the term *pull-down menu* is used.

On the screen of the Macintosh are windows. Each program that runs on the computer runs inside a window. Each window can be resized or overlaid on top of other windows.

The combination of pull-down menus, windows, and a mouse is called a graphics-based user interface as opposed to a text-based user interface. All the information needed to control the computer is on the computer screen. Nothing is hidden with a graphic interface; everything looks exactly as it will when, for instance, you print out a letter or drawing to a printer. This kind of interface is called "WYSIWYG" (what you see is what you get).

Children and adults can easily adapt to this graphics-based user interface because it allows easy access to computer programs. The icon-oriented system allows the user to select little pictures (icons) on the screen to control the computer. For instance, if a person wants to use an animation program all he or she has to do is insert the software into the computer, find the icon, place the cursor on the icon, and double-click the mouse button.

SOFTWARE

MacPaint™, VideoWorksII, and MusicWorks™ are the creativity software programs I have integrated in art therapy sessions. They all take advantage of the graphics-based user interface of the Macintosh computer. Software and hardware work together like a record and record player. Creativity software can transform the Macintosh computer into a paint canvas or drawing pad, an animation stand or a composer's sheaf of music.

MacPaint is a drawing program that uses the mouse to "draw" on the screen of the Macintosh. It is an all-purpose paint program. Its ease of use enables a user to become a computer graphics artist with no prior experience.

MusicWorks is a music program that enables the user to place notes on a music staff and hear the results instantly. It can be used as an electronic piece of sheet music by cutting, copying, pasting, or changing notes of a composition. It can also be used to compose an original piece of music. The program is manipulated by the computer's mouse. With movement of the mouse the user places the cursor on notes and carries them to the music staff or places music in a graphic keyboardlike grid.

VideoWorksII is an animation program that also lets the user draw work and control the movements of the characters created. One can animate more than 24 different moving objects at the same time, add sound effects, and make the computer talk! The software lets you animate pictures in real time or in frame-by-frame increments. It also includes a program that lets the user create quick and easy slide show presentations on the computer.

Together these three programs provide a comprehensive set of creativity tools that clients can use to make art and express their feelings. Because of the unique user interface, children or adolescents who have never used a computer before can easily learn and adapt to new skills, such as drawing and animating objects on a computer screen or composing melody lines.

One of the key elements in these particular creativity programs is that any action done on the computer can be undone by the user. That is to say, if a client draws a line or places a note down on the staff and doesn't like it, the client can undo it and take the line or note away without any other consequences. This feature provides the security to experiment and try things out that one might not do on paper or canvas due to a fear of making mistakes.

Another key element of this software is that it works in real time. This means that as the user places notes down on the staff, the notes are heard instantly. As the user records the movement of the mouse on the screen, the recording plays back instantly, both visually and in sound. The user can even change the drawing being animated, while it is animating. These kinds of features allow children and adolescents with emotional and behavioral problems to make quick changes easily without conflict, embarrassment, or frustration.

PROGRAM

In order to give clients a sense of control over their environment I provide a milieu in which individuals can make their own choice as to the kinds of materials and tools they desire to work with. This allows the therapist to witness one's initial gestalt toward new media and tools. In the art therapy room the computer, drawing, music, and animation software are available along with other tactile art media, both two- and three-dimensional. As individuals enter the room they are asked to choose whatever art media they desire to work with. Some clients work on long-term art projects, while others create new artwork during each session. Some children and adolescents work primarily on the computer; others choose to work with a variety of art materials. Depending on the age, size of group, and gender, a variety of computer responses and work ethics takes place in art therapy. Working individually with clients on the Macintosh versus working in groups does not necessarily speed up the learning process. Children and adolescents tend to enjoy teaching each other new computer skills. It not only builds their self-esteem but gives them the opportunity to interact with peers on a level different then they are used to. In the long run, I have found that individual computer art therapy sessions seem to allow the therapist and client a greater opportunity to interact and follow through on specific themes and therapeutic goals.

Therapy using computers consists of clients mastering the tool and talking about created products—drawings, animations, and music compositions. Having the ability instantly to play back an animation sequence, look at a drawing, or hear a song on the computer is an important step in the thera-peutic process. Looking at work on the computer, session to session, allows individuals to review personal issues in an enjoyable way. Children and adolescents enjoy talking about their computer work, because they produced it themselves and feel good about having mastered the computer. A high percentage of children and adolescents are immediately drawn to computers. Many are familiar with other kinds of computer systems to play games and do school work with. Because of the graphic user interface, children and adolescents can adapt to the more sophisticated features offered by the Macintosh while still perceiving the process as enjoyable.

Children and adolescents with behavioral and emotional difficulties are able to control their hyperactive, manipulative, or destructive behavior in mastering the computer. It provides a world for them to build new sets of learning skills in which they can transfer their way of thinking about them-selves and others. The computer provides categories more useful than "good" or "bad" and allows people to make their own decisions. In creating their own world, clients can build an environment in which they can be successful and feel positive about their achievements.

Because of their acting-out behavior, children and adolescents with be-havioral and emotional problems tend to be treated negatively in their school surroundings. Often they are unable to achieve successfully in such school surroundings due to their emotional insecurity. In art therapy, the computer can create an environment that is creative, smart, and friendly. It is like a teacher who does not get mad about mistakes, but gives individual attention, and lets clients work at their own pace. Working with the computer can enhance a student's self-esteem because the student is in control and can achieve intellectually while focusing on creative problems, in an environment without conflict. The software programs are challenging and interesting, so they hold the client's attention. Clients with learning disabilities are able to concentrate and work longer on drawings at the computer because there are a variety of creative possibilities to be explored and because the computer is simple to use.

Slow learners have very little difficulty learning how to control the com-puter and are intrigued by the limitless possibilities. Children and adolescents who are overly dependent on the therapist's attention when they are using other art media do not need extra attention while working with the computer and do not become frustrated by having to learn the necessary procedures to make the computer work.

One can be very articulate about the work one produces on the Macintosh. Drawing on the computer in "fat bits" mode allows an individual to draw an image pixel by pixel (dot by dot). "Fat bits" magnifies the drawing area so one can work in detail.

The ability to draw pictures on a computer and have them move around the screen is intriguing to a child or teenager. The ability to express an idea in pictures that move around like cartoons also creates a feeling of empowerment and fascination. According to Anthony Reveaux (1977):

> Animation is the art of ideas in motion. It can choreograph the actions of recognizable, everyday objects or zoom off into abstract spaces of fantasy. Even more special is its ability to change from one domain to another, to combine the real and the unreal, all breathing with the rhythm of thought. It can be audio-visual love poetry of mixed metaphors and transformations, logical comparisons and impossible puns. Animation is a syntheses of the design of painting articulated with the tempo of music and, like the dance it's most alive when in motion. (p. 2)

As art therapists we look at personal imagery on paper and ask our clients and ourselves, "What is the image doing and saying?" We question the placement, action, and movement of the object. Through these observations we seek to reveal a personal story to begin a dialogue with our client.

With the Macintosh computer and VideoWorksII, storytelling can be enhanced through viewing moving pictures. This nonstatic approach encourages clients to express what is going on in their minds visually and in motion. Unlike static images, animation sequences can be played back on the computer and viewed like cartoons. Like dream sequences, they tell a story in pictures and deal with many layers of consciousness. With this new tool come new ways for individuals to begin thinking about some of the difficult issues they face. Shooting-rockets, aliens from space, exploding bombs, rolling tanks, and animated love poems are just a few of the animated imageries created by clients in art therapy using the Macintosh computer. Enthusiasm in understanding this new technology offers clients and therapists innovative approaches for learning, listening, and thinking about personal problems.

CASE EXAMPLES

CASE EXAMPLE 1: RANDY

Randy (fictional name), a 7-year-old Hispanic male, attended art therapy sessions for 2 months. He came to individual sessions once a week, for an

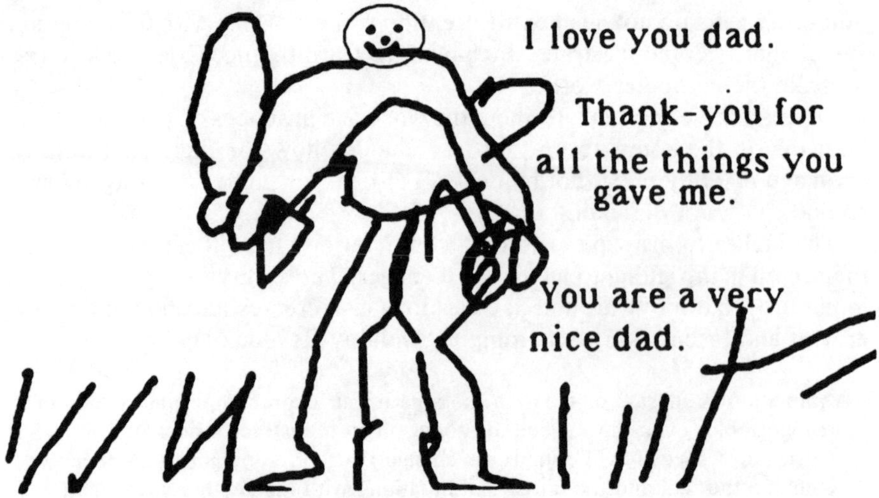

I love you dad.

Thank-you for all the things you gave me.

You are a very nice dad.

Figure 15.1. "Goldi Locks and the Three Bears." Randy used MacPaint to draw a picture of his father with huge muscles.

hour. Randy was sent to the psychiatric facility because he set fire to his mother's home and set toys on fire at his father's home. He had become increasingly unmanageable at home with his mother and his behavior had deteriorated at his elementary school, where he was in first grade. His parents were separated and had been apart for 4 years. His father worked days as a mechanic and his mother worked evenings as a waitress.

Randy feared the limits that his father set and begged for limits from his mother. He got anxious to the point of physical illness with his father and provoked his mother sometimes to tears with his behavior and verbalizations. Randy had frequent nightmares and was often preoccupied with violence and violent play.

In art therapy, Randy was immediately drawn to the computer and was exceptional at working with it. He could sit for a full hour drawing and animating pictures. He was able to follow directions and control the programs without any help. He understood the different features available and would retain what he learned from previous sessions. Randy commented that he thought he was getting good at the computer and was impressed that he had so much control over it. He recognized words from the menu bar and had no difficulty resizing windows, working in the paint programs, using various "edit" and "undo" features, and "saving" his work. Randy used the animation software like an electronic puppet stage. He quickly learned how to animate pictures in real time. He created his own characters, and had them carry on a dialogue.

In Figure 15.1 Randy used the drawing software to draw a picture of his father. Next to his drawing he wrote, "I love you dad. Thank-you for all the things you gave me. You are a very nice dad." Randy drew huge muscles on his dad's arms.

Figure 15.2 shows three sequences taken from an animation Randy produced. He named it "Never Ending Story." The animation begins by having a policeman go toward a dragon. He used MacinTalk™ in Video-WorksII to have the police say to the dragon, "I am sorry, dragon, I have to fight you." Next a little boy comes out on the screen and the computer says, "I like going everywhere, I like God, God is a good guy, I like dragons." Randy included many different sound effects in his movie by selecting the choices from the sound menu.

Randy's creations provide a good example of how a computer and creativity software can help an emotionally troubled child work out frustrations, fears, wishes, and anxieties. Because the computer is so easy to use, Randy was never bogged down trying to save documents to disk or making backup copies. Randy was able to create art and little movies and have fun at the computer while not even realizing that he was going through therapy. By the fifth session, Randy was discussing some of his issues over setting fires. A sense of security, self-esteem, and trust had been growing over the weeks. A combination of feeling positive about himself and trusting his therapist supported an environment for personal growth and communication.

CASE EXAMPLE 2: SAM

Sam (fictional name) is a 17-year-old White adopted male. He was hospitalized at the psychiatric hospital because he wielded a knife and threatened to cut his wrists. He had previously been hospitalized because he did in fact cut his wrists. Sam was adopted at the age of 3½ months. He had a problematic early childhood, a history of poor adjustment in school, and had been in self-contained behavioral disorder programs. Sam's parents requested residential funding for him because of his inability to function in their home.

Sam attended group art therapy sessions, once a week, for 3 months. From the very beginning he was interested in using the computer to produce animation, and he maintained good behavior in working with peers.

Sam spent 5 weeks on his first animation sequence. He named it "The Search for Moby Dick." He worked primarily in "fat bits." This allowed him to be very articulate about his drawings. Sam also brought in pictures of ships to look at for reference. In "The Search for Moby Dick," (Fig. 15.3), a ship appears from one corner of the screen and the whale comes out from the other. At the same time, both objects move toward each other. Before they meet the computer says, "There she blows! Get ready for attack." When the ship and the whale meet head on, the ship explodes.

VideoWorksII was a software program for Sam to master and a tool that allowed him to produce narrative stories. He was extremely proud that he

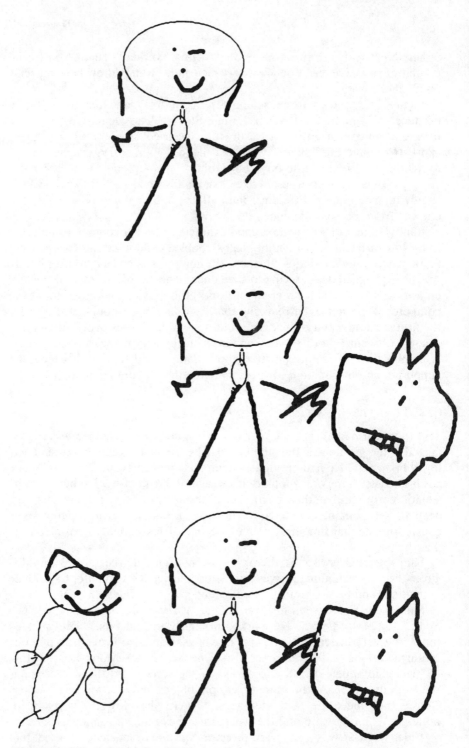

Figure 15.2. "Never Ending Story." Randy said the animation was about a policeman chasing a dragon.

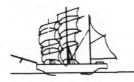

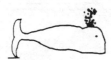

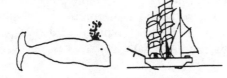

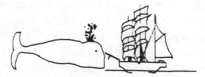

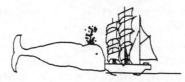

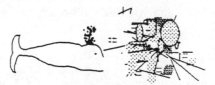

Figure 15.3. "The Search for Moby Dick." Sam worked primarily in "fat bits."

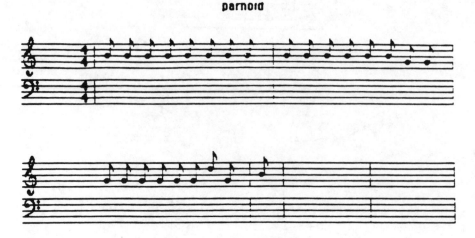

Figure 15.4. The music score Sam wrote, "Parnoid" (sic).

had completed a goal he had set. These accomplishments built his self-esteem, and were an encouraging force in motivating him to produce further animations. Sam's primary therapist interpreted the ship as Sam's mother and the whale as his father. He also commented that his mother and father had marital problems. Perhaps Sam was expressing his family problems metaphorically.

Soon after Sam completed his animation, he mentioned that he had a rock band and he wanted to write some music for it. He used the music program to do this and named his song "Parnoid" (sic). Figure 15.4 shows the music score Sam wrote. This was the first sign Sam gave that permitted us to begin talking about some of his personal problems. The environment was now safe enough to begin discussing some of his paranoid feelings.

This last animation sequence Sam produced was a drawing of a mountain range with many different paths. He named it "What A View." Figure 15.5 shows six sequences taken from the animation. Sam drew a mountain range and a small black dot to represent a person. The movement in this animation is of this person traveling up one of the paths.

While working on his animation Sam talked about his love for the outdoors and about living on his own. Shortly after "What A View" was completed, Sam ran away from the hospital. Unfortunately, he left the psychiatric center before resolving his problems. It would be unfair to draw a direct corollary between Sam and the dot traveling up the path, but it should be suggested that Sam may have been unconsciously reflecting his wishes to be free and on his own.

CASE EXAMPLE 3: DAVID

David, (fictional name), a 12-year-old White male, was at the psychiatric hospital because he allegedly set a fire in a restaurant. Actually David had

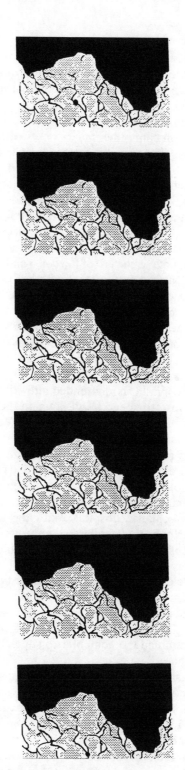

Figure 15.5. "What a View." Sam drew a small black dot to represent a person. In the animation the dot travels up the path.

been lighting pieces of paper in the restroom and then throwing them in a toilet, where the fire would go out. David had what he called a fascination with fires and admitted to having set at least four. David claimed he had another person living inside him, who made him do bad things.

David's hospitalization cannot be understood without an overview of his earlier experiences. In 1978 he and his mother lived in an apartment building which had three fires in a brief period of time. During the third fire David and his mother safely left the building, but David's mother returned to rescue children who were still inside. She saved three children but received severe burns and injuries in the process. She was hospitalized for years and in a coma for many months. David was taken to foster placements, and he thought that his mother was dead, since she was in a coma.

David's mother eventually came out of the coma and gained enough strength to leave the hospital. David's first contact with her was traumatic, since he had been under the impression that she was dead. Eventually their relationship was reestablished to the extent that they were permanently reunited.

In David's social assessment from the psychiatric hospital, it is noted that his fire setting, in light of his history, should be seen as his attempt to master a tremendously traumatic experience rather than a repetitious pattern of sociopathic conduct.

At the psychiatric hospital David attended individual art therapy sessions for 2½ months. He chose to spend a full hour on the Macintosh computer each session. He was patient, enthusiastic, and had excellent control over this tool.

David discussed his familiarity with using computers for doing math and other homework. He drew pictures on the Macintosh fluidly and immediately discovered different options that the software programs provided.

Much of David's imagery on the computer was a reflection of his feelings about living at the psychiatric hospital. With the animation program he produced animated cartoons that exhibited humorous and serious overtones. He became quite fluent with the software and would produce one or two different animation sequences each session.

The first animated cartoon was about a prisoner being captured and running away from jail. David said he was the person who wanted to get out, that is, out of the hospital. Figure 15.6 shows four sequences from an animation David named "Star Chaser." He drew a birdlike animal chasing a boat/car. David programmed the computer to say, "Let's get him. Get him now, let's get out of here."

In "Red Bomb Flash" (Fig. 15.7), planes are chasing each other. David also programmed the computer to say, "Get him now. Let's get out of here."

David named Figure 15.8 "der5r 2,0000." The six sequences display a cartoon of a man throwing popcorn at a robot. David was quite articulate about his drawings and made sure the timing of the sound and animation was correct. This animation reveals his sense of humor and his understanding of sequential movement.

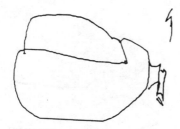

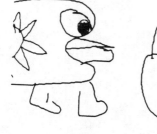

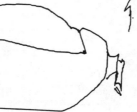

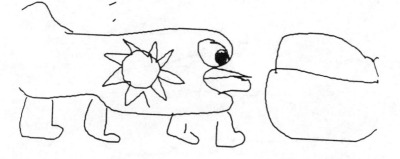

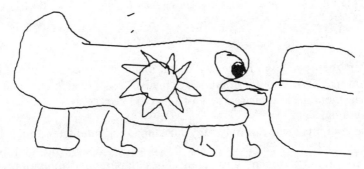

Figure 15.6. "Star Chaser." David used MacinTalk to program the computer to say, "Let's get him. Get him now, let's get out of here."

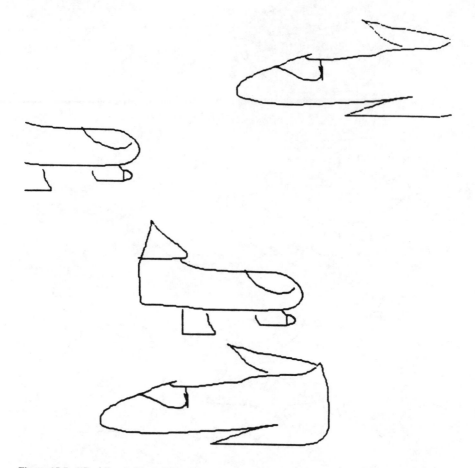

Figure 15.7. "Red Bomb Flash." David programmed the computer to say, "Get him now, let's get out of here."

In art therapy David fantasized about machines, robots, and computers. He said that his computer at home got mad at him. He also commented that when he went back to his real school he would be able to work on computers all day long.

The computer was not only fun, intriguing, and intelligent, but it became a friend to David. He became animated while making his cartoons and enjoyed watching them move and talk. The computer and animation software provided David the means to transform some of his fantasies onto another medium outside of himself.

In the sixth session, David discussed his fears about being alone, seeing ghosts, and having nightmares. He was beginning to open up and feel comfortable enough to talk directly about his problems. It was recommended to

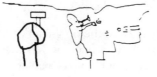

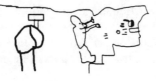

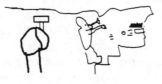

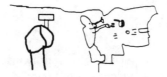

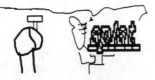

Figure 15.8. "der5r, 2,0000." Six sequences taken from an animated cartoon of a man throwing popcorn at a robot.

his primary therapist that he have the opportunity to continue working with creativity software and computers once he left the hospital. This tool provided a safe and fulfilling environment for David in which he could be creative, grow intellectually, and feel positive about his development.

DISCUSSION AND RESULTS

The Apple Macintosh Computer along with drawing, animation, and music software allows clients to be successful in art production, master the computer hardware, and control their environment. Providing these tools gives clients with behavioral and emotional problems a sense of self-satisfaction while allowing them to participate in a unique, stimulating, and creative learning process. Creative and developmental growth in eye-hand coordination, visual motor skills, logical reasoning processes, creative decision making, and interpersonal relationships can all be enhanced through the use of the Macintosh.

Continual use of computers and creativity software by children and adolescents with learning disabilities produced positive changes in their behavior. The results included increased attention span and development of visual expression, music expression, self-confidence, creativity, and communicative skills. We've seen that children and adolescent clients can benefit from this technological arena of easy-to-use computer hardware and software. Whether or not computers advance art therapy techniques now lies in the hands of art therapists.

CONCLUSION

Art therapists using traditional art therapy techniques may find implementing computers and creativity software in their sessions to be both educational and therapeutic for their clients. The modality used will differ depending on the therapist's approach. This difference of orientation will help expand the multifaceted usages of computers in our field and advance us into new arenas. New software programs are constantly being produced for creative purposes. These new tools can make our work and our lives more exciting and interesting. Software stores, friends who own computers, computer user-group meetings, and computer magazines are just a few resources for information on computers.

In the future, computers will become even more friendly and easy to use. The Apple Macintosh currently provides an easy way to represent inner thoughts with pictures. These new computer art therapy tools will help many clients open up and find the creative talent inside themselves. Sometimes it takes a modern tool like a computer to stimulate clients today.

GLOSSARY

Backup copy.   A second copy of computer information, usually stored on disks.

Creativity software.   Contrasted with business or video game software. Examples: MusicWorks, VideoWorksII.

Cursor.   An indicator on a computer's screen that marks the position at which interaction will happen.

Disk.   A magnetic recording device used to store computer information.

Edit.   To change, alter, or improve any type of computer information.

Hardware.   The physical electronic elements in a computer. Like the record player. See *software.*

MacinTalk.   A program that turns words typed on the Macintosh computer into speech that can be heard from the computer.

Macintosh.   A portable computer manufactured and developed by Apple Computer.

Menu.   A list of available options from which the user can make a selection.

Menu bar.   The bar located at the top of the Macintosh's screen showing a list of menus.

Mouse.   A device that can move a pointer or cursor (see *cursor*) on a video screen. Moving the "mouse" on a flat surface (at or near the keyboard) moves the cursor or pointer.

Pixel.   A picture element; the smallest dot that can be produced on a video screen. The number of pixels that can be produced across and down the screen is a measure of the screen's resolution.

Programming.   The process of developing software.

Real time.   A term used to describe a computer program that appears to produce the end result as soon as inputs are received, as opposed to a program that stores the inputs for later processing and display.

Saving work.   Storing computer information on a disk.

Software.   Like the record on the record player. See *hardware.*

Undo.   To take back the last action that has occurred on the computer.

User interface.   The manner in which the user relates to the computer or to the program running on it. The Macintosh's interface is also known as "user friendly" in that it easily moves at the command of the user, helps the user out, and provides the user with various options and devices to achieve his or her objectives. Hardware devices such as a touch screen or mouse or software devices such as menus or icons are additional parts of the user interface.

Window.   The screen itself or portion of the screen that displays the program. Windows can be resized or overlapped or overlaid.

WYSIWYG. "What you see is what you get," the instantaneous result of working on a computer.

REFERENCES

Aker, S. (1986, May). Child's play. *MacUser,* pp. 83–88.

D'Ignazio, F. (1984). Babes in Microland. In S. Ditlea (Ed.), *Digital deli: The lunch group.* New York: Workman.

Gardner, H. (1982). *Art, mind, and brain: A cognitive approach to creativity.* New York: Basic.

Nathan, J. (1985). *Micro-myths.* Minneapolis: Winston.

Reveaux, A. (1977). *The art of animation.* Chevron Gallery Catalog Essay. San Francisco: Chevron Gallery.

Turkle, S. (1984). *The second self: Computers and the human spirit.* New York: Simon & Schuster.

CHAPTER 16

The Marriage of Art Therapy and Psychodrama

JEAN PETERSON IN COLLABORATION WITH LEIGH FILES

During 15 years of training and working professionally as an art therapist, psychotherapist, and psychodramatist, I have become increasingly aware of the rich cross-fertilization possible between the fields of art psychotherapy and psychodrama. Although I firmly believe that our most effective learning comes through direct experience (i.e., through action), I would like to conceptualize in writing the foundations of psychodramatic art therapy, the marriage of art therapy and psychodrama.

I will discuss some of the central concepts of Jacob L. Moreno, M.D., the founder of sociometry and psychodrama, particularly relevant to art therapy. I will then describe psychodramatic art therapy techniques appropriate for use in different phases of group process. Although many of these techniques may be adapted for use in individual art therapy, the focus of this chapter is on group art therapy, as psychodramatic process is essentially group oriented.

HISTORY AND CONTEXT OF PSYCHODRAMA AND SOCIOMETRY

The founder of psychodrama and sociometry was Jacob Levy Moreno (1892–1974) (1946; 1959; 1969). For Moreno, change in society itself is the ultimate goal of individual therapeutic change. In *Who Shall Survive?* (1953), he proclaims: "A truly therapeutic procedure cannot have less an objective than the whole of mankind" (p.3). This removes therapy from the realm of a sometimes over precious involvement with the intricacies of each isolated individual psyche and places the individual always in the context of relationships.

Moreno was himself an artist, deeply involved in theater, and a poet. His original Theatre of Spontaneity fully utilized the powerful contributions of the visual arts through the spontaneous creation, in the moment, of settings, masks, and costumes.

In the theatre for spontaneity, because of a lack of standardized and rehearsed plays repeated in the same fashion every night, a new postulate automatically resulted: to invent a form of backdrop or background which could be adjusted to the dramatic scenes as they changed from day to day, indeed, as it changed within one performance a hundredfold, and which creates a correspondingly flowing, adaptable and momentary background. The idea was simple. It consisted in impromptu settings, a number of wooden pieces in various sizes, colors and forms. We also used impromptu drawings. The impromptu painter steps upon the stage and illustrates before the audience the coming scene and continues as the scene develops. It is the return to the clapboard, refashioned to the requirements of the stage. Lasting and solid materials, as leather, glass, wood and cardboard, are covered with white lacquer upon which drawings with carbon can be made. At the end of the scene the drawing is washed off.

The actors were dressed and made up in accordance with the role; the masks were cut and painted in front of the public. An impromptu tailor was used who improvised costumes out of simple materials for the scenes to come. (Moreno, 1947, p. 69)

Some of the richness of creative imagery and the powerful ceremonial, ritual quality provided by this use of art tends often to be lost, as psychodramatists have tended to become more clinical and psychodrama itself has become at times more "conserved" and less creative. The marriage of art therapy and psychodrama can infuse psychodrama again with its own original heritage of involvement with the arts. This involvement can also be expanded by creative application of the valuable resources now available in the growing field of art therapy.

This marriage with psychodrama also broadens and deepens the scope of art therapy beyond its sometimes limited self-image as having to do primarily with "interpreting drawings" and with individual process cut off from the therapeutic context of sociometric group process. Art therapy is expanded through a perspective that sees all art making as essentially a mode of enactment. Art products from this perspective are also utilized as props, in the fullest theatrical sense, for ongoing in-depth psychotherapeutic enactment. Art objects can be taken *further* into full personal and interpersonal enactment by the art makers. The art therapy process is not limited to drawing, painting, and sculpture. Activities such as mask making, environment making, and costuming are included. In an enactment framework, art therapy incorporates the use of any objects in the human and nonhuman environment that facilitate the unfolding of healing enactment.

In recent years, in the field of the creative arts therapies there has been some movement toward a more organic and unified view of the role of the arts in therapy, which can serve a vital role in reconnecting the often sterile and fragmented "scientific" mental health professions with the ancient and eternal cross-cultural process of healing. Over the centuries of human history, this has always involved the arts, transformative enactment, and the group or community as integral to the process of healing. The power of Moreno's view of the basic healing principles of spontaneity and creativity and his creation in psychodrama and sociometry of an excellent system through which healing as enactment can take place is being recognized by some creative arts therapists (McNiff, 1981). Psychodramatists, too, need to broaden and deepen their conception of healing enactment to utilize more fully the contribution of the arts.

SPONTANEITY–CREATIVITY: CENTRAL CONCEPT IN MORENO'S THOUGHT

The major link between the creative arts therapies and psychodrama is the crucial centrality in Moreno's work of spontaneity–creativity. Robert Siroka, a leader in the field of psychodrama, has summarized Moreno's concept of spontaneity–creativity as follows:

1. Spontaneity-Creativity is a process of energy distribution, development and exchange which involves responding in novel adequate ways to both old and new situations.
2. Spontaneity can be developed and trained.
3. Spontaneity is differentiated from impulsivity by a different level of cognition which can scan the immediate perceptual field and take new data and environmental shifts and consequences into account while maintaining a heightened sense of originality.
4. Moreno's theory is that spontaneity and anxiety are inversely related, i.e., to the extent you are anxious, you are not spontaneous; to the degree you are spontaneous, you are not anxious.
5. Spontaneity is not automatic but needs to be "warmed-up." (Siroka, 1982, p. 1)

Moreno's theory, then, is a positive one that maintains creativity as central to human nature. Creativity is crucial to human survival. It leads humanity to respond constructively to new situations, an essential capacity in a constantly changing, always somewhat unpredictable world. The more spontaneous and creative the personality the better it can cope with the flow of new problems life is sure to present. The therapeutic process is essentially training for spontaneity–creativity, or, more broadly, training for life. The modality of therapy Moreno developed suited to this goal is psychodrama in the context of sociometry and group psychotherapy.

Much of traditional psychotherapy is aimed largely at reducing anxiety. In general, excessive anxiety is seen in terms of psychopathology and the reduction of anxiety as movement toward health.

Psychodrama, instead of having the goal of reducing anxiety, seeks to increase spontaneity. It is not so much a question of psychodrama being contradictory to traditional therapeutic approaches. The difference is largely in the methodology of treatment and the basic attitudinal approach.

PSYCHODRAMA AS AN ACTION-ORIENTED PROCESS: THE RELEVANCE OF AN ACTION FOCUS FOR ART THERAPY

It says in the Book of Genesis, "In the Beginning was the Word." In psychodrama, "In the Beginning is the Act." Spontaneity is about getting people moving; it has to do with the readiness to *act*. Action is central; doing, not thinking or describing. The individual is the creator—of his or her own play, or, in an art therapy context, of his or her own painting or sculpture. The responsibility for self is retained always by the client (the protagonist in psychodramatic terms). The role of the therapist (the director in psychodramatic terms) is to protect and facilitate the active self-actualizing process of the client. Psychodrama as an action method is very compatible with art therapy, for art making is also an active process. Art making, artist's art or client's art expression, like psychodramatic action, stimulates the free flow of thoughts and feelings and increases spontaneity. In classical psychodrama the action takes place on the stage; in psychodramatic art therapy the stage is the paper and paint, the clay, or other media. Art-making action can also serve as a warm-up for further psychodramatic action in a group. For clients who are severely depressed and find any kind of total bodily action extremely difficult, the smaller "stage" of paper and crayons, for example, can be a less threatening entry or warm-up into physical and psychic action.

PSYCHODRAMA AS A GROUP-ORIENTED PROCESS: THE RELEVANCE OF A GROUP FOCUS FOR ART THERAPY

Before turning to specific examples of psychodramatic art therapy, it is important to focus on psychodrama as a *group*-oriented process. Much art therapy work is done in groups, and skill in utilizing group process effectively is essential to our profession. Unfortunately, this is often a weak spot in art therapy training. I have seen too many art therapists using an extension of an individual therapy model in a group setting. Moreno, who originated much of the work in group process and group psychotherapy, developed an approach that maximizes the use of *the group as the agent, not merely the setting of therapy*. A group psychotherapy situation is not one therapist and a group of patients, but a group of people each of whom is the therapeutic agent of the other, with the designated therapist–leader serving primarily as catalyst and facilitator. What makes a group "work" is the sociometry, the complex network of multilevel relationships among group members.

The two most important forces influencing the sociometry of a group are transference and tele. *Transference*, briefly, refers to the degree to which we see another person not as himself or herself but, through a process of projection, as someone else with whom we have had an important relationship. Moreno considers transference to be a special psychopathological outgrowth of the general interpersonal process that occurs. This process is known as *tele*. Tele loosely corresponds to what are popularly called "vibes." According to Moreno:

> Normal individuals show selective affinities for some persons, and some persons may show selective affinities for them in return . . . this preference for another individual or the preference of another individual for him is in the large majority of cases at least, not due to a symbolic transference, it has no neurotic motivations but *is due to certain realities which this other person embodies and represents.* . . . A complex of feelings which draws one person towards another and which is aroused by the *real* attributes of the other person . . . such a process is called a *tele-relationship.* (1946, p. 229)

Tele appears to be a "given" factor, perhaps based on some as yet undiscovered aspect of individual chemical, physiological, or metaphysical makeup. However, it is possible to expand one's ability to recognize and respond to tele-relationships through increasing one's overall spontaneity level. This in turn also facilitates the process of un-training and working through transference responses (Moreno, 1953). This training for spontaneity is, as I said before in relation to creativity, the primary therapeutic goal. The group therapist understands the structure of the telic and transferential networks in the group and uses this understanding to facilitate the growth of each group member. The primary lines of interaction in a psychodramatic group are often between and among group members and not necessarily from therapist–leader to group members. Indeed, a sociogram involving leader-to-group interactions without interactions within the group would indicate an exceedingly immature and dependency-reinforcing situation. This situation must be guarded against by art therapists, as we sometimes tend to see ourselves as central, the expert "insight givers."

THE THREE-PART STRUCTURE OF PSYCHODRAMATIC GROUP PROCESS

There are three parts to the psychodramatic group process: (1) the *warm-up* phase; (2) the *enactment or action* phase; and (3) the *integration and sharing* phase. This structure applies not only to classical psychodrama, but to any therapeutic group process. It is essential for every psychodramatic art therapist to understand this three-part structure.

The Warm-Up Phase

Moreno speaks of the warming-up process as "the operational expression of spontaneity" (Moreno, 1953, p. 42). "Spontaneous states are brought into existence by various starters. Subjects put their bodies and minds into motion, using body attitudes and mental images which lead them toward attainment of that state. This is called the *warming up process*" (Moreno, 1946, p. 223).

In group process the warm-up phase encompasses the early stages in the overall life of a group, the beginning period of each group session, and the thoughts and feelings each group member brings with him or her into the group. The goal of the warm-up is to bring each person into the "here and now" of the group so that all are psychically present. Warm-up techniques are directed toward helping group members relax, loosen up, get in touch with themselves and each other, feel comfortable in the group, and open channels for spontaneity–creativity. Simultaneously personal discomfort, self-consciousness, and anxiety are reduced. In art therapy groups this process often involves verbal sharing about past experience or inexperience with art media, beginning with nonthreatening, playful, exploratory uses of materials that put little or no emphasis on a finished product. The aim is not only to warm up each individual, but to warm up the group, encouraging free interaction, stimulating the sociometric processes in the group.

The Enactment or Action Phase

It is beyond the scope of this chapter to present all of the important principles and methods of psychodramatic action. I would like briefly to discuss three major dimensions with which a psychodrama director is concerned: time, place, and role. Full psychodramatic action requires these three dimensions to be concretely established.

Time

In psychodrama all action takes place in "the moment." Moreno (1969) defines this as differentiated from "the present":

> The present is a universal, static and passive category. . . . as a transition of the past to the future it is always there. The present is a *formal* category in contradiction from the moment which is a dynamic and a *creative* category; it is through a spontaneous-creative process that the formal category of the present attains dynamic meaning, when it turns into a moment. (pp. 268–269)

All events, past, present, or future, are enacted in the psychodramatic moment.

Place

Establishing place, the setting of the action, helps to "ground" the protagonist. Recreating the scene physically on the stage, or in art media, mobilizes and intensifies the feelings and thoughts associated with the scene. This warms up the protagonist to be "in the moment" rather than just to talk about the situation.

Role

Role theory is one of the foundations of psychodrama. Moreno states: "Role can be defined as the actual and tangible forms which the self takes" (1946,

p. 153). A basic premise of role theory is that human personality develops along many simultaneous dimensions (roles). Psychopathology reflects a distortion of one or more of these aspects or personality and also "often represents a compensatory expression of one facet of the personality primarily due to a lack of development of another" (Blatner, 1973, p. 125). Psychotherapy from the viewpoint of the role theorist emphasizes the expansion of a person's *role repertoire,* the ability to function in a wide variety of roles that can complement and balance each other. This role expansion goes hand and hand with spontaneity–creativity training.

The psychodramatic method provides opportunity for group members to enact many different roles: as protagonist, through role reversal (changing roles with the important figures in one's psychodrama); and as auxiliary egos (persons chosen sociometrically to enact the roles of significant figures). In the role of another, enacting certain behaviors we may personally judge and/or feel threatened by can free us to experience emotional expression and behavior (e.g., expression of hostility) that we cannot yet incorporate as ego-syntonic.

The enactment phase of the group flows from and builds on the warm-up. A protagonist emerges from the warm-up process, ready to explore further some area of his or her life. The specific actions of the psychodrama director and the psychodramatic art therapist may vary, but the basic role is the same—a guide and facilitator for the protagonist's own intrapsychic or interpersonal exploration, a guide who encourages active exploration. Psychodramatic art therapy techniques most appropriate for art therapy groups that include verbal psychotherapeutic exploration follow. The same theoretical framework, however, remains valid for art therapy emphasizing the studio art experience. Here the art therapist's awareness of the internal psychodramatic process involved in artistic creation is important, even though this may not be verbalized.

The Integration and Sharing Phase

This is the final phase in psychodramatic group process. In classical psychodrama it follows the completion of the protagonist's enacted drama. The first concern of the director is to help the protagonist reintegrate into the group after having exposed aspects of his or her inner life. This is accomplished through asking group members to speak personally, opening themselves in return and sharing with the protagonist how his or her drama touched feelings in the lives of group members.

The integration–sharing phase is particularly important in art therapy groups for several reasons. Art making can be a very intensely involving individual process, sometimes giving the individual a feeling of isolation. Reconnecting each individual to others in the group through a personal sharing process is therefore vital to break this sense of isolation. The need for sharing is also magnified in art therapy because there are always multiple internal psychodramas occurring simultaneously while all group members are involved in their own art-making action. The media, color, line, form, and the imagery that emerges all serve to mobilize thoughts and feelings. Some nonverbal dialogue occurs through interaction with the media. It is useful to think of having multiple protagonists and give everyone the opportunity to share verbally as well as visually something of his or her own personal experience in the art process.

Another reason for the emphasis on sharing in art therapy relates to the tendency in the field toward analyzing and interpreting art products. Though there is certainly a place for diagnostic, analytic thinking about artwork, the place for it is usually not, to my mind, verbally within the therapy process itself, group or individual.

In a psychodramatic art therapy group, clients are encouraged to respond to each other and to each other's artwork. A sharing of responses, impressions, and personal associations is encouraged. Direct analysis, interpretation, or questioning is most often related to the personal experience of the interpreter or questioner. When this person can be taught to make a response in the form of sharing personal experience he or she derives more direct cathartic benefit. The protagonists are less likely to feel defensive and more likely to be able to apply aspects of the other's situation to their own and come to their own insights and self-interpretations.

This concentration on sharing is not intended to discount the value and importance in group process of direct interpersonal confrontation, questioning, or cognitive discussion of issues. However, one of the significant differences between psychodramatic art therapy and other approaches to art therapy is its emphasis on a sharing rather than an analyzing–reductive process.

It is important to remember that (1) warm-up, (2) enactment, and (3) integration–sharing is the essential sequence of phases within each group session. It is more important to the group process to allow adequate time for warm-up and sharing than to have major dramatic enactments. With group art therapy processes, as stated before, this is especially true because in this situation there are multiple protagonists experiencing internal psychodramas. The length of the sessions (1½ to 2½ hours is recommended), the size of the group, the specific population, and the level of warm-up determine how much can be included in a single session.

Looking at the entire life span of a group (weeks, months, years), there is also a sequence in terms of which phase is emphasized. Early in the life of a group, warm-up is of primary importance. A session might be focused on warm-up exercises and sharing, with very little depth enactment. As the group begins to "jell" members tend to come in already quite warmed up and more time is spent in enactment and integration–sharing. Toward the termination of an ongoing group, primary attention shifts to integration–sharing with little new material being warmed up or enacted. These are generalizations, but each session remains a unit in itself in which all three phases must be attended to.

PSYCHODRAMATIC ART THERAPY TECHNIQUES

In order to illustrate the broad application of art therapy within a psycho-dramatic framework, I have listed several examples of techniques appropriate to each of the three phases of group process: warm-up, enactment, integration–sharing. These techniques are drawn from my own art therapy–psychodrama practice in several settings: a psychiatric adult in-patient service; a nonresidential therapeutic community; a residential treatment camp for children with special needs; staff training groups of professionals; groups of art therapy trainees; psychodrama groups and classes; and private art psychotherapy groups. Some modification of techniques may be indicated with different populations, and some techniques have application to more than one phase of group process. Many are also applicable to individual work. I hope they may serve as stimuli for the creativity "in the moment" of each therapist who uses them.

Warmup Techniques

1. *Psychodramatic Age Regression to an Early Art Experience.* The aim is to tap group members' general warm-up to art materials and their past experience with art. Ask the group to relax, close their eyes, go back in their minds to a childhood memory of involvement with art, and recreate that experience internally. What are they doing or making? What are their feelings? Who else is involved in the incident? Allow enough silence for images to develop. Ask group members to share psychodramatically, speaking from the role of their child selves in the here and now. Encourage group members to share with and relate to each other's memories. Facilitate expression of both positive and negative past experiences with art.

2. *Images Expressive of Present Feeling State.* The purpose is to open communication about how members are feeling as they enter the group. Ask group members to relax, close eyes, and tune in to how they are feeling. Encourage them to allow an image to appear in their mind's eye. If they were a color or had color, what color would they be now? What shape, form, texture, size, medium? Would they have movement or sound? Allow enough silence for internal images to develop. Ask group members to share their images. For a group new to art media, begin with verbal sharing. This may spontaneously create a desire to draw, paint, or sculpt the image. A group more comfortable with art media may move immediately to a visual sharing through art expression. When art materials are used, facilitate fast, spontaneous expression and return quickly to the group for verbal and visual sharing of images. The goal is to help group members warmup and connect to each other; they should not go deeply into themselves before they feel related as a group.

3. *Warmup to the Art Space.* This is used when working in a space with

a wide variety of art materials and equipment. Have the group get up, walk around, explore the space, look at various media, poke into closets and cabinets, get a sense of what materials are available and where they are. Give a tour of the space, pointing out where various materials are kept. Encourage people to take responsibility for getting out their own materials, choosing their own work space, cleaning up. All these activities are *actions* that get people moving, warming them up to more spontaneous involvement.

4. *The Group Scribble Game*. This is used to promote sociometric interaction and spontaneous flow of imaginative images. Have group members take a stack of paper and crayons. Ask them to move around the room until they find someone they would like to make contact with—a sociometric choice. Ask pairs to sit together and play Winnicott's (1971) Squiggle Game. One person makes a free spontaneous scribble and gives it to the other, who then creates an image out of the scribble. Then partners reverse roles and repeat the exercise, continuing rapidly through several sequences. Encourage partners to talk to each other about the process and the projected images. Have the group change partners, again choosing sociometrically, and repeat the process. This can be continued several times before the group is called together for general sharing.

5. *Fast Feeling Drawings (Sculptures) and Sociometric Placement*. Have group members take a stack of paper and some drawing implements (or several lumps of clay). Ask them to make a series of rapid images in response to affective words (Denny, 1972) such as *love, fear, joy, freedom, anger*. The leader begins the series, then encourages group members to suggest words. Complete the series by asking group members for a final image expressing their own present feeling state. Share and compare images to build group cohesiveness and illustrate the strong relationship between affect and qualities of art expression. Then ask group members to choose an image, their own or someone elses, most expressive of some aspect of themselves at the moment. Have members place these images on the floor next to the other(s) they feel most related to. This is one form of "action sociogram," substituting artwork placement for direct interpersonal choices (e.g., "Put your hand on the shoulder of the person you feel closest to.").

A variation on this is to do pre- and post-sharing sociometric placement. Have members choose one of their drawings that best represents them in the moment. Then, before any verbal sharing, ask the group to look at all the images and place their drawings sociometrically. After verbal sharing about the images, give the opportunity for anyone who would like to change the placement of his or her image and share about this.

As the art process and imagery involved in an art exercise become more involved, the line between the warm-up and action phase of the therapeutic process becomes blurred. As previously stated, all art-making processes are essentially enactment, involving internal psychodramas in the interaction of the artists with thoughts and feelings stirred up by the images created and intensified through the qualities of the art media and the activity of the art-making process. The next techniques listed can readily be extended into further exploration through externalized psychodramatic enactment.

6. *"Draw a Place That Is [Has Been] Important to You."* The purpose is to facilitate open personal communication among group members about their lives. When images are complete, have group members share about their places, where they are, what is important about them, feelings brought up by the action of creating the place on paper. Depending on group needs, you may vary the directions, e.g., "Draw a place where you felt really good," or "Draw a place from your life that gave you trouble." This may lead directly to the emergence of a protagonist. The drawing itself, or an expansion of it, may be used as "backdrop" to the psychodrama.

7. *"Draw the Floor Plan of the House [Apartment] Where You Grew Up."* Here the psychodramatic functions of "setting the scene," establishing place and time, are directly brought into play. The individual is asked actually to draw the scene of innumerable childhood interactions and events. This action stimulates and intensifies feelings related to the scene and warms the individual up to dealing therapeutically with childhood issues. Because of the intensity of this technique, allow for adequate sharing from all group members. This process leads easily to further psychodramatic action. The action may be taken further through media as well, by suggesting group members make another image exploring a specific room in their house or a specific memory that has been aroused (Fig. 16.1).

8. *"Draw a Significant Person in Your Life."* The "empty chair" is a classic psychodrama warm-up. An empty chair is placed on the stage. The group is directed to allow a person from their life to appear for them in the chair. From this flows a process of sharing, dialogue, and role reversal with the people in the chair, and the emergence of a protagonist for full psychodrama. In an adaptation using art media, direct the group to look at the empty paper (or unformed lump of clay) before them until a person from their life appears; then use the media available to create an image of that person that expresses the essence of the relationship. This warm-up process can be moved into further action in several ways. Group members can introduce the persons they have emotionally brought into the room. When it is evident that a person has "unfinished business" with the person portrayed, the image can be placed before him or her as he or she is asked to address the person directly. To move a step further into psychodrama, have group members give their image to the person in the group who could best play the role of the other for them. This taps the sociometry of the group, identifying chosen auxiliaries. A one-way verbal cathartic expression can thus be expanded to a dialogue involving a spontaneous auxiliary and role reversal. A possible final step would be a full psychodrama involving scene setting, other auxiliaries, and so on.

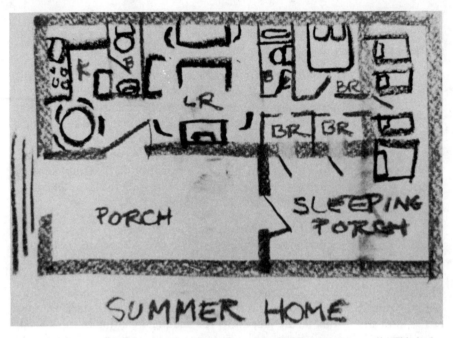

Figure 16.1. "Draw the floor plan of the house [apartment] where you grew up." "This is the summer house where I went with my family every year. We all slept together on the sleeping porch."

9. *Mask Making.* Wearing masks has, throughout all human culture, had a magical power to enable us to become someone "other" or "more" than we experience ourselves as being. Simple masks can be made easily and quickly with simple art media of many kinds (e.g., paper plates, scissors, markers, crepe paper, yarn) to be used in many ways. Group members can make masks of significant people in their lives (as in preceding exercises), of specific emotions, of fantasy or mythological characters that intrigue them, of persons or qualities they fear. An endless variety of self-persentations and role reversals is possible using these masks.

10. *Costumes and Hats.* Mask making can be augumented or substituted with the use of creative costuming to enhance role playing. All that is necessary is a trunk full of various lengths of fabrics of many designs, colors, and types and a miscellaneous collection of distinctive garments, hats, belts, and so on. Hats and costumes can also be made using crepe paper, staples, construction paper, feathers, and the like.

Enactment Techniques

1. *Shift from Verbal Expression to Nonverbal Art Expression When Spontaneity Is Blocked in the Verbal Mode.* In the process of psychodrama, or

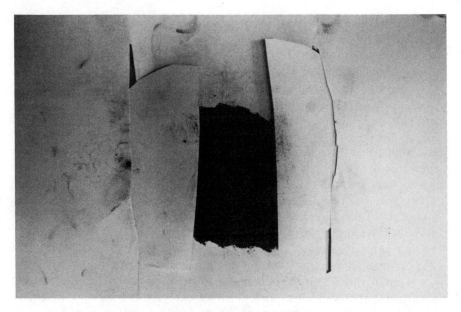

Figure 16.2. Going inside or behind psychodramatically. "That's my 'black hole' behind the trapdoor. I'm afraid I'll get sucked into it, so the trapdoor protects me."

in psychotherapy of any kind, a person may become stuck. The psychodramatic procedure in this situation is to change one of three major dimensions of time, place, or role. A further option is to change the mode of expression. This may be done through use of movement without words, or through expression with art materials.

2. *Use of Art Media as the Stage of Action.* When a person has created an image indicating possible further action, the therapist may remove that paper (or lump of clay), replacing it with another and directing the person to portray "what happens next." This process of "scene changing" can be continued until some resolution is reached in the action.

3. *Going Inside or Behind Psychodramatically.* People often portray blocked or evasive images—for example, walls they cannot go over or through, a box or enclosure they or someone or something else is within, the facade of their house, a face with no expression or a stereotyped expression not reflective of the client's true feelings. In such situations it is effective to change the scene by actually going behind or inside the image. The therapist may turn over the paper on which the first image is drawn and direct the person to express what is going on behind, or, in the case of a wall-like image, provide scissors actually to make a hole in the wall to look through. Add new paper underneath on which the view of the other side can be drawn. If the person cannot cut through the wall, encourage the fantasy perspective of peeking over the top (Fig. 16.2).

4. *Completion of or Change in the Image*. In sharing about an art product, a person may become aware of new feelings and express an "act hunger" to make an addition or change in the image. The therapist supports the enactment of the desired change in the moment.

5. *Doubling Through the Media*. The therapist or another group member warmed up empathically to the protagonist may work alongside with art materials, taking a supportive internal role of psychodramatic "double." The auxiliary may double through the media or verbally as well. For example, with a client who begins to pound clay and then stops abruptly or makes some comment about "getting out anger," the double may begin pounding as well, very gradually increasing the intensity of both nonverbal and verbal expression. The role of the double is to enact what he or she senses the protagonist to be feeling but not expressing. This encourages the protagonist's further expression of feeling.

6. *Create a Cartoon Story*. Direct the group to tune in individually to a situation they are currently dealing with and draw a cartoon sequence about it, writing in verbal and internal dialogues between the characters. Sharing these cartoons may lead to enactment of one of the situations with live, sociometrically chosen auxiliaries.

7. *A Group Cartoon Sociodrama*. Group members are often dealing with similar issues and roles; for example, they may be patients in the same hospital or students in the same school. This situation lends itself to sociodrama as well as psychodrama. Sociodrama is the exploration of common social roles rather than a single protagonist's interpersonal or intrapersonal roles. Sociodramatic action can be initiated through the creation of group cartoons around a common theme, for example, being in the hospital. One person begins the cartoon, setting the scene, and others take turns spontaneously, adding elements, characters, dialogue to express their perceptions of the situation. Follow by sharing and discussion of the issues portrayed.

8. *Nonverbal Dialogue Drawings*. This technique is effective as a modality for the exploration of problematic interactions between group members, or when group members have a need to make close contact but seem unable to verbalize feelings directly to each other. The group members involved are given one piece of paper to share and are directed to engage nonverbally in a diaolgue through art media, responding genuinely from their own feelings and the expressions of the other(s). When the art communication is complete, verbal sharing and discussion follow.

9. *Social Atom*. This technique is based on Moreno's concept of the social atom (the network of important relationships in a person's life). Adapted as a psychodramatic art therapy technique, the procedure is to direct group members to imagine that a piece of paper represents their "life space." They are to place themselves somewhere in the center of their world and place around them all the persons whom they experience emotionally to be within their life space, irrespective of geographic distance, death, or other physical factors. Persons whom they feel closer to should be placed closer to them

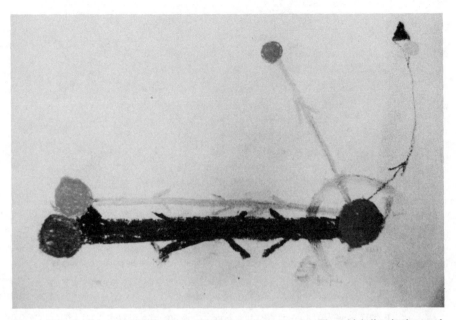

Figure 16.3. Social atom. "This is my life the way it feels now. That thick line is the good feelings between me and my friends. They go both ways. The circle around me is my protection. Mom and Dad are way off in the corner—not very good [feelings between them] right now."

on the page; those who are more important to them should be made graphically larger. Classically in sociometric procedure, females are indicated by circles; males by triangles. It facilitates further spontaneity–creativity and more information about the image maker to encourage the use of personally chosen symbols and colors to represent different figures. This procedure warms up group members to many issues concerning significant relationships or the lack of them. The social atom stimulates an extensive internal psychodrama for each group member making an opportunity for full group sharing important. It also leads easily to further psychodramatic action.

The social atom is also very valuable as a diagnostic tool and can be used as a regular intake procedure. A wealth of information can be gathered simultaneously through this one image. In "reading" a social atom, principles of projective drawing techniques apply. Where special graphic attention of any kind is evident—erasures, changes in size or shape of a figure, changes in placement, differential pressure or intensity of treatment—a problematic relationship is indicated. Certain significant figures—for example, mother, father, wife, husband—may also be conspicuous by their absence (Fig. 16.3).

The Ideal Social Atom.

In the manner just described, picture your world of relationships as you would ideally like it to be. This is an effective modification especially used

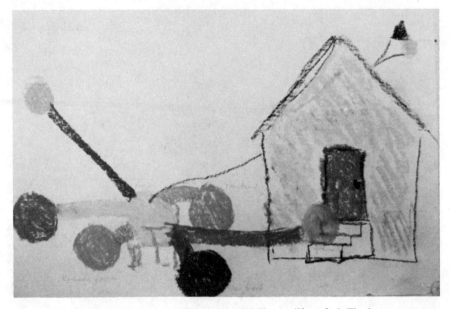

Figure 16.4. The ideal social atom. "This is how I'd like my life to feel. That's me at my new house with all my friends around me. We're having a party. Mom and Dad are in the backyard."

in conjunction with the current social atom. Comparison of the two points to areas where psychodramatic exploration is needed (Fig. 16.4).

The Perceived Social Atom.

This is particularly useful where the focus of therapy is exploration of relationships between clients as in marital or family therapy. In addition to their own social atom, each person is asked to draw the social atom of the other(s) as he or she perceives it. Then both sets of drawings are shared and differences in perception can be discussed and explored. As this process can be quite confrontational it is recommended for use when family members are feeling positive and open with each other.

The Social Atom in Age Regression

Social atoms may be drawn from a psychodramatically age-regressed position as a way of helping group members remember and explore past situations. Allowing people to choose an important past age is usually more fruitful than the director arbitrarily assigning an age to be explored (Fig. 16.5).

10. *Total Psychodramatic Enactment of the Image.* When a client brings in or creates in the group an image especially rich in symbolic significance,

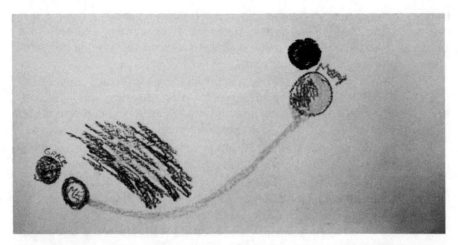

Figure 16.5. The social atom in age regression. "This is how things used to be, before coming here [to therapy 3 years ago]. Mom and I are connected, not Dad. Those scribbles are the "stuff" that gets in the way—the reason I started coming."

the entire image may be enacted psychodramatically, paralleling the process of dream enactment. The protagonist sets up the scene, brings in sociometrically chosen auxiliaries to play the different figures and symbols in the image, and the situation is explored through psychodramatic interaction and role reversal. This process moves beyond the limited technique of an individual group member "gestalting" (speaking from the role of) individual images within an art production.

Integration and Sharing Techniques

The techniques listed here aid in facilitating communication and personal sharing among group members, increase group cohesiveness, and help group members reach closure in the group process.

1. *"Share Through a Graphic Expression What Was Brought Up in You by the Protagonist."* Following intense psychodramatic work, the group is directed to make a quick image expressing their personal response to the protagonist's drama. These images then may be shared nonverbally, accompanied by verbal sharing where appropriate.

2. *"What Gift Would You Give to the Protagonist?"* When the protagonist has expressed particularly vulnerable or needy feelings, direct the group to draw their response and present the picture to the protagonist.

3. *"Make an Abstract Image of How You See the Essence of the Relationship Portrayed."* This may be used when a complex relationship has been explored. It corresponds to the psychodramatic technique of mirroring. Care should be taken that mirroring not be used out of the director's frus-

tration, for example, to "make him see." It is an external technique that can be confrontational and arouse defenses. It should be used only in a supportive group and when there is time to unwind the protagonist's responses to the mirrored relationship.

4. *A Channel for Catharsis in Sharing.* When intense feelings are aroused in a group member by the psychodramatic action, directing this person to express what she or he is feeling directly through art media can provide an immediate arena for catharsis when verbal expression is too threatening.

5. *"Give Yourself a Present."* Group members are asked to draw something they need and/or want to complete the group action for themselves.

6. *Nonverbal Dialogue Drawing.* For sociometric closure, direct group members to move to someone they feel related to through the group process and communicate with him or her through media.

7. *Group Mural.* Full group art expression may be indicated as an expression of group cohesiveness and communication. Encourage a spontaneous flow, rather than working on a prestructured theme, unless the theme emerges naturally from the group process.

8. *Create a Group Environment.* Make available a wide variety of materials (mural paper, colored tissue, fabric, etc.). This creation of a group space fosters group cohesiveness and provides a sociometric post-test as each person selects a comfortable position.

CONCLUSION

The techniques I have listed are only a few suggestions of possible ways of integrating psychodrama and art therapy. Specific techniques, however, are of little value unless they work organically with an evolving therapeutic process in the moment. My main goal in this chapter has been to communicate the importance of seeing psychodrama in its original context of full use of the arts, and specifically to awaken art therapists to utilizing the possibilities of enactment inherent in the visual arts.

REFERENCES

Blatner, H. A. (1973). *Acting-in: Practical applications of psychodramatic methods.* New York: Springer.

Denny, J. M. (1972). Techniques for individual and group art therapy. *American Journal of Art Therapy, 11*(3), 117–134.

McNiff, S. (1981). *The arts and psychotherapy.* Springfield, IL: Charles C. Thomas.

Moreno, J. L. (1946). *Psychodrama* (Vol. 1). New York: Beacon House.

Moreno, J. L. (1947). *The theater of spontaneity.* New York: Beacon House.

Moreno, J. L. (1953). *Who shall survive?* New York: Beacon House.

Moreno, J. L. (1959). *Psychodrama* (Vol. 2). New York: Beacon House.

Moreno, J. L. (1969). *Psychodrama* (Vol. 3). New York: Beacon House.

Siroka, R. W. (1982). *Spontaneity–creativity*. Unpublished manuscript.

Winnicott, D. W. (1971). *Therapeutic consultations in child psychiatry*. New York: Basic.

CHAPTER 17

Six Starting Points in Art Therapy with Children

LENORE STEINHARDT

Children attending art therapy in a semivoluntary setting need to recognize from the outset that there is something in therapy for them to gain. They can easily be scared off and refuse to return. The first phase of interaction between therapist and child client is sufficiently important to warrant an attempt to correlate available art therapy techniques to this beginning stage in order to develop ease in using art materials, and to encourage the child's acceptance of his or her own graphic imagery and graphic ability. To get the work started as soon as possible, the therapist must be able to assess the child's needs and choose an effective starting point, one which will capture the child's interest and help pave the way for the subsequent therapeutic process. In later stages of therapy, when a secure bond of trust exists between child and therapist, there is time to allow for developing appropriate intervention techniques through the work itself. But at the start, there is no time for experimentation to see what works.

Children begin therapy at different levels of internal organization and differ in their readiness to accept control of the art activity or responsibility for the outcome. Art therapy issues, such as the relevance of a nondirective approach versus a structured approach, are crucial as the therapist gauges a child's beginning anxiety, willingness, or resistance to work in art. Since children start off in unique psychic places, they must be approached individually and enabled to perceive themselves as able to choose and create situations appropriate to their needs.

In this chapter I present six interventions that I find effective in facilitating interaction between art therapist and child client at the earliest stage of therapy. As techniques, they are often used in the therapeutic process. In this chapter, however, the emphasis is on their function in this early phase and variations on their use that prove helpful in engagement. The interventions are: simultaneous graphic mirroring of the client's artwork; a nonverbal "conversation" drawing; the Squiggle Game invented by Winnicott (1971); a directed scribble drawing; child acting as graphic secretary for the therapist;

and therapist acting as graphic secretary for the child. Brief case studies illustrate child and therapist interaction through these techniques.

FIRST INTERVIEW

The art therapy setting described here is located in a children's therapy center serving the school population of Ramat Hasharon, Israel. It is a free service of the board of education and the local educational psychological service. Art therapy groups are run as after-school special creative arts activities, removing some of the stigma from the fact that the children's emotional and behavioral dysfunctions have brought them here and the purpose *is* therapy. In contrast to those adults who are self-motivated to seek therapy, children do not begin therapy voluntarily, but are referred after testing by school psychologists. Remaining in therapy is essentially voluntary, however.

The first face-to-face meeting between therapist and child often is in the presence of the child's parents and siblings. This is a meeting set up after both child and parents have been briefed by a school psychologist that art therapy is recommended for the child. Parental attitudes vary. Some are upset at their child's being singled out for therapy. They often fear exposure of their role in causing the child's problem and at times find some excuse not to leave the child alone in the room with the therapist in subsequent sessions. Other times they wait outside ready to enter at the first small noise. This broadcast of uncertainty about therapy and therapist is usually picked up by the child, whose collaboration with the fearful parent may become manifest in a reluctance to trust the therapist.

Other parents who are aware of a problem come willingly, perhaps relieved to transfer responsibility for solving the child's problems to someone else. Some of these parents may not find a single good word to say about the child during the first interview. It is likely that during the course of therapy they will refuse to see improvement or admit any changes for the better, as obvious as they may be. Other parents seem amenable to therapy, profess bewilderment as to the causes of the dysfunction, and view the therapist as a magician who somehow will change things. There are also those who grasp an opportunity to obtain a free art class for the child and refuse to recognize it as therapy (Oaklander, 1978). The child's own attitudes are influenced by parents, psychologist, and previous experiences in art. The therapist has received reports from both teacher and psychologist about the child and has to come to her own conclusions. Choreographing all these attitudes, the therapist uses personal sensitivity and joins with family members in listening and appraising their relationships with one another. They are also very likely appraising the therapist.

After conversing with the family, the focus of attention is given to the child. I begin by asking questions pertaining to routine matters such as school, class, phone number, and address. I then invite the child to look around the room and to investigate the materials and objects it contains. The child is asked how the room seems and what he or she likes best. I also ask if the child prefers working alone or in a group, with boys or girls, with noisy or quiet children, and which days of the week are preferable. It is anticipated that by this time the child feels respected for being able to choose and can sense the therapist's nonintrusive support. If this is achieved, it is hopeful that both child and family will view art therapy as a pleasant activity rather than a punishment for being bad or different. Thereafter, a suitable arrangement is made to see the child alone for two or three sessions before placement in a group of four children or fewer who will meet weekly throughout the school year. My final emphasis is on the child's responsibility to attend regularly and punctually. If two sessions are missed without prior notice the child's membership in the group is discontinued.

FIRST INDIVIDUAL SESSION

I do not engage the child in art activity in the presence of the family, reserving this for our time together. I hope that the child comes to the first individual session with favorable memories of the previous meeting and with a sense of excitement, expectation, and willingness to explore new areas. Usually, a first session is characterized by a quality of subtle examination, an attempt to sense what will be created through the therapist–child interaction. Contact begins slowly and cautiously, the child presenting a "mask" of behavior, sometimes compliant and polite, sometimes belligerent or obstinate. Often these behaviors change radically during the course of therapy. As contact and trust grow, the children often become willing to reveal their greatest difficulties.

Creating a magic space in the therapy room is effected in large part by the variety and allure of art materials. The ideal room contains paper, paints, oil pastels, easels, clay, small pottery trimming wheels, plasticene, musical instruments, recording equipment, puppets, toys, and natural objects. Any of these may be used during a session; however, I tend to promote oil pastels because of the wide choice of color, the flow and spontaneity that is possible, the easy cleanup, and the fact that I can work in this medium comfortably with the child. Few children can resist a new box of 36 or 48 colors arranged in exquisite rainbow order, and large, good-quality white paper (20 by 27½ inches), materials generally not available at home or at school.

During this session my goal is to augment the child's perception of me as a supportive, nonintrusive individual, respectful of the child's innate self-directedness and feelings. I also wish to establish the ground rules for making art expressive and spontaneous rather than creating stereotyped subjects. As do most people, children view the blank page with a variety of responses, from direct and enthusiastic plunging in, to hesitancy and reticence, to outright resistance and fear of art. Still, the only place to start is precisely where the child is.

ART MAKING IN ART THERAPY

The art therapy experience is distinctly different from any other art experience that children may have encountered at home, school, or elsewhere. Most children making art have been exposed to the conventional subject matter often admired by adults, such as a bowl of fruit, a wine bottle and apples, birds flying into the sunset, or the stereotyped cartoon characters readily accepted by children. Wishing to draw such a safe subject, the child can fall into the trap of attempting to execute an accurate replica of a subject and fail, often resulting in frustration. When such an attempt is successful, the child may become bored halfway through, finding it difficult to finish mechanically something that did not develop through personal involvement.

A technique in which the outcome is unplanned and spontaneous is often an ideal method for beginning work in a noncommittal way, enabling the child to experience creation from formlessness and the excitement of the work becoming *more*, both artistically and as a reflection of the emergence of the child's inner self. The creative act is an encounter between artists and their world (May, 1975), something sparked from an internal impulse. Unconscious experience suddenly assumes symbolic form on paper and reveals to us messages from deep within the self. Using an open-ended approach at the start of therapy establishes the value of a client's expressive potential and its acceptance by the therapist.

Art techniques are valuable in therapeutic work with children when they actually provide a framework conducive to self-expression, regardless of the degree of accommodation or resistance that accompanies the child's art. Making effective use of techniques entails correlating them to the child's ability or inability to organize the work, control its content and form, both physically and emotionally, and assume responsibility for the outcome. Wadeson (1983) observes:

> There are art therapists who plan activities in advance and do not deviate from them, who eagerly seek out techniques that others have used. Therapy cannot be a lesson plan or series of exercises. What gets lost is the art therapist's sensitivity and responsiveness to the client's ongoing process, and often to the relationship as well. (pp. 50–51)

Thus using techniques should derive not from the therapist's agenda but from the client's expressive potential (Wadeson, 1983).

Children may initially view the art therapist as a kind of art teacher. This perception quickly changes as the art therapist determines the degree and type of his or her own participation in allowing the children to control their mutual interaction, whether directly or indirectly. The art therapist is an active observer, reflector, or semiactive participant in the child's process and art, and is also in process himself or herself. As Winnicott says: "Psychotherapy is done in the overlap of the two play areas, that of the patient and that of the therapist" (1971, p. 63).

SIX TECHNIQUES

The usual interaction between a child and an authority figure may sometimes be defined by noting who tells whom what to do. In a therapeutic interaction, the child is given a position of leadership and from the first moment is enabled, in a nonthreatening way, to assume control and responsibility for the work, or share this with the therapist. Some children need a stage of organization prior to assuming control or responsibility. Thus in choosing an effective starting point, the therapist assesses the child's self-assurance or anxiety, attitude toward giving or taking directions, attitudes about art, and levels of internal organization. In each of the six interventions presented, the therapist functions as a mirror or self-object, whether directly or indirectly, always enabling the child to lead the way.

Order of Presentation of the Techniques

The six techniques presented here are arranged in an order indicating the type and amount of control and responsibility a child is willing to take during the session. Table 17-1 can be used as a guide for choosing a certain art task based on the child's attitude and behavior.

A child willing to draw freely needs no technique. Oaklander (1978) says that "the very act of drawing, with no therapist intervention whatsoever, is a powerful expression of self that helps establish one's self-identity and provides a way of expressing feelings" (p. 53). The first technique, a nonverbal simultaneous graphic mirroring of the child's artwork in process, allows the therapist to provide an empathic sense of silent support and begin contact with the child. The second technique, a joint nonverbal "conversation" drawing, may be useful in working with children who are responsive to art materials but for various reasons lack a subject to draw. Together with the therapist, a drawing and its surprise outcome are shared. The third technique, the Squiggle Game, employs line and color to create unexpected images, with the unpredictable outcome shared by child and therapist. This may suit a child unable to commit himself or herself to subject matter and also unsure of art materials. In these first three interventions, the child has participated both graphically and in directing the course of action.

The fourth technique, the directed scribble, frees the child of a feeling of responsibility while scribbling according to the therapist's directions. Seemingly told what to do at first, the child may later agree to find and develop an image in the scribble. Some children may be unable to organize themselves and begin work at all. Here, it may be of help to use the fifth technique,

TABLE 17.1 Characteristics of the Six Techniques

Child's Attitudes and Behavior			Suggested Techniques	Type of Interaction		
To Therapist	To Art Task	Attention Span		Verbal, Non-verbal	Who Directs Work	Who Executes Work
Cooperative	Independent, responsible, enthusiastic	Prolonged	Graphic Mirroring	Non-verbal	Child	Child—therapist mirrors
Cooperative	Hesitant	Good when supervised	Conversation drawing	Non-verbal	Child and therapist	Child and therapist
Cooperative to ambivalent	Hesitant	Good when supervised	Squiggle Game	Non-verbal	Child and therapist	Child and therapist
Ambivalent	Ambivalent, needing guidance	Good when supervised	Directed scribble	Verbal	Therapist	Child
Ambivalent, disorganized	Disorganized and chaotic	Brief guidance necessary	Child as graphic secretary for therapist	Verbal	Therapist	Child
Resistant, detached	Resistant, blocked	Prolonged when supervised, guidance necessary	Therapist as graphic secretary for child	Verbal	Child	Therapist

where the child becomes a graphic secretary for the therapist, drawing according to the therapist's directions. Although the interaction is ostensibly controlled by the therapist, her directions and choice of subject matter will derive from hints gleaned from the child's associative conversation. If for some reason the child is totally unable or unwilling to draw, the therapist may use the sixth technique, and become a graphic secretary for the child, drawing a picture according the child's specific instruction. Here the child remains in control although not executing the work physically. In these last three interventions, the child has either participated graphically while being directed by the therapist or given directions but not drawn at all.

Thus in choosing an effective starting point, the therapist will assess the child's beginning self-assurance or anxiety, attitudes toward giving or taking directions, attitudes about art making, and levels of internal organization. The children are respected rather than confronted for being themselves. The work is accepted rather than interpreted, allowing a sense of contact and trust to grow.

1. Non-verbal Graphic Mirroring

When a child shows willingness to draw without direction, the therapist can *be with* the child as an active observer, offering to participate in the session nonverbally by "copying" what the child draws. Some children think that my graphic mirroring is strange since copying is usually a secretive, unacceptable activity. Making it open and valid somehow implies a high value on the emerging drawing as well as placing the child in a position of leadership as I follow, and giving a feeling that he or she is not alone in this activity. I may explain that I will get to know the child better through copying. I have never been asked not to copy, nor has any beginning self-consciousness on the child's part seriously inhibited the drawing. I respond on my own paper to the child's choice of color, pressure on the crayon, speed of execution, and spatial distribution as well as noting attitudes toward me as I mirror.

Occasionally I introduce some change of color or detail as a deliberate statement that we are not the same person. We may have similarities but we each have separate and unique identities. Reinforcement of our separate selves avoids the threat of merging or being engulfed yet enables the child to benefit from the feelings of support and validity derived from being mirrored.

In the first session of a small group I may mirror everyone on my own single sheet of paper by drawing some element from each child's work. A guessing game may ensue as to what I copied from whom, while the representation of each group member as unique, although part of the same unity, is symbolized.

RINA

Seldom in a first individual session does one witness the entire sequence of establishing contact, creating trust, and finally drawing forth a willingness to reveal deep personal difficulties. When all this is telescoped into an hour's time, the great force that a first meeting can contain is demonstrated.

Rina, a tall, beautiful, intelligent 14-year-old, was failing all her classes. Her opening conversation was sweetly sociable and fastidious as she described her helplessness at coping with parents, teachers, and false friends. Her family, English-speaking immigrants, had lived in Israel for 5 years and remained socially attached to the English-speaking community. Fearing that Rina's poor schoolwork would prevent her from being accepted to high school, they brought her for psychological testing. The results indicated that her problems were emotional and connected to the tense relationship between her parents. Rina was referred for individual art therapy while the entire family received family therapy. After 13 sessions both Rina and her family terminated therapy in preparation for leaving Israel for another country.

Rina liked to draw, and her first picture of a powerful and formless, frightening monster (Fig. 17.1) surprised me with an intense sensation of frenzy and brutality very different from her gentle facade. This powerful "thing" from another planet had no stomach, no feelings, and thought that people were ugly. On the reverse side of the paper I asked her to draw the side of the monster that no one could see (Fig. 17.2). The result was a sad and formless mass of scribbles. I had participated by copying or mirroring both aspects of the monster as she drew them. I believe that my nonverbal sharing of her experience provided the initial sensation of support and validation that she needed for her explosion of emotion projected into the "thing" she drew. She was then able to become both sides of the monster as she wrote down what each side had to say, without inhibition. She underlined words that applied to her own feelings about life, indicating anger, disgust, and fear. The monster had provided a tangible form into which she had projected her helplessness, as well as the immense power that was her own and could now be reowned by her and used positively. Rina's schoolwork showed immediate improvement and subsequent art therapy proved beneficial.

2. Joint Nonverbal Conversation Drawing

Assuming that a child is not resistant to art materials but has a problem with subject matter, the therapist can establish new criteria for work by suggesting a "conversation" between the two using color, line, and form. There is no goal in mind other than sharing the space of the paper and seeing what happens.

Starting off, the therapist chooses a color that seems to fit the moment and makes a line that feels appropriate. The child does the same and the process continues as each responds to the other's graphic expression. Kaplan (1983) describes this procedure with an adult, where both therapist and client take turns until they both feel finished. With children, it may become obvious after a while that the child prefers to continue alone, and then the picture

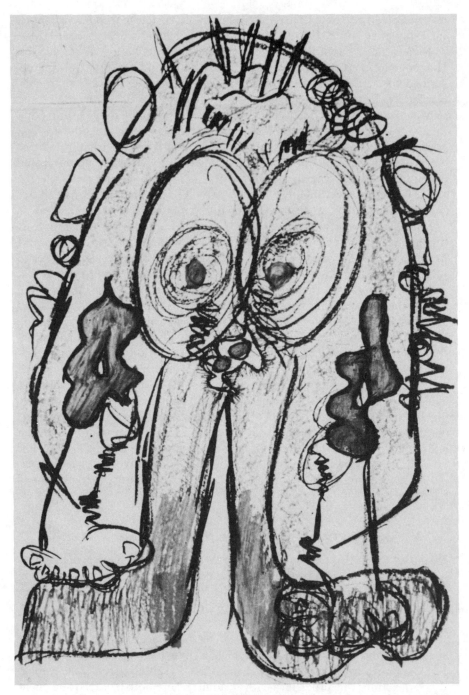

Figure 17.1. Rina's monster.

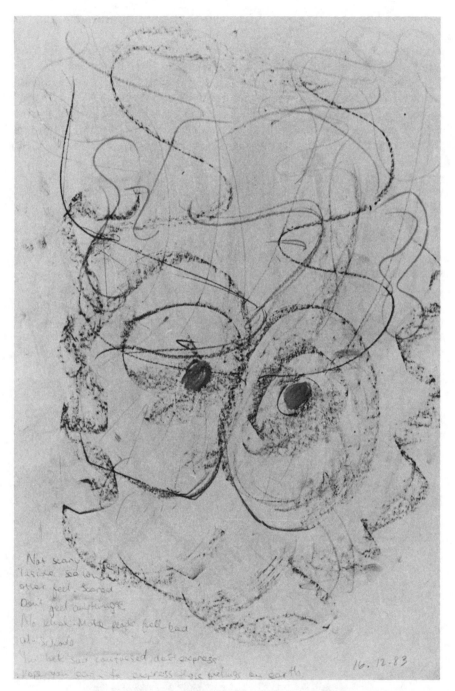

Figure 17.2. The weak side of Rina's monster.

is given to him or her to develop. The child's attitude toward authority gives form to the developing interaction. One child remains in a corner, unresponsive to the therapist and regarding any attempt at contact as an intrusion. Another child genuinely enjoys an interaction of mutual response and surprise, or perhaps turns the game into a power struggle, challenging the therapist at every turn, invading and destroying as in war. The work can be signed by both participants, dated, and titled. Saving and dating all work sets the precedent of valuing artistic statements for their truthful integrity.

The therapist's role in the drawing is not autonomous, but once again an empathetic mirroring of the child. In reflecting the child's emotional progression in the game and then relinquishing the work to him or her, the child's need for limited merging with a "good parent" is gratified while he or she retain individuality and a sense of control of the interaction.

AVI

Avi, 9 years old, was the eldest of two sons in a family of second-generation welfare recipients, with one parent being a narcotics addict. During Avi's first session with me and an assistant, we did a three-way conversation drawing with Avi deciding to turn the paper at intervals so that each person could get another view of the work. I knew that Avi had artistic talent, but his thoughts and speech were unfocused, and he seemed remote and possibly depressed. I wished to convey to him that nothing in particular was expected of him in the art therapy room and that he could enjoy an art experience

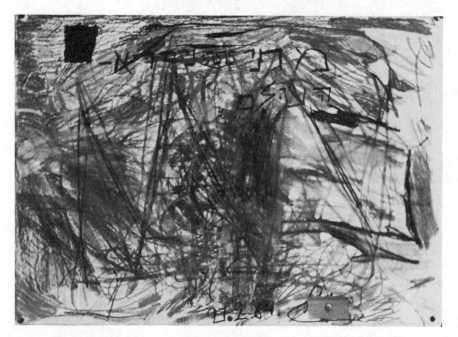

Figure 17.3. Avi's conversation drawing, "When Was the World Created?"

with two adults who would be his equals in the interaction. I also hoped to give him a sense of leadership as he controlled the group work. Avi told us when he wished to continue alone. As he drew he spoke, using the words *kill, murder,* and *death.* With hot pink, orange, red, blue, and black, he finished the picture, which remained abstract. He titled it "When Was the World Created?" (Fig. 17.3).

ORA

Ora was a 12-year-old girl of low self-esteem and low intelligence who had never drawn before. She was the only child of a father who was his family's sole survivor of the Holocaust and a mother of Sephardic origin who was now in a mental institution. Ora was cared for by an uncle and aunt as part of their large family. As with Avi, I wanted Ora to feel that nothing specific was expected of her. Because she had no experience in art, I felt she also needed my participation to begin work and become accustomed to art materials, while feeling less responsible for the work, which we shared at the start. During our first session, she enjoyed our noncommittal interaction on paper and soon began to see her own images in the lines, mostly angry faces in rows. She continued drawing alone, emphasizing a large, threatening central image, and called her picture "Anger" (Fig. 17.4).

Both Avi and Ora used most of their first art therapy session for maximum development of their artwork as art. For them this was a new experience in persistence and prolonged concentration, and a step toward individuation

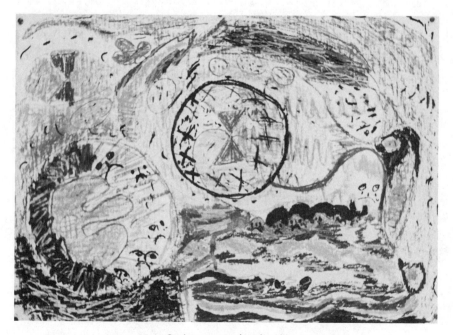

Figure 17.4. Ora's conversation drawing, "Anger."

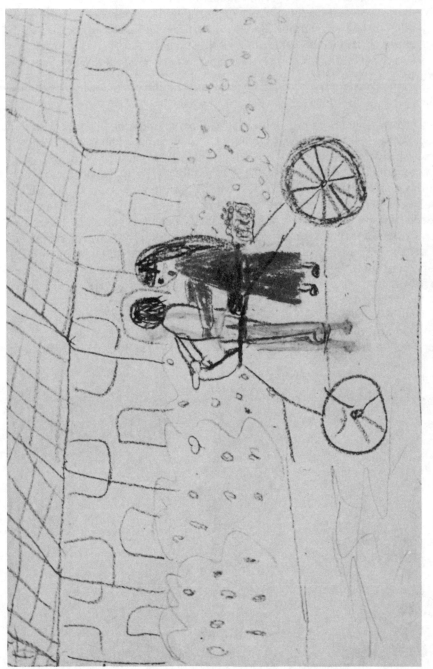

Figure 17.5. Nira's drawing of a couple riding a bicycle, begun by a squiggle.

and a sense of self-worth. At this early stage I try to encourage the most complete artwork possible for the child in order to provide an emotional satisfaction that in later stages may be achieved through verbal insight. The artwork becomes a personal confirmation of the child's newly expanded ability. This in itself is therapeutic.

3. The Squiggle Game

Winnicott (1971) introduced the squiggle into his interviews with children, describing it as making "some kind of impulsive line drawing and inviting the child whom I am interviewing to turn it into something, and then he makes a squiggle for me to turn into something in my turn" (p. 19). The Squiggle Game is a noncommittal game, introducing an element of challenge and visually inaccurate whimsy, yet having some connection with reality. A child ambivalent about art materials and wary of abstract approaches may be enticed by the squiggle. The child may also feel less burdened by responsibility for the outcome of the work when shared equally with the therapist. And the squiggle can always be useful when a child cannot get started drawing.

When playing the game on one large paper several times, the child may find a connection between squiggles and create one picture. Or the paper can be first folded into eight sections, and in each a squiggle can be made alternately by child and therapist and then developed. In case a child sees an image in his or her own squiggle (which has been created for the therapist), I allow the child to finish it. I also wait for the completion of all squiggles or a finished picture before attempting to follow with a story sequence created by the child (Gabel, 1984). The child's story is written down as dictated by him or her with no changes, and then recorded on tape by either child or therapist. Replaying the tape effectively reinforces noncritical acceptance of spontaneous creativity and the self that produces it. Hearing one's own words again provides the opportunity to focus on one's self.

NIRA

Eight-year-old Nira was an apathetic, complacent child whose divorced parents remained on friendly terms. From the first session she had me make a squiggle to start off her pictures. Later she began with spontaneous squiggles of her own. In many of her pictures Nira developed the theme of two people doing something together—swimming, bicycling, hiking, or sleeping in bed (Fig. 17.5). Nira's mother had participated in a parents' group and had shown a desire for reunion with her ex-husband. Nira's pictures so frequently depicted couples in activities her parents liked that I suspected that this was a reflection of her mother's longing to remarry her husband, as well as of Nira's own similar wishes.

RONEN

Ronen, 12 years old, was the second of three children in a family who had just left their kibbutz. Ronen had previously attended a special school for children with organic problems and had also received therapy there. He was diagnosed as slightly dyslexic and unskilled at reading and writing due to minimal brain damage. He showed difficulties in understanding instructions, copying from the blackboard, writing from dictation, and copying geometric forms. Despite this, his visual understanding was good and he was highly motivated toward good execution, usually causing extreme slowness in his work. His excessive self-criticism caused him to erase constantly and correct his work. His family was very defensive, apathetic, passive, and severely critical of the environment and the school system.

Although Ronen was friendly during our first session, he compared the new environment unfavorably to his old one, complaining that the old school was better and that other therapy rooms were less cluttered and filled than this one. He preferred order and neatness. The therapist wished to make him feel comfortable, to form contact and avoid placing him in an anxiety-producing testing situation. She chose the Squiggle Game as a way to enable Ronen to relate to new material spontaneously. However, she first developed a 10-minute verbal warm-up using the Squiggle Game principle of providing a partner with a stimulus to complete. She suggested a word such as "playing field," or "television" for which he formed any sentence he chose. He alternately did the same thing for her. Then, in writing, Ronen was asked to complete sentences beginning more personally. For example, he completed the words "my family" with "is getting organized," and "my school" with "is violent." He now could approach the same sequence in art with enthusiasm and curiosity, free of anxiety as he already knew what was expected of him.

The therapist folded the paper into eight sections and drew the first line (Fig. 17.6). Ronen, after great deliberation, found a face and took a long time coloring it in. In the second section Ronen made a line for the therapist but then indicated that he would like to complete it. On the third and fourth sections he made a squiggle and again took the turn for himself, finding a cat's face. However, he severely criticized the colors he chose as not suitable, and asked the therapist to make squiggles in the fifth and sixth sections, complimenting her as he discovered many possibilities. His slow and intense execution prolonged the work. The fifth and sixth sections were completed during the second session and the seventh and eighth sections during the third session. In these last four, all but the last were begun by the therapist's squiggles. In all, the color is rich and many layered, the entire space filled up. The last section, begun by his own squiggle once more, is the most spontaneous and the one he enjoyed most for its unexpected outcome. Separate titles were given to each unit: "The Cat That Got into Trouble," "Lion Statues Guarding the Palace," "Confusion," and "The Mexican," each separate and ordered within its own space, and secure in its own borders.

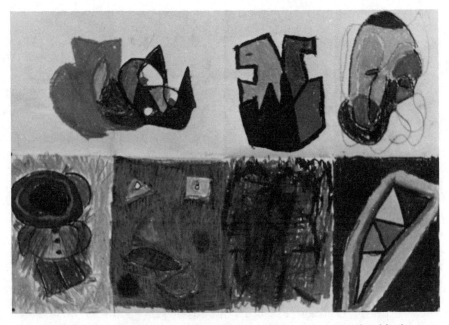

Figure 17.6. Ronen's squiggle game with the therapist; eight sections completed in three sessions.

4. Directed Scribble

Ulman states, "Possibly the scribble drawing, where imagery is projected into random lines that record rhythmic movement, is art therapy's most famous technique." Originated by Florence Cane, it was later adopted by her sister Margaret Naumburg, who "developed it to great advantage through her systematic use of her patients' verbal associations leading to interpretation of personal symbolism appearing in the graphic material" (Ulman, 1983, pp. 122–123).

As a child in the New York Public School System in the forties, I can testify to the later decline of the scribble into stereotyped filling in which Edith Kramer laments (1971). No matter how many times we drew scribbles, most of us found only "fish" in the crossed forms. Missing from the teacher's unimaginative instructions was an awareness of each child's natural rhythm and emotional range. The scribble can provide a personal semistructure that enables the client to approach art spontaneously and uniquely, providing that the line traveling around the page does indeed share the client's own rhythm and emotion. In a first session, a client's willingness to enter into a spontaneous body movement warm-up may be curtailed because of shyness or physical inhibition. Therefore a certain amount of suggestion can aid the child in creating a rhythmic movement that will be transferred to the paper. The directed scribble can be used when a child needs to share responsibility with the therapist such as in the squiggle, but is still unable to work without some direction at first. Although it is possible for the child to scribble with the therapist on a single paper, it may be preferable for the child to work alone so that the image chosen for development later is solely the child's own.

The child is asked to choose a color that feels "right" and hold it above the paper (20 by 27½ inches) wherever it feels comfortable. The hand holding the color descends and lands on the paper in some movement, such as a leaf falling, a feather drifting, a bird flying, a fish swimming, a stone rolling, or anything else that comes to mind, such as a sound, a color, or an emotion. Or I talk about the color that touches the paper and slowly becomes a line moving with low energy in any direction, quietly, gently, gaining force, moving quickly or joyously now, angrily or perhaps nervously jumping all over the page, slowing down, gliding calmly until it comes to rest. As I speak, the child draws with eyes open or closed and changes colors if so desired. When I have finished I ask the child to continue awhile alone, remembering the lines that felt good before, repeating those he or she wishes until it feels right to stop. Then the page is turned in all directions until an area of interest worth developing becomes apparent. When the picture is finished, a story or title is written on it and read. Speaking *as* the picture in the first person is effective, but may be rushing things for a first session.

I have used this method in a first session with two children and an assistant, the immediate goals being to start group interaction, to give a sense of equal participation of all group members, and to encourage a spontaneous result begun by a noncommittal approach. We all do the directed scribble on one paper, freely continuing after I have finished speaking. Then each participant (child or therapist) chooses an area of the picture that seems attractive, not necessarily his or her own, and develops the image. Or one can create a movement or body sculpture that describes it. A group movement sequence can be developed to end the session. Choosing someone else's area creates the beginning of group communication through the positive feedback of being selected, and working together on the scribble with some direction enhances group cooperation with little individual risk. I have also used the directed scribble in normal art classes with large groups of adolescents. Here I may ask for just a title to describe the art statement.

KAY

Kay was a pretty 10-year-old girl whose wide and pale face projected a sense of pleading and great suffering. Her upper body was heavy, hunched, and constricted, suggesting an old woman, while her legs were comparatively thin. Always dressed in black, she appeared distressed when spoken to and barely could move her lips or utter a sound in brief answer. Kay's parents had been divorced for 5 years and the father had remarried. Although Kay had attended four different schools in 4 years as the family moved from place to place, her school record was good. Now she shared one bedroom of a large apartment with her mother and 17-year-old brother. Her maternal grandmother and an unmarried uncle used the two other bedrooms. Kay's mother was often away from home and Kay was responsible for caring for her diabetic and difficult grandmother. She was also forced by her brother to "do things" for him. Another older brother was in the army and came home infrequently.

During Kay's first session with the art therapist and the dance therapist, her presenting behavior was compliant, like a child used to taking instructions. Despite her almost total silence and physical inhibition, I sensed Kay's need for personal contact and chose a directed scribble as suitable for working together with some verbal direction. Both therapists mirrored Kay's gentle, hesitant line and cautious use of color as we suggested movements such as an ant crawling slowly, a river gently flowing, a leaf lazily drifting. Kay was also encouraged to contribute her ideas to this sequence. Then each person developed an area near herself in color. Kay was asked to choose a title and wrote "Oceans and Continents" in black. In the picture (Fig. 17.7) Kay's area is central, her isolation respected and mirrored by the therapists' areas in far corners.

As trust developed, she expressed her intense fears and feelings of entrapment in her artwork. As her paintings revealed more, she replaced her black clothing with lighter hues and extended her relationships with the girls in the group to the outside. She now revealed many appalling details of her daily life, such as her brother's sadistic demands on her at knifepoint, her distress at being responsible for her grandmother, her fear of telling her

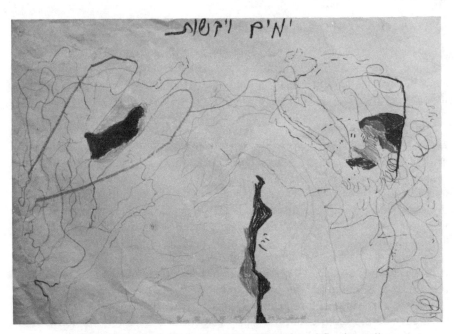

Figure 17.7. Kay's directed scribble, "Ocean's and Continents."

mother or anyone about her distress, and her desire to run away from home, possibly to her father.

After a meeting with her mother and the school psychologist, the home situation changed considerably. The grandmother and uncle took a separate apartment, Kay got her own room, and she began to speak up in family discussions, asking questions rather than just being the passive recipient of instructions or demands. Upon conclusion of the art therapy group at the end of the school year, Kay was referred to individual therapy for continued support.

5. Child Acts as Graphic Secretary for Therapist

Highly anxious children may be unable to organize their thoughts and activities for more than a few minutes. Having the child draw for the therapist something that the therapist asks for may aid in focusing, containing, and organizing the child within one subject for as long a time as possible at this stage. It is not an attempt to teach, give compulsory instruction, or actually extract a gift. Fears may intrude even upon a child's most sincere efforts to concentrate, to do something by direction for himself or herself. At first the therapist's efforts may be largely to set benign limits and give form to the activity, which is frequently interrupted by the child's disjointed thoughts and fears. Giving a gift drawing to the therapist may correlate with a child's need to placate authority figures so as not to be abandoned by them. Cues for the therapist about what to ask for come from the child's associative speech during their interaction.

6. Therapist Acts as Graphic Secretary for Child

At age 82, Henri Matisse had his secretary paint bright colors of his choosing on paper. He then cut them into shapes and directed her to place them in accordance with *his* inner vision, on a wall. His illness prevented him from doing most of the work himself, but did not extinguish his creative illuminations (Duthuit, 1962).

Almost every child has had an "inner vision," one subject above all which he or she dreams of drawing, yet is not able to attempt alone. Very self-critical children resist art because of self-doubts about using materials or drawing well enough. Some manipulative children make a show of starting and immediately throw down crayons in despair, complaining that they can't do it and beseeching an adult to do it for them. Clearly, being manipulated into doing children's work for them is an unhealthy precedent. But that child still has an inner vision, and offering to draw according to his or her instructions, even apologizing in advance that the artistic quality may be imperfect, is often an open surprise. The therapist draws the entire picture by instruction, further stimulating the child's creative imagination by gently asking questions regarding color, size, placement, and detail of the objects requested. Often a child gaining a sense of control asks freely for items that he or she would never have thought to draw alone, containing perhaps a deeper emotional significance as well. The therapist may also be surprised at her own freedom in drawing for someone else. Again, a few sentences dictated by the child to the therapist can enhance the experience. The goal is to get the child working, in any way, and paradoxically the child feels as if the picture is his or hers.

Contact and communication with the therapist begins, and trust and support become a part of the relationship in this special place, the therapy room. The authority person becomes an accepting helper who enables the child to begin just where he or she is, emotionally and intellectually, with no other demands. Although the child at first is unwilling to assume responsibility for determining the form and content of the interaction, conditions are provided for control to be taken indirectly. The next time it may be easier to attempt doing something by oneself.

Children Who Have Difficulty with Spontaneous Techniques

The work of organically impaired children often resembles a scribble. This may be the limit of their motor control and may represent the best they can do. They may consciously yearn to do something precise and organized and conventionally acceptable and may call their own work disgusting and ugly. Sometimes it is not possible to help them find pleasure in spontanteous approaches such as scribbles or conversation drawings. Serving as their graphic secretary, therefore, provides an expressive experience in art, otherwise unattainable for them.

CONCLUSION

Meeting an art therapist for the first time may be a new and potentially stressful situation for children, as they do not usually enter therapy of their own choosing. They have been tested and referred for behavior that others have labeled emotionally and socially dysfunctional but that for them may be the only possible coping mechanisms for surviving in their world. Often aware that they have been labeled problematic, they are acutely sensitive to the way the therapist presents himself or herself and art therapy, and anxious to know what will be expected of them.

The first mutual interaction between art therapist and child client sets the stage for the subsequent therapeutic process and lays the groundwork for art making in therapy as distinct from any other art experience the child may have had. Alone with the child, the therapist must know his or her options—which techniques are appropriate at this early stage and which alternative among these suits each child. Willingness to work alone or in partnership with the therapist and levels of internal organization of the child guide the therapist in his or her choice. Even in instances of outright resistance, the therapist can transmit the belief that the child's expressive potential can and will emerge when provided with a supportive framework within which assumption of responsibility is nonthreatening.

The six interventions presented in this Chapter are not theme centered but rather provide the structure within which therapist and child begin their mutual interaction and play. They emphasize a more spontaneous, open-ended approach to art, providing an experience that may extend the child's range of achievement, reinforcing acceptance of graphic ability and truthfulness in art making, and finally allowing the child to begin formation of a new self-image, knowing himself or herself in a new way. In any case, sensitivity and caution are necessary when choosing. In later stages of therapy the same techniques may be used for other purposes, such as helping a child through a creative impasse, emphasizing the excitement of allowing internal symbolic messages to surface into images, or just having fun through making art.

REFERENCES

Duthuit, G. (1962). Matisse's illuminations. *Portfolio & Art News Annual*, *5*, 84–99.

Gabel, S. (1984). The draw a story game: An aid to understanding and working with children. *The Arts in Psychotherapy*, *11*, 187–196.

Kaplan, F. (1983). Drawing together: Therapeutic use of the wish to merge. *American Journal of Art Therapy*, *22*, 79–85.

Kramer, E. (1971). *Art as therapy with children*. New York: Schocken.

May, R. (1975). *The courage to create*. New York: Norton.

Oaklander, V. (1978). *Windows to our children*. Moab, UT: Real People Press.

Wadeson, H. (1983). The art in art therapy. *Art Therapy*, *1*, 50–51

Winnicott, D. W. (1971). *Playing and reality*, Middlesex, England: Penguin.

Ulman, E. (1983). Roots of art therapy: Margaret Naumberg (1890–1983) and Florence Cane (1882–1952)—A family portrait. *American Journal of Art Therapy*, *22*, 122–123.

CHAPTER 18

"Barrier" Drawings for Depressed Patients

SUSAN BUCHALTER-KATZ

Patients often describe their depression as a living hell, or all encompassing. There is a pervasive sense of emptiness described as unbearable by many patients. Patients share feelings of intense loneliness, even in a room full of friends. They usually are not able to understand the reason behind their feelings of alienation and isolation. These feelings are expressed by a group of patients at the private short-term psychiatric and substance abuse facility where I work.

A high percentage of these individuals suffer from a characterological depression that has plagued them throughout their lives. They are looking for a "magic pill" to make them happy and make their problems disappear. Frequently patients ask, "When will my medication take effect?" or "Why doesn't it work better?" or "Why can't my doctor do more for me?" These people usually take little or no responsibility for their roles in job, family, and relationship problems.

The patients with whom I work are generally middle- to upper-middle-class individuals. They are well dressed and well groomed; often the women wear full makeup and take great care to look attractive. One would never know from their appearance that they are suffering major depression. They put on a mask, often adorning themselves in gold jewelry and designer clothes. One patient explained part of her problem is "having to look perfect." She'd never leave the hospital or home without looking flawless.

These individuals are quick to point out their imperfections, especially when supported or complimented. Remarks such as "But I need to lose ten pounds," "Oh, look how awful my hair is," or "But my eyes are puffy" are commonplace. Many of these people have an unrealistic perception of their inner and outer selves.

I've been working with this group of patients for more than 6 years and have studied hundreds of their artworks. The art in many of the therapy groups I led until recently was spontaneous and nondirective. In these sessions patients were encouraged to draw whatever they pleased. A variety of materials including craypas, markers, and pastels were available for use. Pencils were given only when specifically requested (because they encourage rigidity). Groups were usually composed of five to eight individuals, 90% of whom were female, between the ages of 20 and 70. The sessions lasted an hour, half of which was frequently spent processing and exploring the meaning of the work.

Originally I chose to lead nondirective groups in order to help patients develop decision-making skills, a core issue in many depressions. (Nondirective groups are less threatening than directive groups in that they tend to avoid confrontation.) I didn't want to threaten the patients by asking them to draw specific fears and worries (especially since they were hospitalized for only 2 to 3 weeks). I expected their issues would present themselves in the art or discussion period afterward.

I began to see patterns and recurring symbols in the artwork produced during nondirective groups. The work was often cheery: attractive landscapes and still lifes, beach and ocean scenes, suns, rainbows. Patients took great care in signing and titling their work. Uplifting titles such as "Happiness" and "A New Beginning" were commonplace. The art was complete, for example, a house in the woods surrounded by trees, the sun shining on a meadow filled with flowers. Many symbols were seen repeatedly in these productions; yellow suns, flowers, trees, houses, green grass, blue lakes or oceans, birds, and rainbows. The trees and flowers would appear to be flourishing; houses were outlined but colors weren't filled in. In general, the work seemed superficial; it told a story but usually not that of the patient. The colors were usually depicted in a realistic manner: blue skies, pastel-colored flowers, rainbows the colors of the spectrum (Buchalter-Katz, 1985). When asked if the pleasant artwork was representative of their feelings, they'd say "no." They stated they drew the way they'd like, wish, want things to be or the way things used to be. Patients rarely drew their depressions, anger, or isolation.

I became increasingly perplexed and curious. I thought people suffering from depression would draw empty, lifeless, flat pictures, and that discussion of isolation and fear would predominate group meetings. It seemed strange to observe depressed individuals drawing bright scenes and speaking happily about their pictures. Where were the isolated, unconnected images and lack of color I'd read about?

Another puzzling observation was the connection between the art product and physical appearance of many of the depressed patients. When feeling despondent, many of these individuals took great care to look attractive; this facade was also seen in many of their drawings where their depression is masked by superficial subject matter.

These nondirective pictures, although not accurate portrayals of major depression, serve many purposes. Most importantly, they allow the patients to contrast reality with fantasy. The work affords the opportunity to adapt symbolic hopes for use as coping mechanisms. For example, a nervous patient who drew serene landscapes benefited from examining methods of attaining the calmness portrayed in his work.

The problem I faced was lack of time. The average length of hospital stay was 2 to 3 weeks, and it takes time to cut through thick coatings of "sunny days at the beach" and "blue mountain scenes." Most patients attempt to structure themselves through their art; they need to feel in control and are not willing to break down their barriers and lose that "put-together" facade. I knew that I needed to explore alternate art therapy methods in order to encourage sharing in a more immediate manner. A structured, directive approach was chosen. Patients were now given specific themes such as family and self-portraits to focus upon.

Directive art therapy (suggesting specific themes) improved the quality of the group, increasing participation both artistically and verbally. This contrasted with my original expectations that patients would withdraw and become overly threatened and anxious. Patients usually drew specifically what was asked, and the work became less superficial. The patients were less reluctant to share their work in depth and seemed to enjoy directive art therapy better than nondirective work. Having a ready-made idea relieved them of a burden, perhaps encouraging them to share more openly on paper.

Quite accidentally I stumbled upon the theme of "barriers" or obstacles to recovery. It came up in a verbal therapy group which I also lead. I decided to use the theme later that day in art therapy; patients were asked to draw their barriers(s). When asked to clarify the term, I specified "obstacles to recovery—what's preventing you from functioning to the best of your ability." To my surprise, many patients quickly began sketching. These drawings, even more so than other directive drawings, looked like classic depression, as documented in the literature: fragmented, unconnected, lots of dark colors— especially black and brown. These pictures didn't have the superficial appearance that typified the work generated in the nondirective groups. Many of the pictures were drawn quickly, with heavy, pressured strokes. Some patients appeared to have experienced a catharsis while drawing, saying they felt better, relieved, exhausted. The work frequently represented the depression: what it looked like, felt like, and what factors precipitated it. Confronting one's barriers through drawing appeared to be an important first step toward overcoming them.

The barrier approach inspired many patients to draw their inner selves, helping them break down their facades and examine obstacles in a clear, specific manner. This method proved to be a more direct way of bringing into awareness, and dealing with, frightening, confusing, and upsetting issues. For the first time patients began to take responsibility for their depression and help themselves in their treatment. The barrier method encouraged patients to begin to explore their roles in family, job, and relationship problems. In fact, patients sometimes drew self-portraits as a response to the barrier theme. People were rarely depicted in spontaneous work.

These barrier drawings displayed more negativity; the group members often drew how they experienced life, as opposed to the way they'd like their lives to be.

A casual comparison of barrier and spontaneous drawings suggests differences in symbolism and drawing approach:

Barrier Drawings	Spontaneous Art
People depicted	People rarely represented
Lack of color	Bright, colorful art
Negative themes	Cheerful images
Realistic issues	Optimism, wishes
Empty at times	Frequently complete
Sometimes fragmented and unconnected	Usually connected
Structured, rigid	More flow noted
Pastels rarely used	Pastels used frequently
Abstraction used	Abstraction rarely used
Labeling	Labeling rarely used

(It is of interest to note that pastels, which allow for more flowing movement, are rarely used in barrier drawings.)

Barrier drawings led to more in-depth discussion than spontaneous work, partly because of the rich symbolism. Through observation and introspection, patients were given the opportunity to explore the characteristics of their barrier, for example: Does it appear insurmountable? Can they climb over to, under it, break through it? How large is it? Is it taking up the entire page or a small portion of the page? How long do they think it will stand? What is it made of (steel, sand, wood, etc.)? How do they feel upon viewing it (angry, hurt, frightened, strong)? What color is it? How does the color reflect barrier strength? Does the artist describe feeling helpless while actually drawing a weak, tiny obstacle? Discrepancies such as these can be explored, the goal being to find methods of dealing with the barrier and overcoming it.

By analyzing their barriers on paper, patients increased their objectivity and gained a new perspective. The barrier drawings presented the opportunity for practicing decision-making and problem solving-skills. Questions such as When did the barrier go up? Who built it? Where? and How long has it been up? are helpful. The process of drawing the barrier was cathartic; often patients were able to share feelings they'd kept locked up for many years. It is interesting to note how quickly the patients began to drop their defenses in contrast to work in nondirective therapy. Patients were more likely to use labeling in barrier drawings. It seemed to be their way of maintaining structure when faced with sharing genuine concerns, which often made them feel fragmented. Depressed patients usually want to control their environment since they feel controlled by outside forces. I rarely saw labeling in other art forms of the depressed individual.

I found it fascinating to observe the characteristics of the barrier and spontaneous drawings. In order to study further similarities and/or differences between the two pictures, and to understand better the patient response to the two styles of presentation, I decided to combine the approaches. Patients were first asked to draw a spontaneous picture, and then a barrier drawing. I kept in mind that the nondirective art might serve as warm-up for the directive work. My goal was for patients to compare the two pictures and to use the differences (generally a fantasy and reality theme) to help clarify their sense of self and direction in therapy. I hoped group members would more readily share their obstacles to recovery.

They were allowed to choose large or small sheets of paper and work with pastels, craypas, markers, crayons, or colored pencils (if requested). These groups consisted of five to eight individuals (50 to 60% female), all ages, starting from age 17. Patients were encouraged to sign and date their completed work. Drawing stopped when the majority of patients finished their pictures. Group members were usually amenable to drawing two pictures at one sitting. It is important to note that patients volunteered to attend the group; it was rarely mandatory.

CASE EXAMPLES

NANCY

Figure 18.1, "Sunrise" (spontaneous), and Figure 18.2, "Wall" (barrier), were drawn by Nancy, a female patient in her thirties. She was attractive, well made up, and a world traveler. She masked her depression by wearing a lot of gold jewelry and dressing glamorously. She had recently traveled to Europe, hoping to overcome her depression. This patient had been battling bouts of depression since her early teens. Her parents were wealthy and gave her expensive gifts, sending her on trips when she felt poorly.

This was her first hospitalization, although she had been seeing psychiatrists for a number of years. Nancy had gone to an Ivy League college, majoring in English literature, but she hadn't enjoyed school. An A student, she had high expectations for herself. She was either unable to live up to her expectations, or when she did indeed achieve goals, she wasn't satisfied and discounted her accomplishments. She stated she had a lot of acquaintances but few close friends. She desired to be married but seemed to avoid close relationships with men. Nancy came to the hospital because it was becoming increasingly difficult for her to function. She was sleeping and eating poorly, watching television most of the day. She felt she might hurt herself if she didn't seek help.

Nancy stated that "Sunrise" reminded her of Paris. "It was beautiful

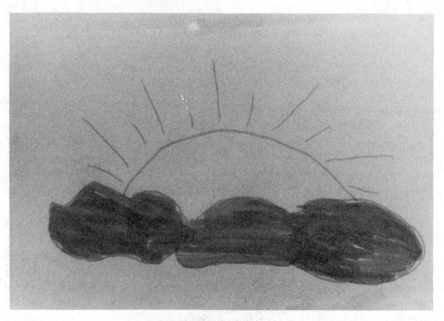

Figure 18.1. Sunrise.

there . . . I'd like to go back." The sun was outlined but not colored in. The cloud under the sun was emphasized and drawn in turquoise, "my favorite color." Nancy smiled as she spoke about the picture, stating it gave her a "good feeling." One group member remarked that the picture seemed to be floating. Nancy remarked, "Perhaps that means a feeling of freedom." She chose not to share the meaning of the darkened cloud when asked to do so by a fellow patient. She denied the possibility of disturbing or negative symbolism in her work, wanting to speak only about pleasant subjects. Most of Nancy's other spontaneous works were bright and cheerful, much like the image she presented to the group.

In discussing her barrier drawing, "Wall," Nancy seemed more somber. She drew the wall, filling the entire page, and explained, "The bricks are heavy and indestructible." (I have noticed that sometimes patients relate walls to anxiety and/or low self-esteem; as they progress in therapy the bricks may begin to tumble down.) She stated, "I drew a wall. I would have drawn it bigger if I had more paper—it's all encompassing. The black rectangles are not windows," she volunteered. "They mean I'm imprisoned." Nancy stated that the wall symbolizes herself; everyone in her life criticizes her and she "tries too hard," and "loves too hard." She stated she smothers people and therefore keeps her barrier up.

Nancy spoke coarsely, cursing quite a bit, as she discussed her barrier. (She didn't curse when describing her spontaneous picture.) She admitted

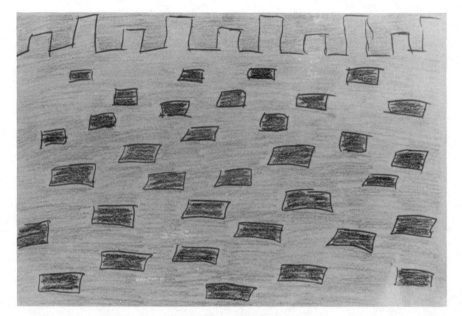

Figure 18.2. Wall.

that her manner alienates her from others. She was upset about breaking up with a boyfriend after a 1-year relationship. Nancy stated that he tortured her emotionally and caused her great pain, but "he also made me feel good, that's why I stayed with him." She acknowledged that she must gain self-esteem and self-acceptance. When asked, Nancy stated that she felt uneasy while viewing and discussing her picture. She hoped her barrier would become smaller or begin to crumble in the near future; there was a lot of work to be done.

Nancy hadn't shared nearly this much in other art or verbal groups. She explained that the drawing helped her express herself, and she was able to remove her mask by narrowing her art to the barrier theme. When asked to compare the different drawings, she remarked that she liked the barrier picture much better, since it allowed her to release pent-up emotions. Nancy chose to use crayon for the barrier picture and large, thick markers to design the spontaneous picture. She explained that the markers flowed smoother— "It took more work to draw the wall."

Many other group members were able to relate to Nancy's wall drawing. The idea of putting up a wall around themselves for protection seemed prevalent. One patient stated, "If the wall comes down, you're vulnerable; it's much safer to keep it up." Another group member related the wall to the story of the three pigs: "The pig who built the brick house, the sturdiest one, was able to best deal with the wolf."

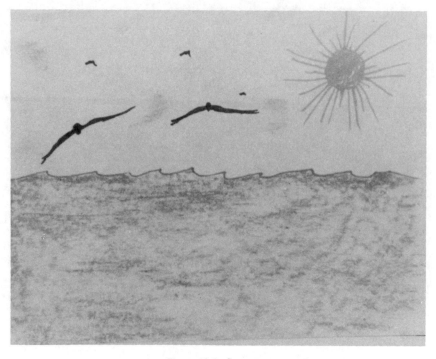

Figure 18.3. Seascape.

TRUDY

Figure 18.3, "Seascape" (spontaneous), and Figure 18.4, "Abstract" (barrier picture), were drawn by a young woman in her twenties. Trudy was attractive, dressed stylishly, and obviously took great care with her hair and makeup. She was attending graduate school, majoring in special education, and working part time in a department store as a cashier/salesperson. Trudy was somewhat overweight, and this troubled her. She had a very low opinion of herself; she saw herself in an unrealistic manner as "tremendously fat." She continued to eat a lot of food during her hospital stay.

This was Trudy's first hospitalization; she felt the breakup with her fiancé of 2 years had precipitated it. "It was the straw that broke the camel's back." Although her fiancé blamed the breakup on her rigidity and their constant bickering, Trudy blamed it on her weight: "If I was 10 pounds thinner he never would have left me." Trudy disliked her job and complained about "loud and abusive customers." She saw herself as a victim: Her supervisors at school and work treated her poorly, her fiancé had left her, graduate school was very difficult. She found it increasingly difficult to function, stating she felt more and more tired, also hating how she looked—"obese and ugly." Trudy dyed her hair and got a permanent, but "it didn't help." She stopped going to classes and was put on probation at work. She

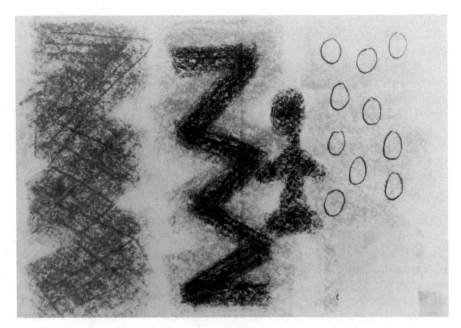

Figure 18.4. Abstract—barrier.

shared an apartment with another student who urged her to seek psychiatric help. Trudy reluctantly took her friend's advice and checked herself into the hospital.

Trudy did not appear shy; she shared in groups, but in a self-deprecatory manner. She wouldn't accept support of any kind from others. She viewed herself as a total failure, with "no future." In contrast to this negative description, Trudy's spontaneous picture, "Seascape," was optimistic and represented "freedom" for her. She saw the birds as her fiancé and herself, flying on their honeymoon. She described the picture as a warm, sunny day: "We are in Florida, having a wonderful time. The water is blue and warm; we'll go for a swim later."

Trudy's barrier drawing looked quite different. It was drawn with a lot of pressure; at one point Trudy broke the black pastel when drawing the dark zigzag line. She took twice as long drawing the barrier picture, frequently stopping and staring at her work; she appeared totally immersed in it. Trudy chose the smaller sheet of paper for her spontaneous design and the larger sheet for her barrier picture; she needed to "spread out." Trudy included black and red in her barrier drawing, while her spontaneous work consisted of brown birds, blue water, and a yellow sun. "The red and black had to be there," she stated. "They are angry colors." She related the zigzag design to her ambivalence about life, and anger about losing her fiancé. She drew herself in black next to the black design. Trudy stated she was angry with herself for "allowing Robert to leave; I could have stopped him, but maybe I was afraid?" Trudy drew the circles last, remarking that they were friends she used to know. "I guess I stopped keeping in touch, too bad." Trudy slowly began to see her role in her depressions and relationship problems. One group member pointed out that Trudy drew herself in "mid-air, just black, no real face or legs . . ." Trudy admitted to feeling "just like that, faceless, invisible." She began to discuss her low self-esteem as well as methods to improve the quality of her life. The group encouraged her to take a more realistic view of herself.

KATHY

The next set of pictures was drawn by a single female in her early thirties. She lived with her mother and socialized little. She had been in and out of psychiatric facilities for the past 10 years. Kathy had been raised primarily by her mother; she had been abused verbally and frequently beaten by her stepfather from ages 8 to 12. Kathy felt her mother had ignored these beatings and ridicule because she was afraid of losing her husband. Kathy's stepfather eventually left her mother, moving to the Midwest with a younger woman. Kathy felt she was her mother's scapegoat, receiving blame for her stepfather's decision to move away. Her mother demanded that she do most of the household chores; she was never satisfied with Kathy's work and constantly criticized her. "She didn't let me be a teenager." Kathy remarked that her mother made fun of her appearance, grades in school, and friends. Eventually Kathy stopped bringing home her friends and now had only two acquaintances whom she rarely saw outside of work. She explained that she didn't like living with her mother, but claimed she doesn't earn enough money for her own apartment." She spent her weekends "chauffeuring her mother and elderly aunt around town." She complained but allowed herself to remain in the same situation year after year. Kathy said she would like to have a boyfriend but she's too shy, and that she'd like to change jobs but her benefits are too good.

Kathy is well groomed, somewhat overweight, and moderately attractive. She is almost 6 feet tall and very quiet. She doesn't volunteer information readily, but shares when asked questions. During this therapy group patients were encouraged (with Kathy's approval) to ask questions about her artwork and life in order to encourage Kathy to open up.

Kathy generally attended art therapy, drawing landscapes, speaking little about her art or herself. Figure 18.5 shows a typical landscape, "part of a farm visited when I was a child." She stated the picture looked "serene; I'd love to be there." When asked whom she'd like to have there with her, she replied, "no one." Kathy remarked that the picture looked like "an escape. I wish everyone would leave me alone. I'd like to build a log cabin and live there forever." Kathy ignored the jeers of group members who

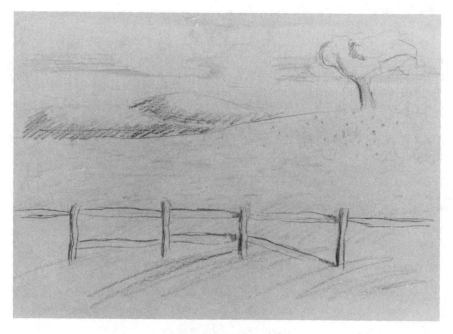

Figure 18.5. Landscape.

insisted she was being unrealistic and working hard to avoid dealing with her issues. Kathy drew this picture with crayon, in a meticulous manner.

Kathy drew her barrier picture (Fig. 18.6) with black, which she didn't use in her spontaneous picture. She drew quickly, almost as if she needed an immediate release. Kathy didn't stop drawing her spiral even when her marker began to run out of ink. Drawing from the inside out, she described her barrier as a volcano. She was able to relate the volcano to herself: "I'm ready to explode." She remarked, when asked, "The barrier drawing is ugly; I don't like to see myself like that." She was able, after this remark, to discuss her home and job situation and how disgusted she was with her life. Group members were very supportive of her and helped her to feel comfortable with sharing. When contrasting the two pictures, Kathy stated, "The spiral is me; the farm is where I'd like to be." Wadeson (1971) has noted the recurrence of the spiral symbol as an image of entrapment in the art of depressed suicidal patients.

JOHN

John, a man in his late twenties, was separated from his wife and was filing for divorce. He was trying to gain custody of his 3 year old daughter. John had never been hospitalized before although he said he had suffered other debilitating depressions. He stated that somehow he had always been able to "pull himself out of it." John was married for 6 years, a "stormy rela-

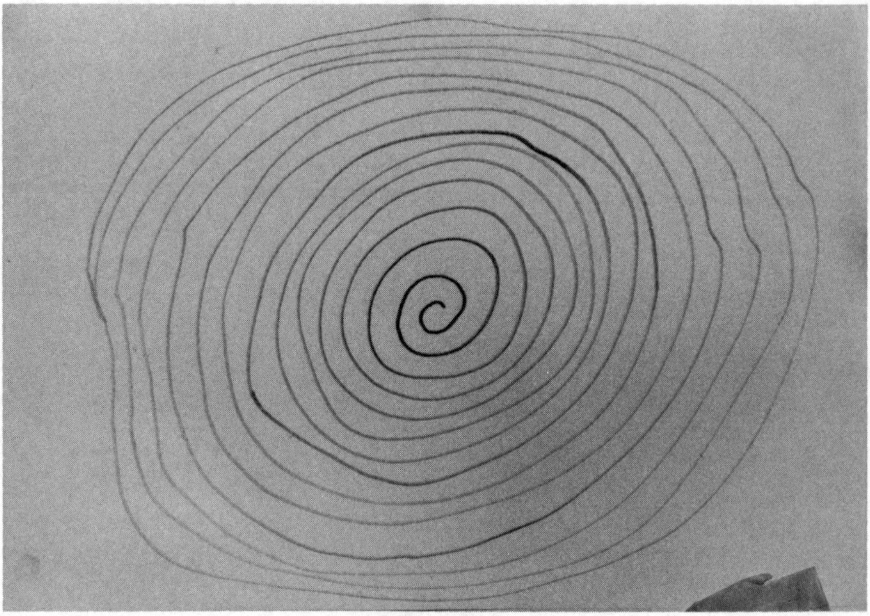

Figure 18.6. Spiral—barrier.

tionship." He had difficulty communicating with his wife, who had been seeing another man for almost a year. John knew about this relationship but hoped his wife would tire of this man and return to him. Most of the year he handled the situation by ignoring it, pretending everything was fine.

John worked full time as an accountant; he also did most of the housework and shopping. He explained that his wife was extremely sloppy, throwing her clothes on the floor and leaving them in whichever room she happened to be at the time. There was so much dirty laundry piled up that he had to wash, dry, and iron his clothes in the morning before going to work. His little girl frequently wore clothes from the day before and ate peanut butter and jelly sandwiches for dinner. He characterized his wife as a poor mother, lazy and self-centered, yet he was still willing to stay with her if she would have him.

John had few friends, stating he preferred to be alone. He explained being shy at parties and other social events, a "wallflower." He loved his daughter very much and had decided that for the first time in his life he was going to fight. He would try to win custody of his little girl. This fight frightened him very much. The thought of the battle he was about to embark upon left him nonfunctional; he was unable to get out of bed in the morning, unable to carry out his daily routine. John's parents brought him to the hospital.

Reluctantly attending art therapy, John said that he couldn't draw, but was willing to give it a try. Figure 18.7 is typical of much of his work, and of the spontaneous work of many depressed individuals. He drew a house

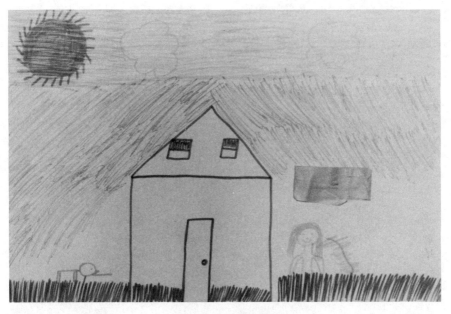

Figure 18.7. House.

outlined but not colored in, green grass, a yellow sun, and blue sky. He drew his daughter next to the house. He stated, "No one is in the house; Mary [his daughter] is smiling; she's waiting for me." He continued, "We'll have a picnic with our dog, George [lower left]." John related the picture to "happy times," and hope for a future with his daughter. He didn't share his anger at his wife or the turmoil he was experiencing.

John drew his barrier picture slowly and carefully (Fig. 18.8). The barrier is himself; he even looks a lot like the picture. He stated that he's preventing himself from living, describing himself as "a wimp." When asked by another patient, John spoke about his floating head: "That's me but I'm detached from my body; I know how to better myself but I don't." He related his lack of neck or body to his inability to take action, to help himself. The picture encouraged him to explore further important issues in his life, such as his lack of self-esteem and the custody battle to come. In a later piece of work he drew a similar barrier picture (smaller head and this time his body was included) to represent his readiness to fight. When asked to discuss this later picture, he laughed at his portrait: "It looks just like me, I'm going to change." John's spontaneous picture depicted hope; his later barrier picture represented action.

SUBSEQUENT BARRIER DRAWINGS

The barrier pictures act as a more immediate route to exploring and expressing issues. Depressed patients often must be pushed to share genuine

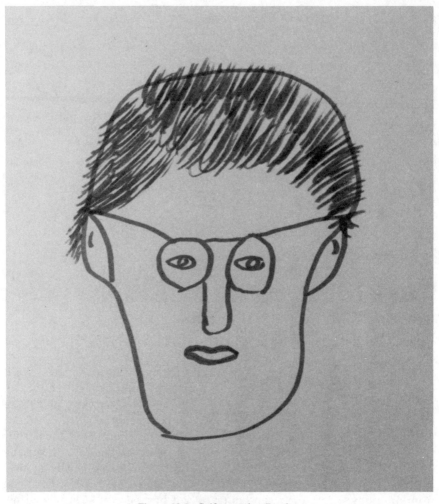

Figure 18.8. Self-portrait—Barrier.

concerns. It's difficult for them to transcend their walls of isolation. As a result, I decided to present the barrier theme frequently in group and individual therapy. Patients are asked to sign, date, and put the pictures in a folder. Once a week a review group meets to provide the patients the opportunity to examine these pictures and look at progress, regression, and/or changes. This gives the patients a tangible record of their therapy work and reviews issues needing to be explored.

DISCUSSION

In my experience, barrier drawings have proven to be a more direct route to conscious and unconscious material than spontaneous art when used with depressed patients. Spontaneous art frequently allows the patient more defense and takes longer to work through in therapy. Barrier drawings are less concrete and less connected than spontaneous art. The colors used are darker and the theme is more often of a somber nature. The work is more genuine.

The work described was conducted with a population of depressed patients at a private psychiatric facility. It would be of interest to determine whether similar observations may be obtained from different populations of depressed patients, such as those in a state or city hospital. Questions arise from this methodology, such as: What differences and/or similarities in symbolism can be seen between barrier drawings and other directive themes, such as family portraits? Do the barrier and spontaneous drawings vary significantly during different stages of therapy? Is there a correlation between the type of artwork produced and the number of hospitalizations? Is there a specific relationship between the amount and type of antidepressant medication and the artwork produced? What role does color play in these pictures? It would be helpful to study the barrier drawings systematically throughout the course of therapy, perhaps a daily barrier drawing. A controlled study in which one group of patients worked on spontaneous drawings and the other group drew barrier pictures might prove interesting. This study might be used to explore the following questions: In which group would patients appear to improve faster? Would there be a difference in length of hospital stay? What would this possibly mean in terms of patient recidivism?

Much research is needed to understand more fully the nature of the depressed state and how art therapy can be of help. I believe that the methodology introduced in this study is useful in helping the depressed patient explore problems; it gives the art therapist a tool for encouraging an art product that truly reflects the nature of the depression. I plan to continue experimenting with directive therapy groups, emphasizing barrier drawings, hoping to gain further access to patient material.

REFERENCES

Buchalter-Katz, S. (1985). *Observations concerning the art productions of depressed patients in short-term psychiatric facility*. New York: International Universities Press.

PART 3

Art Therapy Training

HARRIET WADESON

The future of a profession is in its training. Beginning with a scattering of courses and apprenticeships in the 1950s and 1960s, art therapy training became formalized in graduate programs offering master's degrees in the 1970s. An annual Art Therapy Educators' Convocation began in 1978. Toward the end of the 1970s the American Art Therapy Association established a procedure for approving training programs that meet its guidelines for education and training.

Although art therapy preparation was in this way becoming more standardized, in no way has it become regimented. Within the framework of meeting broadly defined standards, there is much diversity, with different training programs approaching the profession from various theoretical perspectives and differing emphases.

As the profession continues to grow and develop in ways described in the previous pages of this book, training needs develop as well. These developments constitute a two-way process. Training programs create student practicum placements in new kinds of facilities with new populations of clients. The result is the development of training to meet the new needs. Thus training both develops new opportunities and seeks to meet their challenges.

Often as well, it is the training programs that stimulate new thinking in the field, for both students and faculty. It is here that ideas are developed and tested. Unlike the clinical setting where the art therapist often works in isolation from other art therapists, the training program provides a forum for stimulating perspectives on the profession, as students and faculty exchange and challenge ideas.

Much of this sort of evolution becomes manifested as training programs change their structure, course offerings, emphases. These developments are not necessarily reported in the literature. As a result, the chapters in this section comprise an area of innovation, but do not necessarily represent the direction of art therapy training.

Although submissions for chapters in this book were received from art therapists with varied backgrounds from all over the country (and other countries as well), to our surprise those dealing with art therapy training emanated primarily from our own program at the University of Illinois at Chicago. I believe one reason is our continued exploration and development of broader uses of art making for professional and personal self-processing. Each of the chapters describes an ongoing process of art expression for a different aspect of training.

Barbara Fish has risked knowing herself more fully as issues for her patients evoked responses in herself that she did not understand. We also are the beneficiaries of her insights as she openly shares with us the self-revelations generated by her artwork in her chapter, "Addressing Counter-transference Through Image Making." She began this work as her thesis project while in training and has continued its development in her professional work. Indeed, it is surprising that art therapists who encourage their clients toward self-understanding through art expression do not utilize it themselves as a routine examination of their own work in ways similar to those described here.

Another bold project was undertaken by co-editors Jean Durkin and Dorine Perach as a component of their practicum supervision. Each had a field supervisor who was a graduate of our program. Fortunately, they too were interested in self-examination through image making and sharing. Fortunately as well, they were bold and adventurous enough to accept the invitation (and challenge) to examine the supervisory relationship through an ongoing artmaking and sharing process. This innovative and daring collaboration is reported in the chapter "A Model for Art Therapy Supervision Enhanced Through Art Making and Journal Writing" by Jean Durkin, Dorine Perach, Joanne Ramseyer, and Ellen Sontag. Their conjoint processing of art therapy supervision by student and supervisor provides an excellent model for those willing to trust both the art process and one another in the supervisory relationship.

The five authors represented in these two chapters are especially generous in opening to us their own sensitive and vulnerable recesses that were exposed in imaginative self-confrontation.

Finally, the chapter I have written, "The Art Therapy Termination Process Group," though not designed specifically to utilize art expression for self-processing, makes use of this modality to examine the difficult and significant issues in termination. This course is unique in its scope, following a dual track of handling separation and ending treatment with clients and the parallel process of the student's completing training, dealing with the separations involved, and transitioning to becoming a professional.

It is neither accidental nor coincidental that the three chapters on art therapy training embody art making as a significant vehicle in the preparation of the art therapist. It is paradoxical indeed that the distinctive essence of art therapy—art expression for the enhancement of human growth—is utilized so little for the development of the art therapist. The training program with which all the authors in this section have been connected has striven to apply the art therapy process itself to the development of the art therapist. The training models described in this section, therefore, reflect a congruence between the content of art therapy education and its process.

CHAPTER 19

Addressing Countertransference Through Image Making

BARBARA FISH

As an art therapist, I have found that my images may be utilized as an effective way to uncover and address the countertransference issues that often occur and interfere with therapeutic work. I am writing this chapter with the hope that other art therapists will be encouraged to use their own images to monitor and explore themselves within their therapeutic relationships.

LITERATURE REVIEW

Countertransference is barely addressed in the art therapy literature. This parallels the paucity of information available in psychoanalytic literature. Transference is discussed by both art psychotherapists and those who view art as therapy (Agell et al., 1981; Kramer, 1971; Naumburg, 1966; Wadeson, 1980). Because of the significance placed on defining the role of transference in art therapy, it would appear that countertransference is an issue worthy of exploration as both a clinical and a personal issue.

The lack of information about countertransference may be due to the intimate nature of this kind of self-exploration. It is not surprising that I have not found a discussion of the uses of image making to elucidate countertransference issues in either art therapy or psychoanalytic literature. In discussing this process with other art therapists, it has become clear that few use their own image making to explore problematic aspects of their therapeutic relationships. Those who do appear to find the process fruitful (Wadeson, 1987).

DEFINITION

An individual involved in a therapeutic relationship brings to that relationship unconscious feelings about other relationships as well as unresolved issues from his or her past. The displacement of these feelings onto the therapist is called transference. Countertransference refers to the therapist's reactions to the patient that are based on the therapist's unconscious issues. When countertransference is not addressed, the therapist may remain unaware of his or her own issues, allowing them to interfere with effective therapeutic work. I view transference as an important part of the therapeutic interaction within the art therapy session.

Transference is addressed as it occurs. It is not discouraged or redirected. Transference may be addressed through choice of media, exploration of images, interaction, and interpretation. It is also clear that I can do effective therapeutic work only with an understanding of my own countertransference issues. This self-exploration has become a crucial part of my work as an art therapist. Through visual exploration of my own countertransference issues, many of the dynamics within the art therapy sessions that appear unclear are elucidated. My responses to the patient are viewed in the context of the interaction. Those that are inappropriate responses to the relationship or are overly intense are cues to look for countertransference issues.

Image making may be used to explore and clarify the dynamics of the therapist involved in countertransference reactions toward the patient. This work may be approached on two levels. First, the therapist may use images to explore confusion on his or her part within the therapeutic relationship. Second, once countertransference is identified, images may help put unresolved issues back in context, allowing the therapist to continue the work of therapy more effectively. When working with patients, it is important to remember that the special qualities of our tools as art therapists are ones that we may use effectively for our own insight, growth, and healing.

THE FACILITY

The countertransference issues explored here developed within the therapeutic relationships with hospitalized psychiatric patients. The ages of patients on the unit ranged from 13 to 80. Patients had a wide variety of diagnoses including schizophrenia, bipolar disorder, borderline personality disorder, depression, conversion disorder, obsessive–compulsive disorder, anorexia nervosa, and psychosomatic disorders.

The facility is a university medical center. It is a teaching hospital, and many problematic cases are admitted for reevaluation. The treatment approaches used are psychopharmacology and psychotherapy. Patients are seen daily by their psychiatrist for medication management and psychotherapy. They are also assigned a primary nurse or mental health counselor for additional support. The milieu approach is also stressed. Patients' length of hospitalization ranges from 1 to 4 months. Art therapy is offered as an adjunctive treatment. The focus of individual art therapy is developed in conjunction with the treatment team.

METHOD

I drew images when some aspect of the relationship with the patient became unclear. My assumption is that this lack of clarity suggested the presence of countertransference. The most common response that I had to a patient that initiated image making was confusion. I also produced images when the direction of therapy became unclear. When my affect was overly intense or inappropriate in relation to the patient, I saw that as a cue for image making.

When possible, I drew immediately following the art therapy session. At times, my image making did not appear to be necessary until several hours later, when the session appeared problematic. In some cases, I drew images following the patient's discharge to clarify issues that were unresolved. I explored my images on my own, as well as taking them to supervision and my own therapy.

CASE EXAMPLES

The following are two case examples that illustrate the use of the images of the art therapist in clarifying countertransference. In all cases, image making helped to illuminate the dynamics at work during the sessions. At times, the issues were realistic responses to interpersonal dynamics. At other times, countertransference was apparent.

PAT

Pat, a 30-year-old White, middle-class, unemployed woman, was admitted for hospitalization for obsessive–compulsive behavior and anorexia. She had had one previous psychiatric hospitalization 6 months previously with a diagnosis of anorexia nervosa.

Pat is the youngest of five siblings. One brother, her twin, was killed in an automobile accident 2 years before. Pat lived with her mother who has multiple sclerosis and is confined to a wheelchair, and father who retired a year before the patient's present hospitalization. Pat left high school as a sophomore to stay home and care for her mother. All other siblings are married and have families.

Pat seemed like a small frightened child. Her clothing was disheveled. She seldom washed her hair. She compulsively picked at her fingers, clothes, chairs, or anything that was soft and upholstered. During her hospitalization, she spent a great deal of time by the sink in the day room. One month before leaving she developed a ritual of kissing the faucet nine times periodically. Pat also had compulsive behavior around the bathroom. She had difficulty flushing the toilet and stood nude before the mirror for hours every night.

Pat was admitted to the psychiatric unit soon after I began working there. She was referred to art therapy at my request. I felt drawn to Pat without understanding why. This was one of the questions I attempted to explore in my image making. I was curious about Pat and I liked her. I hoped that art therapy might help relieve her anxiety. I saw her in individual art therapy weekly throughout her 4-month hospitalization. In addition, she sporadically attended art therapy group, which was offered three times a week.

During the course of Pat's treatment, her behavior on the unit remained fairly consistent. Within art therapy sessions, however, there were significant changes. Initially Pat's images appeared rigidly drawn and highly defended. Pat was unable to leave the day room spontaneously to attend art therapy sessions. Much of her time was used getting ready to come to the session. Her affect was depressed and anxious. She appeared shy and childlike. Pat looked as though she wished she were invisible.

I drew Figure 19.1 in supervision. My intention was to draw the patient. Once the image was produced, I tried to stand it against the wall. The paper fell. I tried again. The paper fell again. I became furious. Why wouldn't the paper stand on its own?

The clarity of the analogy was powerful. The drawing was about the patient's need for control. My control issues became startlingly clear. The paper could not be held responsible for not being able to stand or lean, and neither could the patient.

It is interesting to note that the figure in my drawing has no mouth. This is an aspect of the image that I noticed some time after I drew this picture. I am not sure of its meaning. This is especially interesting in the light of Pat's prior diagnosis of anorexia nervosa.

Previously, I had come to get Pat for individual art therapy sessions without notice. After drawing this image, I started to make appointments with her. We contracted that we would set up sessions on Monday and she would be ready to leave the day room at the appointed time. Once Pat felt more in control, she was much less resistant to coming to sessions. She was never more than 5 minutes late to our meetings.

I drew Figure 19.2 depicting Pat and myself and our relationship after her first month in treatment. Initially Pat was represented as a tiny child with me towering over her. The next section represented the same small figure pulling me off balance. This is where my control issues come into play. Following that, I am represented with my back to Pat who has grown larger than I am. An angry line divides us. Next I have turned back to Pat. She has decreased in size, but a line still divides us. Finally I am represented sitting in a chair leaning toward Pat. There is a rope that is attached to the back of my neck and a stake in the ground to keep me from falling toward Pat. In sessions when I feel that I am losing objectivity or that I am inconsistent without apparent reason, I feel tension in the back of my neck. It is my cue to sit back and look at the dynamics of the session. The rope attached to the back of my neck in this image represents this tension and my need to be aware of my countertransference issues.

It is important to note that Pat never faces me in this drawing. All of the movement is mine. I felt as though I was reacting to her with extreme ranges

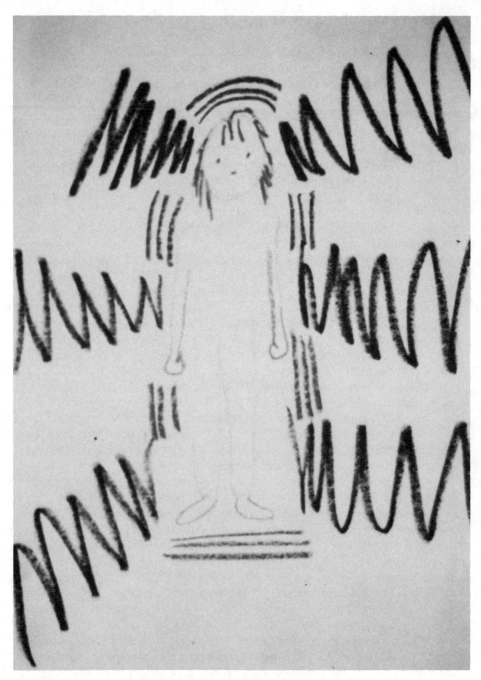

Figure 19.1. My impression of Pat, drawn in supervision.

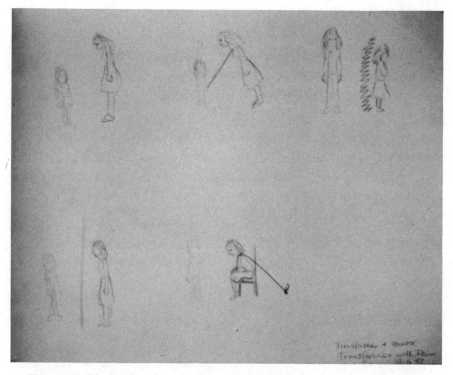

Figure 19.2. My drawing of the dynamics with Pat within our therapeutic relationship.

of affect, feeling either overinvolved or distant and angry. This indicated countertransference. I also noticed that I did not represent myself wearing a lab coat. I always wore one on the unit. All other drawings I have done representing myself with a patient show me wearing a lab coat. My projected identification with Pat came from a relationship outside the clinical setting. In my image, we were no longer art therapist and patient.

Through this image, I became aware of how much Pat and my relationship with her reminds me of myself and my sister. The need to remain in control demonstrated by Pat is very similar to my sister's needs. By engaging in a power struggle with Pat, I was reenacting the dynamics of my relationship with my only sibling.

I felt out of control and manipulated by Pat. I felt the need to help and protect her. When this was not successful, I felt powerless, frustrated, and angry. This is a pattern that has been consistent in my relationship with my sister.

With this realization, I felt freed from my anger and frustration with Pat. I was able to address Pat's needs and function in a way that was helpful to her and to bring my own need to explore my relationship with my sister to a place that would be helpful to me.

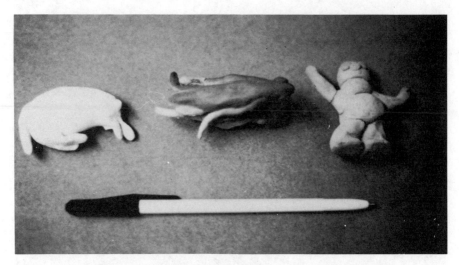

Figure 19.3. Pat's three clay sculptures, created over time.

Figure 19.3 is a sequence of three clay figures that Pat produced over a month's time. She used clay in a careful and controlled manner. She stated that she found it relaxing and requested clay often. The figure on the left was produced first. Pat described this as a "poor little thing." She stated that the figure was an "it" and "it" couldn't even stand up.

The center figure was described by Pat as a tadpole. During this session, I worked with clay as she did. This session was observed by my supervisor. I worked with the clay to defuse the focus from Pat and her image, as well as to alleviate my anxiety about being observed. I made several nondescript flat forms. Pat took one of these and placed the tadpole on top of it. She stated, "He can rest there."

Pat's increased comfort with the relationship and the medium are demonstrated by her image and statement. At this point, she was able to attend sessions on time and stated she felt more comfortable and relaxed while making images.

The figure on the right is a little man. He is represented with eyes and a nose, but no mouth. His arms are held out and up like a child who wants to be held.

Pat requested that I use clay with her in the session following the production of the center form in Figure 19.3. I began working in sessions with her because it appeared to make her more comfortable.

Figure 19.4 was produced in the session before my vacation. Pat made one of the "lizards"; I mirrored by making another. Together we made the base. She asked me to put the two lizards on the rock together. Then she stated, "Two lizards sitting on a rock talking about their problems. What

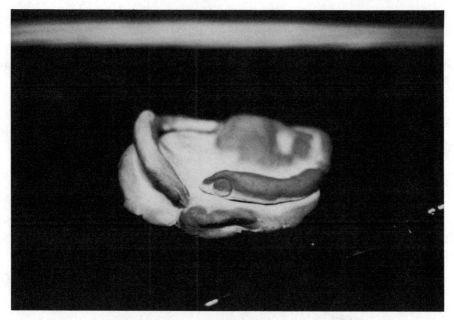

Figure 19.4. "Two lizards sitting on a rock. . . ."

will happen if one jumps off and swims away leaving the other all alone?"
We then addressed her issues regarding my vacation. I reassured Pat that I
would return.

The awareness of my countertransference issues allowed me to develop
a therapeutic relationship with Pat, enabling her to use art therapy in a way
that was valuable to her. Once I recognized the power struggle, I was able
to use that energy to support Pat instead of using the therapeutic relationship
to address my issues. My own need to understand this issue with my sister
was addressed outside of my therapeutic relationship with Pat although Pat
assisted in my recognition of the need for this work.

RICK

Rick, a 21-year-old middle-class, Black, single male, was hospitalized for
the first time following seclusive, bizarre behavior and paranoia. Prior to his
hospitalization, he was a freshman in college, living with his sister. He is
the youngest of six siblings, all of whom are successful professionals. Both
parents are deceased. Rick's mother died when he was 14. Rick's father
died 1 year prior to his hospitalization.

Upon admission Rick was extremely agitated. His major complaint was
that his mind was being controlled by a machine. He had difficulty concentrating and sitting still. His diagnosis was process schizophrenia.

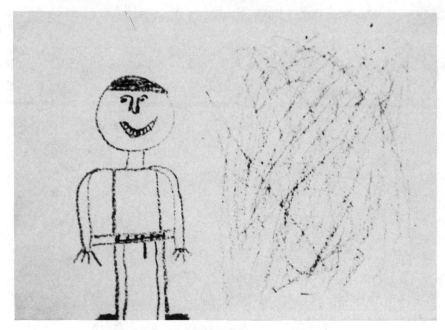

Figure 19.5. Rick's self-portrait, early in treatment.

Rick responded poorly to medication. When his medication reached therapeutic range, he became extremely agitated and rigid. For this reason he had several trials on various medications to determine which he could tolerate with the least agitation.

Rick was referred to art therapy because of his increasing complaint of not being able to feel anything any more. It was hoped that use of media would help him regain some affect. Rick was seen in group art therapy three times each week during his 4-month hospitalization. He was seen individually for art therapy throughout his last month in the hospital.

Figure 19.5 is a self-portrait drawn by Rick. The figure is drawn with the legs attached far apart and arms barely attached to the torso. A line is drawn vertically between the legs, which may represent Rick's penis. Rick drew his head as a round circle with his hair as a caplike form. No ears are represented. His mouth is smiling with teeth showing. Rick drew his hands with four lines attached to his arms. The belt on this figure extends past the torso to the arms. Rick drew the feet attached to the side of each leg. Rick stated this was a picture of himself but did not discuss the image further.

Rick became anxious following the drawing of this self-portrait, but was able to remain in the session by producing the scribble drawing on the same page. Rick had made scribble drawings in prior art therapy sessions as a warm-up exercise. He had stated he enjoyed doing them and found them relaxing. Rick may have tried to relax by drawing this scribble after his self-

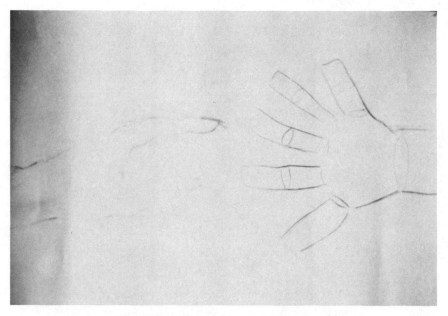

Figure 19.6. "Barbara, I can't feel any more."

portrait. The scribble may also have reflected Rick's feelings of anger and/or disorganization. He left the session following the scribble drawing before discussing his image.

As Rick's thoughts became more integrated, he expressed concern about his loss of function. There was despair in the way he talked about being a burden to society. Rick's mourning for his old self moved me deeply. I was overcome with a panicked sense that I had to change things. I had to make things better. This feeling carried into my sessions with Rick.

I drew Figure 19.6 after a session with Rick in which he stated, "Barbara, I can't feel any more." After doing the drawing, I looked at it for a long time. I knew it was important, but I couldn't understand how. Over time, two realizations have come into focus. First, my feelings were aroused about a physical problem that I have, which only recently has been brought under control. My feelings of being limited, tainted, and not the same as before are similar to Rick's. His mourning aroused my own.

Secondly, the image of the two hands reaching toward each other reminded me of Michelangelo's painting in the Sistine Chapel of God and Adam. My rescue fantasy became clear. This time it was to rescue myself. If Rick did not have to come to terms with his limitations, neither did I.

These realizations enabled me to be more objective within the therapeutic relationship with Rick. Instead of needing to help him rid himself of his pain, I could support his mourning and sense of loss.

Rick drew another self-portrait (Fig. 19.7) shortly before his discharge.

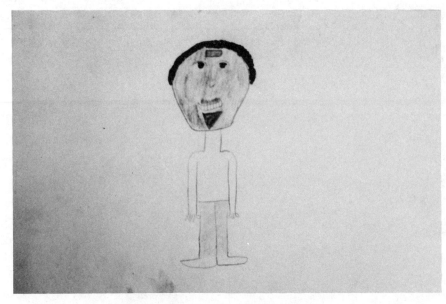

Figure 19.7. Rick's self-portrait late in treatment.

This drawing looks more like Rick than his previous self-portrait (Fig. 19.5). The hair, mustache, and beard look like his own. The head remains enlarged without ears, but is now drawn as a more headlike shape. The outlines of the body are drawn in a way that makes the arms and legs appear connected to the body. The fingers are now outlines instead of being represented by the lines themselves as in Figure 19.5. The neck remains elongated as in his earlier self-portrait. This figure floats in the center of the page. Rick represented himself in Figure 19.5 as standing on the bottom edge of the paper. This self-representation is more integrated than Figure 19.5.

In discussing Figure 19.7, Rick stated that the block in his head made it impossible for him to think. Rick explored his feelings in relation to his limitations. He became more able to represent these issues within art therapy sessions as my need to make things better lessened.

I drew Figure 19.8 after Rick was discharged. He is represented walking out the door. I am represented in a cloud of confused feelings. I felt sad to see him go. I felt left and abandoned. We had built a significant relationship. I felt the loss of someone important to me.

I was worried that Rick was not ready to leave the hospital. I thought I should have done more. Termination and his regression in relation to it brought an increased sense of my loss, as well as echoes of previous personal and interpersonal losses.

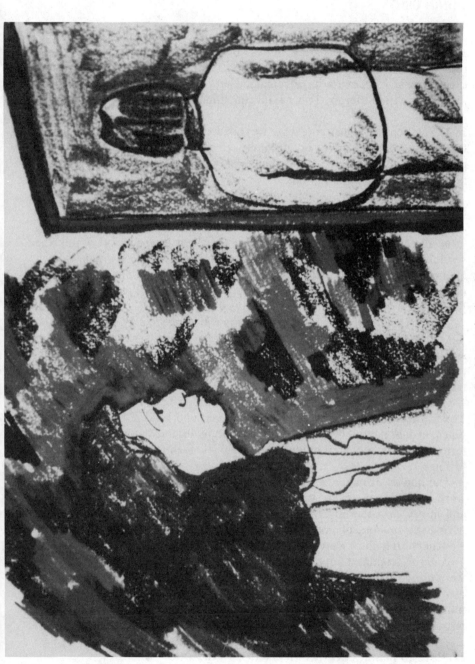

Figure 19.8. My termination with Rick.

387

CONCLUSION

Through my study of addressing countertransference issues through images, I have gained an increased awareness of the importance of understanding one's issues while working with patients. With the increased focus on my own images, I believe I have remained more sensitive to recognizing my responses within therapy that have been stimulated by my own unresolved problems.

The patients I have represented evoked countertransference responses that have to do with issues of autonomy. In all cases, my responses to these patients involved my own dependency and control issues developed in significant relationships in my past.

These patients were dealing with their own anxiety, feelings of powerlessness, dependency needs, and loss of functional ability. These are focal concerns for me, and ones to which I respond powerfully.

In all cases, image making led to a greater sense of comfort within the sessions. Drawing was soothing and helped me to feel more organized following a session with a patient who was disorganized or confused. Focusing on my own imagery also turned my attention to myself and what I needed. I felt self-nurtured and attended to, as well as monitored.

An unexpected result of this exploration is that new patients often remind me of images that I have done while treating others. This recognition of similar issues may facilitate better work. The early recognition of countertransference enables less obstructed therapeutic work to begin early in the relationship.

One of the problems I encountered was the difficulty of objective self-exploration. At times, images were significant and I did not know why. At times, insight did not come quickly and therapy fumbled along. Often, countertransference appeared hidden under realistic feelings such as fear or confusion.

The impact of many of these images indicated unconscious processes at work, but I was unable to trace them. I discussed my images in supervision and in my own therapy. Insight came through those supports, as well as during the process of image making and my reflection on the images immediately after they were drawn and over time.

A more structured approach to image making may be helpful. The images were drawn when a session felt problematic. Using images as part of my own standard process notes may lead to other insights including countertransference issues of which I am not yet aware. These may include countertransference issues with which I am comfortable. Because of the displaced affect associated with countertransference, positive issues should also be explored to permit effective therapeutic work.

It would be of interest to continue this work over time. Working with many patients would lend insight into whether countertransference can be a response to the psychodynamics of various diagnoses or the personalities of specific individuals.

Kohut (1971) suggests the use of the therapist's unresolved issues as a motivating force in creative work: "I believe that true psychoanalytic creativity may be motivated by the urge to investigate certain psychological areas that have remained incompletely elucidated in the personal analysis" (pp. 318–319).

It is my view that a creative use of self as an art therapist will lead to greater insight and an ability to increase the understanding of the wide range of uses of visual imagery for therapeutic use. The tools of our trade, image making, have much potential for art therapists, as well as for art therapy patients and clients.

REFERENCES

Agell, G., Levick, M., Rhyne, J., Robbins, A., Rubin, J., Ulman, E., Wang, C., & Wilson, L. (1981). Transference and countertransference in art therapy. *American Journal of Art Therapy, 21,* 11.

Kohut, H. (1971). *The analysis of the self.* New York: International Universities Press.

Kramer, E. (1971). *Art as therapy with children.* New York: Schocken.

Naumburg, M. (1966). *Dynamically oriented art therapy.* New York: Grune & Stratton.

Wadeson, H. (1980). *Art psychotherapy.* New York: Wiley.

Wadeson, H. (1987). *The dynamics of art psychotherapy.* New York: Wiley.

CHAPTER 20

A Model for Art Therapy Supervision Enhanced Through Art Making and Journal Writing

JEAN DURKIN, DORINE PERACH, JOANNE RAMSEYER, AND ELLEN SONTAG

Art therapy supervision is usually conducted in a traditional manner in which the supervisee presents case material and artwork to be examined verbally, rather than utilizing the rich resources of the art process, thereby applying the essence of art therapy to the supervisory process. Because art therapy is a new field, art therapists have worked around the mental health practitioner model, struggling to find ways to integrate the art therapy process or artwork into supervision. Art therapy interns are often assigned to placements in which they are supervised by social workers, psychologists, or other mental health professionals and spend much of their supervisory hour learning pragmatic and theoretical issues regarding client dynamics, case management, agency policies and procedures, and broader aspects of the mental health system. In many instances, the student may be called upon to educate the supervisor about the art therapy process. For the art therapist who is accustomed to using the rich process of art making professionally and personally, the traditional model of supervision may result in an experience that neglects the importance of the art making.

Two student–supervisor dyads decided to examine the supervisory format of art therapy, incorporating the exchange of journal writing and art making throughout the internship to discover a more appropriate model of supervision and its impact upon the supervisory process. In both dyads, the supervisors were art therapists. This chapter describes the experience from the perspective of both dyads, and from the roles of both supervisor and supervisee.

REVIEW OF LITERATURE

Little has been published concerning the supervision of art therapy students and art therapists. Those who have ventured into this territory include the following:

Marion and Felix (1979) state in their article concerning the relationship between art therapy interns and their supervisors:

> Because there is a notable lack of literature specifically addressing supervision in art therapy, the art therapy supervisor often molds his or her identity from traditional fields, as well as from personal experience. Art therapy training, however, presents many unique situations in which traditional roles must be questioned. (p. 37)

These authors emphasize that during on-site clinical supervision in art therapy, one is called upon to be as "flexible as the discipline itself, adapting to a variety of situations; prepared to be rater, participant, mentor, therapist, observer, teacher and even student" (p. 37).

Wilson, Riley, and Wadeson (1984), in their three-part article "Art Therapy Supervision," address specific phases of art therapy supervision as beginning, middle, and termination. Wadeson suggests that "the fantasy tapping process of art therapy can be useful in supervision as well. Students can be encouraged to make pictures of their images of being a professional and in this way confront some of their fears" (p. 105). Wadeson (1987) furthers this idea by suggesting: "The supervisee can illustrate clients, her relationship with them, problematic staff relationships, images of the facility in which she works, feelings about her work, career goals, and so forth" (p. 284).

Although these articles address the special attention and sensitivity needed on the part of the supervisor in exploring with the intern the art produced, no articles or suggestions have been written about both supervisor and student creating and using the art itself to understand further the dynamics of the supervisory relationship. Based on our interest in breaking new ground in this area, we agreed to bring the tools of the trade into our supervisory relationships. In our explorations we hope to view the roles art making and journal writing can play in developing a supervisory model unique to the art therapy process and how it affects the relationships.

FORMING THE MODEL

The objectives of this chapter evolved over the course of a 9-month internship. Initially we entered into our working relationships to examine how the exchange of artwork and journal writing would affect the supervisory relationship. The exchange of journal writing was suggested by the students, based on Yalom and Elkin's book, *Every Day Gets a Little Closer* (1974). In this book, a therapist–client team published their journal entries, which they had exchanged during the course of therapy, and which had significantly enhanced their therapeutic relationship. These exchanges often revealed differences in their perceptions of a certain session, illuminated many transference–countertransference issues, and permitted them to record many thoughts and ideas post-session that may have been easily forgotten or lost.

We felt that journal writing would record the self-reflective process generated by the artwork, and agreed to shape Yalom and Elkin's model to fit
our individual needs in supervision. By adding art making to this model we
gave each other the freedom to choose either mode to process our experiences. Both dyads agreed to set up their own schedules to review the art
and journals at regular intervals.

As time went on the process evolved. Each of us found journal writing
and art making useful to a different extent. We mutually discovered that this
model brought interpersonal richness to our relationships, cut through to
the core of many issues very quickly, and permitted access to three modes
of communication: visual, verbal, and written.

What follows shows different ways this model was utilized. This process
reveals separate and overlapping discoveries: individually, between student
and supervisor, and between the two dyads. Having clearly felt three separate phases of supervision as described by Wilson and colleagues (1984),
we will present the narrative of these experiences in chronological order.

DYAD A: JOANNE RAMSEYER, M.A., SUPERVISOR, AND DORINE PERACH, STUDENT

Background Information

Dorine and Joanne worked together for 9 months at New Images, an outpatient, psychiatric rehabilitation program serving the chronically mentally
ill. The program is operated as a psychosocial clubhouse and clients are
referred to as members. Supervision took place formally an hour each week.
During the course of the week other time was spent informally on logistical
matters. Art making was done at home during the first 2 months. Dorine
kept a journal consistently through the year (about once a week) and Joanne
used journal writing as a way of reflecting back on longer periods of time,
about once every month.

After 2 months of this routine, the supervision format changed and art
making was incorporated into the supervision hour, which immediately followed a group Dyad A co-led. They continued the format of writing at home
and when time allowed created additional artwork, which they continued to
exchange.

The Beginning Phase

Joanne

When Dorine approached me with the idea of exchanging journals throughout
her internship I was intrigued by the concept of mutual self-disclosure in
the supervisory process, and hoped it would contribute to a richer working
relationship between us. Because of her initiative and willingness to take
risks in our relationship, I respected Dorine from the outset. She seemed to

radiate a lively curiosity and creative energy that paralleled my own drive to explore uncharted territory. I looked forward to the challenge of working with her, yet I had reservations regarding her proposal.

This was my first experience in the supervisory role and naturally I felt insecure about exposing my inexperience or other "less-than-perfect" parts of myself to a student who would be looking to me for role modeling. I also anticipated potential boundary problems because Dorine was enrolled in the same art therapy program from which I had graduated. I was sure that our informal setting and the journal experience would intensify the difficulty of maintaining a professional distance.

I knew it would be necessary to examine my fears and insecurities more carefully, and if the experience was to be personally meaningful it would be essential to add art making to our venture. The use of art making for personal and professional development was an integral process in my life that I wanted to encourage Dorine to cultivate. Besides personal art making, I had been looking for additional ways to incorporate art therapy into the work setting. I frequently created artwork about clients and co-workers and brought it into my own supervision to use as a springboard for discussions. This had always felt one-sided, though, since only I was actually using the art therapy process. Mutual art making and journal writing to facilitate supervision would be an excellent opportunity for experiential learning for both of us. In spite of my fears, I decided to "dive in," and a unique interpersonal and professional adventure began.

During the initial stage of our relationship I used art making frequently to examine my desire to "do things right," my exaggerated fears of boundary problems, and my feelings of inadequacy as I struggled to develop new skills. Searching for role models from my past, I reflected upon my previous supervisory relationships, and several pictures emerged expressing unresolved anger about some supervision experiences as a graduate student.

Figure 20.1 is an image depicting angry feelings directed toward a supervisor who withdrew abruptly from our relationship after our first conflict developed. The imagery expresses both anger and the feeling of the relationship "shattering." I had idealized this person, and her unwillingness to explore and share her responsibility in our conflict had robbed me of the opportunity to work through my feelings and develop a more realistic relationship. It had left me feeling frustrated, and in my journal I wrote about the need to remain aware of the potential destructiveness of my new role. Creating more artwork and writing about other supervisors who had behaved destructively put me in touch with my own power and control issues. I wrote, "My worst fear would be to stifle Dorine's creativity" (as one supervisor had clearly attempted to do to me early in my training).

My wish to be the "perfect" supervisor was unrealistic and I knew this, but I wanted Dorine to walk away from her internship at least having experienced the possibility for resolving conflicts on my part. I would eventually have to come to terms with my limitations and continue to explore

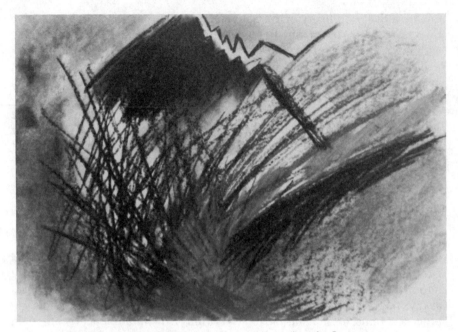

Figure 20.1. Feelings toward a past supervisor, by Joanne.

power issues—work that would be uncomfortable and difficult for me at times. Somehow the artwork and writing were already making this less painful than it might have been. Rather than share this art and journal writing with Dorine, I brought them to a supervision class, and the resulting dis- cussions and support helped me to adjust to the difficult transition from supervisee to supervisor.

Dorine

As I walked into New Images the first day, feeling curious, hopeful, yet a little unsteady, my nagging self-doubts and lack of confidence followed close behind. What if I fail? Such an outcome was unbearable to think of, let alone to say. I told myself, "Stay centered, be there for the members . . . sweat a little, learn, and don't be so scared." I entered a facility where I knew they wanted a student intern, where the clients loved art therapy, where it was accepted and supported by staff, and where I had been matched with a supervisor who was enthusiastic about being assigned a student intern. I knew from the beginning that she took her role as supervisor seriously (she even enrolled in a supervision class to understand her role better). I antic- ipated the sharing of art and writing would ask much from both of us. I wrote, "I know I will be exposed to you, as you will to me." I was also fearful that Joanne would "expose my true self and discover that I'm an impostor playing out the 'good student' role."

I began my internship with a few specific goals in mind: really to listen and "be with" the members. I felt certain that these skills could compensate when my newly forming therapist skills felt shaky. Little did I know then how difficult it is to "be with" others, really to hear them. I worked on learning to be curious about their artwork, and to put my interpretations and biases aside. These became important skills I worked on steadily throughout my internship.

Initially I spent much time observing. In my early pictures I explored feelings of how I sensed staff were affected, touched, and changed in some way by working with a population that seemed so draining to me. I questioned how this would affect me and took comfort in the fact that art seemed to permeate the program; it brought creativity and energy into many barren lives.

As time went on I found myself beginning to experience the harsh realities of what it must be like to be chronically mentally ill, and found myself taking these feelings home with me, often reenacting what I had just observed. I recorded, "Sometimes I come home from work . . . and I start acting, like it is my turn to be mad. It is such a weird phenomenon." I questioned my own attraction to working with this population, and my identification with many members. "I am one of them. I know that. I am more like them than different. I am that face, that depression, that lame leg, that car accident, that obesity. But in my closet of disguises, I have chosen to live in both worlds. It's just that the transition from one to the other is very, very hard." The first 2 months' experiences had affected me deeply, and they had also drained much of my energy.

I decided to look closer at how a specific client was affecting me whom I was seeing in both group and individual art therapy. Don, a 34-year-old, very talented chronic schizophrenic man, exuded the message loud and clear that he wanted to get better, but he had no idea how. He often sat, steadily shaking his leg, looking at the ground in an obsessive mode of worry. Don was undergoing medication changes that altered his creativity, interest, and investment in art throughout the year. In Figure 20.2, "The Disguise," I drew Don fiddling an instrument, to represent him playing a tune that no one would ever hear.

I brought the picture to supervision and Joanne helped me explore the feelings underlying the image. The masklike quality of Don's face in the image made it difficult to see who he actually was. The sadness in his eyes evoked a deep sadness within myself that I was just beginning to understand. Joanne helped me become aware of the difficulty of being a presence in clients' lives without feeling the responsibility to "fix them." I learned to lower my expectations for Don, maintain my hopefulness by looking at more of his strengths, and relate to him at his level of functioning. In my journal I later asked myself, "If I can thrive with my sadness, why can't Don?" Though it took many months, I learned to accept Don more clearly and found myself able to reach a point where we could work together without my emotions interfering.

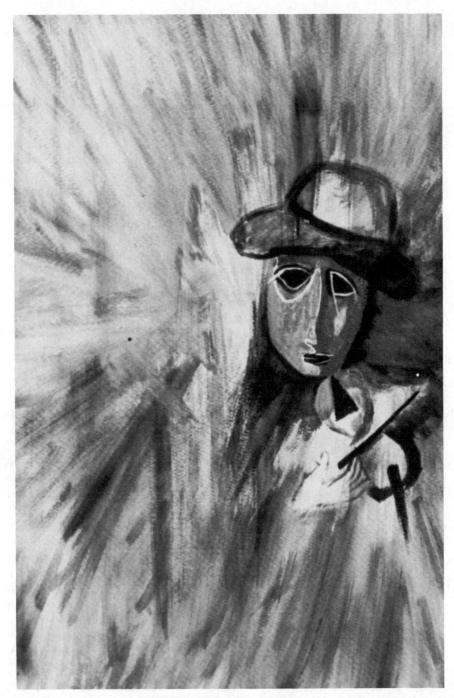

Figure 20.2. "The Disguise," by Dorine.

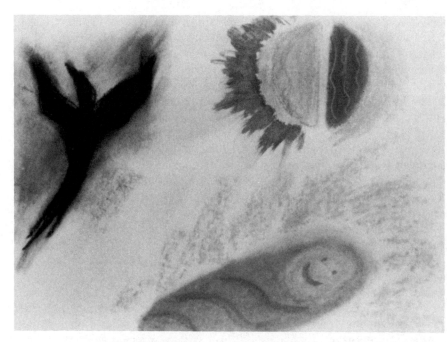

Figure 20.3. Dorine as a "new baby," by Joanne.

Joanne

Important insights emerged during this phase after I created artwork about a staff member with whom I had co-led an art therapy group for a year and a half. Dorine had replaced Phillip, and whenever the three of us were together a power struggle between him and me seemed to ensue. To ventilate my feelings of frustration, I created several pictures and wrote angrily in my journal about the situation. Out of this I discovered that because of my new role and enthusiasm to have a student intern I had become preoccupied with Dorine's presence—much like a new mother preoccupied with the care and responsibilities of a "firstborn" child. Meanwhile I had ignored Phillip, and I sensed that he probably felt rejected. The dynamics of our power struggle became clearer as I realized we had both been competing for Dorine's attention. To explore the situation further I drew Figure 20.3, which led to additional insights.

The smiling baby initially represented Dorine's arrival and the new life and energy I felt she had brought into our program. Studying the image, I recognized that in some ways I envied the childlike joy and excitement she expressed openly about art therapy and our setting. I remembered back to when I had been more like her, and I acknowledged to myself that I had lost some of those enthusiastic feelings with experience. Even though I was happy to move into a new role that represented professional growth, I had been the only art therapist on staff, occupying a special position on our team. Now I would have to share that attention and uniqueness with Dorine. The image of Dorine as a "new baby" took on more meaning and enabled me to identify my feelings of sibling rivalry and envy.

The circle split in half in the upper right-hand corner represents the end of a harmonious co-leader relationship with Phillip. The black bird symbolizes the various losses just described. After reflecting on the picture for several days, I shared it with Phillip, which helped us resolve the conflict. In this way, the use of art making to understand the supervisory relationship expanded into staff relationships as well.

At our first exchange meeting I shared the picture with Dorine, hoping to discuss staff politics, power and control issues, competition, and conflict resolution. I assumed Dorine would understand the complexity of the issues I had expressed. Although we discussed the picture's meaning to me, and Dorine understood, her focus returned to the image of herself portrayed as a baby. She seemed to be insulted, questioning why I had drawn her with her arms bound, "like a papoose."

I realized too late it had been a lot to ask of a new student to understand co-worker politics and my transitional struggles, particularly since Dorine was just beginning to feel some of her inadequacies and inexperience at this stage in her internship. I wondered if this exchange process was going to be helpful after all, as I sensed the beginning of a conflict stirring.

Dorine

Two months quickly passed and somehow the chaos gave way to organization, a process that occurred repeatedly during my internship. The first time Joanne and I exchanged our writings and artwork I remember feeling very exposed. I had filled pages in my journal with positive transference: "Joanne, you seem so together and sure—so open. You seem very colorful to me . . . and very committed and connected to your work. . . . Joanne lights up when we speak about the members." I shared only good things. "I feel at home around you because we are alike in many ways . . . same art therapy roots. . . . My ideas, feelings, thoughts all feel validated, acknowledged, affirmed, understood." I dreaded the day that conflicts would enter our relationship, but for then all was okay.

I was not quite ready to explore the boundary I felt settling between us, which was unclear to me at that time. Due to the informality of the milieu setting I often felt confused regarding how much of myself I should reveal. The staff seemed so open on a personal level and I wanted to become closer to Joanne in some ways, but questioned whether it was my place. Though outwardly I attempted to look relaxed around co-workers and clients, I found myself often feeling awkward and uncomfortable inside.

Joanne received my recorded experience positively and explored the many nuances I could not see in my artwork. I found myself repeatedly surprised at the drawings Joanne presented to me and all that she had written about me. When Joanne showed me her pictures I felt somewhat flattered and important as I realized that my presence was both affecting and influencing her growth.

However, one image that appeared at that exchange did not sit right with me: Joanne's portrayal of me as an infant. I couldn't stop focusing on my arms being bound within the infant's blanket. Although at this time I did not understand the meaning this image held for me, the picture evoked angry feelings but I did not feel ready to convey them to Joanne. Perhaps the conflict-free honeymoon was coming to a close.

Several weeks passed. Two weeks in a row Joanne "took over" a group we were co-leading. Not having expressed the disappointment and anger I felt following these groups, I was reminded again of the image of me as a baby. I decided to create some artwork to explore my feelings. In Figure 20.4, "Breakdown," I attempted to draw Joanne, but it turned out to be about our relationship.

I began the picture by drawing a night scene, reminiscent of what Joanne had painted that day in our group. This was followed by a picture of a bird flying away, representing my wish to avoid conflict—a desire I knew only too well. The next image is a woman with two faces, one looking straight ahead representing Joanne and the other face representing me, looking at Joanne. This particular image helped me realize how difficult it was to be a group leader and hear the members when my attention was focused on Joanne rather than on the group.

Central in the picture is a beautiful show horse, representing Joanne. I wrote, "When around Joanne she seems to be the center of attention, she's funny and fun. And in other times and places that's me—but not here where I tend to stay removed and watch the staff in action." I questioned how much of me wanted to be the star as well. During supervision that day, I became more aware of my envy of Joanne. "What she has . . . I want too." Especially the security of knowing how to be a good group leader and dynamic as well. In the lower left corner is a peasant woman, the Joanne I perceived as having experienced much more of life than I. The two faces of this woman represent the face of Joanne I could see as supervisor and a face looking away, the personal side of Joanne that she might not want to share with me, which I was curious to know. Once more I found myself questioning my ability to accept the boundaries demanded by our professional relationship.

Although I began the picture drawing Joanne, I finished the lower right corner with a picture about myself, restricted like a papoose. I saw myself on fire and furious, envy and anger shining through the red. I questioned whether it could be possible to co-lead with someone who naturally took center stage. Though I felt very nervous about sharing this picture with Joanne, I trusted her and relaxed as she gave me permission to explore what the anger was about. Joanne was sensitive to my discomfort in sharing my

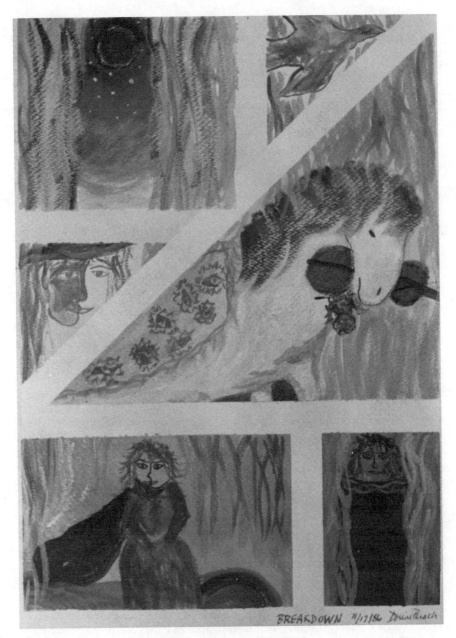

Figure 20.4. "Breakdown," by Dorine.

first negative feelings toward her and helped me to discover several important parts of my picture to explore further. She also took responsibility for "taking over" the group and shared the difficulty of slowing down to work at my level—subjects I sensed were difficult for her to talk about. She added that she was bound to make mistakes in her new role, and empathized with my part in having to make adjustments to her ups and downs as she struggled to learn new skills. Based on my past record of avoiding conflict, without the artwork I might have passed by many of these topics. I later realized how appropriate the title was as my barrier to facing conflictual feelings and maintaining the facade of "everything's okay" began breaking down.

Joanne

When Dorine responded to the "papoose" image (as she referred to it) in my drawing by creating her series of progressive images, I became excited that we were communicating and interacting visually. The artwork allowed Dorine to "show me" how she felt, rather than being forced to put words onto difficult emotions. It also enabled me to appreciate more clearly the depth and importance of her feelings. Our "visual dialogues" were an especially helpful tool at this early stage in our relationship and provided us with rich imagery for ongoing conversations about the concepts of projection, transference, and countertransference, owning our respective roles in conflicts, and accepting our individual limitations.

Throughout her internship Dorine continued to pursue and expand the papoose imagery, searching for a deeper level of its meaning. It was difficult for me to admit to being less than perfect to her, to disclose my control and territory issues. It was also hard to be the target of her competitive envy and anger, yet I knew that it took a lot of courage to reveal her negative feelings to me and I admired her honesty. Our artwork continually opened doors to mutually rewarding discussions about vulnerable feelings that were difficult to articulate. It was an especially rewarding process for me to watch Dorine's professional development and identity unfold through the visual drama of her imagery.

As I suspected, during this phase I shared less about myself through my journal writing, preferring to rely on the familiar and comforting process of art making to writing, which was difficult for me. On the other hand, Dorine wrote fluently, informing me that because she had kept journals since childhood, writing was a natural, enjoyable process for her. I looked foward to reading her journal entries because they became an excellent guide for facilitating her learning. For example, on the surface Dorine initially presented herself as a confident, conscientious, well-organized and creative intern. In her journal, however, I read about the exhaustion she felt from working with mentally and physically disabled individuals; her reactions to being exposed day after day to the painful struggles of mental illness and poverty of our clients and community; her identification with clients; fears of being unable to complete her thesis work in time for graduation; and her desire to be accepted by me and our team.

Our busy schedules had permitted little time for us to discuss these important and typical feelings of an intern's experience since supervision was so often taken up with casework and planning. As Dorine's first quarter came to an end, I felt that we had reached the end of the first phase.

Dorine

After Joanne and I worked through our first conflict, I felt the beginning phase grow to a close. I no longer experienced myself as taking an observing or passive role. In addition I found myself beginning to make progress with clients, feeling their impact on my life and becoming more willing to express negative feelings to Joanne.

Keeping the journal throughout my internship ensured that important ideas that I might not have had time to express during supervision would not be lost. Journal writing was easy for me to do, but I was forever procrastinating about making art. I started each piece with an idea rather than starting more spontaneously and seeing where the art might take me. I found myself not trusting the art to work its way to my issues. Joanne always responded to whatever sort of art product I brought into supervision with enthusiasm, and through her keen interest and observations we explored various meanings of the imagery.

Viewing Joanne's artwork proved to be very illuminating as well. I felt fortunate to have a supervisor who would share her experience of me so honestly. Though it certainly was not her intention, it felt flattering to appear in someone's artwork. I felt important in my role as an intern. In the beginning phase we established an effective working relationship and successfully built a safe place where the exchange of journals and art could take place.

Middle Phase

Joanne

With our hectic work weeks catching up with us, Dorine and I were both having trouble finding time to create artwork after hours. At the beginning of Dorine's internship I mentioned that it might be useful to create art together during supervision, and it seemed an appropriate time to try this. The new structure marked the beginning of the second phase for me. Dorine and I were tackling the challenge of co-leading, and struggling to find a balance given our different levels of experience. Her supervisory hour occurred immediately following the group we co-led so I suggested we make spontaneous drawings for 5 to 10 minutes, and use the rest of the hour to discuss them. We chose to draw about co-leading, group dynamics, and transference–countertransference issues or any other subject that arose. This was exciting because our supervision now paralleled the work we asked of our clients. Because it was Dorine's hour, I generally tried to give her as much time as she needed to explore her picture before I shared mine with her. If issues that emerged in my artwork felt unresolved, I brought them to my own supervision.

By now Dorine and I were absorbed in a working mode of our relationship. Creating artwork together reflected that phase of development. It was also an excellent way to "compare notes" and "debrief" after our groups (where surprises never ceased), and it provided time out from our busy schedules to regenerate through the creative process. As co-leaders, during our group we were one step removed from the powerful process and results of art therapy. By incorporating art making into supervision we found that we too could experience the benefits we had just facilitated for our clients. We both enjoyed the new format, and I began to feel a special closeness to Dorine.

I had often felt alone with my work as an art therapist; in spite of my co-workers' support I never felt they truly understood my love of this process. Dorine's presence filled this void. Our affinity stimulated many rich conversations about art, creativity, therapeutic philosophies, and the struggle to develop one's individual professional identity. This raised important questions for me about the significance and importance of the "mentor" role involved in supervision as well as the student's contribution to the supervisor's growth and learning. While we were still smoothing out the rough edges of our relationship, I felt we had discovered a way to practice art therapy supervision par excellence and felt most in my element during those hours.

Dorine

At last I found myself relaxing in my relationship with Joanne as well as in the group we co-led, which I had begun to experience as full of life and fun. I often left the group experiencing some of my highest moments and feelings of hope for the members as well. I wrote:

> I really enjoyed watching the members explore their art today. During the art making, sort of a collage "round robin," it really felt to me like THIS IS LIFE. Living for the moment, working side by side the person next to you, forming a community, be it for one hour. Somehow it gives me strength and enlivens me. Dipping into our creative souls is an amazing act. Maybe this is the antidote for our society. Using our hands, self-expression, validation, letting go of our inhibition . . . this is when we can experience true freedom. In our art there are no rules, no laws. If we can let go of our insanity for an hour, perhaps it will lead to another. And when I think of all their hope, their courage to endure insanity—all I can think is how weak I am in comparison . . . and they come to me.

These people were affecting my life and I was discovering how important my life's work was to me.

I still found myself taking feelings from work home with me, but I was not drained, as before; instead, I found myself inspired by the clients. I wrote,

> And you, dear members, are the strong ones. You suffer, you scream and move onward. My motivation seems so tangible, and yours? How do you do it? How do you arrive early to your 1000th group therapy session? How do you keep yourself from pulling the trigger?

The paradox was that on a typical day I could experience the devastating realities of their world and yet found inspiration sharing their journey. Joanne identified strongly with many of my feelings when I shared these journal entries with her. I felt in harmony with her at these moments, experiencing us more as colleagues than as supervisor–supervisee.

Co-leading was now taking a back seat as I focused on the difficulty of processing the artwork with members. I often felt frustrated with my newly forming skills as I compared them to Joanne's natural ability and experience leading the group. At these moments I still identified with the papoose picture of months ago and would again feel angry. I returned to the symbol in Figure 20.5 hoping to resolve these feelings further.

I began the picture struggling with the image, allowing the process to lead me to what proved to be an important realization. The blanket emerged to represent my abilities. When unable to accept my limitations or level of development I questioned whether Joanne was holding me back. She questioned whether in some way it was myself. In practicing to break out of the "papoose" (top right corner) I began to see how I was responsible for controlling my abilities, what I might achieve, and how I limited myself. Allowing the art to lead me to the next two images revealed a more settled and comfortable image of me sitting under the blanket, a metaphor for my growing acceptance of myself and my rate of development. Yet as my expression in the last picture shows, I am still not pleased, feeling inexperienced. This series came to represent my progress in becoming aware of both strengths and limitations in becoming an art therapist.

In sharing this picture and my thoughts with Joanne, we acknowledged the different levels we were at and she helped me recognize some of my own strengths I had been overlooking. She respected my request for more time to struggle with processing client's artwork in our group by slowing down her responses. I was relieved to have the permission and opportunity to work at my own pace and thereafter felt less pressure to perform as a student.

Joanne

A picture that I drew near the end of this phase became another turning point in my relationship with Dorine and clarified the underlying tension about boundaries that I had struggled with from the beginning. After an

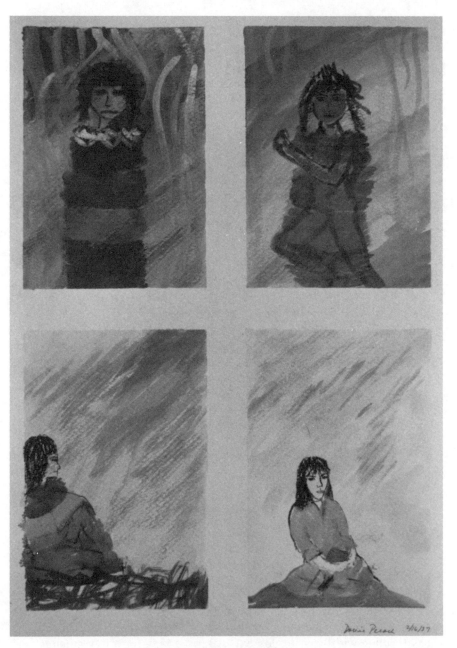

Figure 20.5. Blanket series, by Dorine.

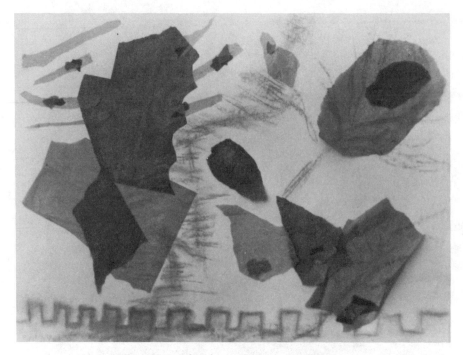

Figure 20.6. Joint picture, by Joanne and Dorine.

interesting group in which members had paired up to work on joint pictures, I suggested to Dorine that we make a joint picture in supervision to obtain a better feel for the members' experience (Fig. 20.6).

I was relaxed about the idea, and began working immediately on one half of the page. I hoped the resulting picture would provide us with a way to discuss some of the frustration I felt at this point with my role as a supervisor. I had grown to like Dorine very much as an individual, but felt my position prevented me from interacting more casually with her as I could with other co-workers. I also wanted to explore her interpretation of my "keeping distant from her," which she had briefly mentioned in her journal.

As we worked, Dorine began pasting pieces of tissue paper closer and closer to my initial image (the three larger shapes on the left side), so I drew a zigzag line across half the page, making a clear statement that I wanted my own space in the picture. Knowing Dorine, I had a feeling she would react by challenging the limit I had just set. She hesitated, and I knew she was struggling with what to do next. After working for a few minutes, she crossed the line by pasting scraps around my image until finally drawing on top of it with chalk. I didn't mind the small scraps of paper she pasted on "my side" because they seemed to mirror some imagery I had placed on the paper that represented our shared creative energy. On the other hand, I disliked her drawing on top of my image—it felt as if she had not respected my need to be separate from her and only emphasized my own difficulty with having to maintain a professional distance between us. Nevertheless, to express my feelings of genuinely liking Dorine and enjoying our affinity as art therapists, I completed the picture by drawing a border on the bottom of the page connecting our two sides.

I proceeded to wipe off the chalk Dorine had drawn on my image and told her I had to do this because it had felt intrusive and it was important, even if difficult, to maintain our sense of separateness and professional boundaries. I sensed Dorine felt rejected, but the picture had relieved the tension I had experienced in *not* having discussed these issues sooner. The picture became a springboard for further discussions about the boundaries of our relationship, the boundaries between herself and clients, and several other school relationships she was feeling uncomfortable about. It was paradoxical and a relief that once I clarified my feelings to her, describing my frustration and reasons for keeping my distance, I became more relaxed in our relationship. It was also an important discovery that the actual *process* of art making had been as useful for working through significant issues as the symbolic content of our previous artwork.

Dorine

The day that Joanne and I created the boundary picture I wrote, "In many ways termination has begun." At one point during the making of the picture, I felt daring and drew over a prominent image of Joanne's, just to see what would happen. In response to her wiping my chalk off I felt pushed away and went home feeling that perhaps it's time to think about moving on.

The next day, we were both feeling somewhat uncomfortable so we processed the joint picture once more. In staying with the image my fears of being pushed away were alleviated as we discussed the importance of settling limits and the limitations of our relationship.

As in the previous picture, my daring nature shone through again in another incident where we worked through a related conflict. Shortly after we made the boundary picture, I handed Joanne an uncensored version of my journal entries. Feeling somewhat confrontational, I wanted to share some of my observations of her; I no longer feared delving into uncomfortable topics and hoped by working through these issues we could once more grow closer.

Joanne responded to this by explaining some of her anger and hurt feelings with me in her journal. When I read her reaction, I realized I had acted insensitively. I became aware of the harshness words can hold and the potential destructiveness of sharing uncensored journal entries.

I wrote in my journal, "I'm going to turn to art for awhile. Words feel too permanent. Knowing you're reading things I wrote months ago that often have been resolved feels wrong. But a picture from 2 months back would have surely adapted itself to the present." Dealing with difficult and uncomfortable topics did not destroy our relationship, but helped us grow closer, and helped me learn to respect our separateness. I also learned to become much more selective in what I chose to share.

Using art for self-processing grew easier for me than it had been earlier in my internship. I was learning to trust the art process more as I experienced it being pivotal time and time again in facilitating many issues.

The Termination Phase

Joanne

During the middle phase Dorine had made rapid gains in her professional development and I had been immensely gratified by our use of art therapy during her supervision hour. My positive feelings about our work together gave rise to the awareness that she was in her last quarter of school and would soon be terminating from our program.

I spent most of this phase reflecting upon the impact Dorine had made on our clients, her unique contributions to our program, and the special role she had played in my own professional and personal growth. I had "cut my teeth" on Dorine as I learned a different set of skills required by the supervisory role. She had, in turn, learned to become more patient with my "mistakes" and inexperience in this role, and had come to accept more fully both my limitations and strengths and her own. In my journal I wrote, "Dorine will always have a special place in my life because of her role as my first supervisee. Letting go is hard."

My reflections led me to think more carefully about the exact nature of our relationship and its function in our professional and personal lives. On a personal level Dorine had brought much to the relationship. I wanted to convey this to her, to let her know how much I had enjoyed her warmth and humor, her motivation to learn and grow, her openness and spontaneity.

Earlier in the year Dorine had made signs of the students' names who shared her office and hung it on her door. One day when she was at school I walked by her office and found her name card lying on the floor. After putting it back, I drew a picture about this moment (Fig. 20.7) to express my sadness and awareness that her absence would leave a void, particularly at work. We had shared and explored much together, using a process we most enjoyed. The door in Figure 20.7 is closed to represent our relationship coming to an end. Although I felt Dorine and I would continue our relationship as colleagues and friends, it was important to acknowledge the ending of our supervisory relationship. I shared the picture with Dorine, and it enabled me to express these feelings.

The exchange of journals and artwork had contributed to a more intimate connection with one another. By the end of this phase I concluded that cultivation of interpersonal mutuality in the supervisory relationship had significantly enhanced and facilitated our professional work. I remembered how little attention had been paid to the actual relationship in my student supervisory experiences, how the focus had been primarily on learning tech-

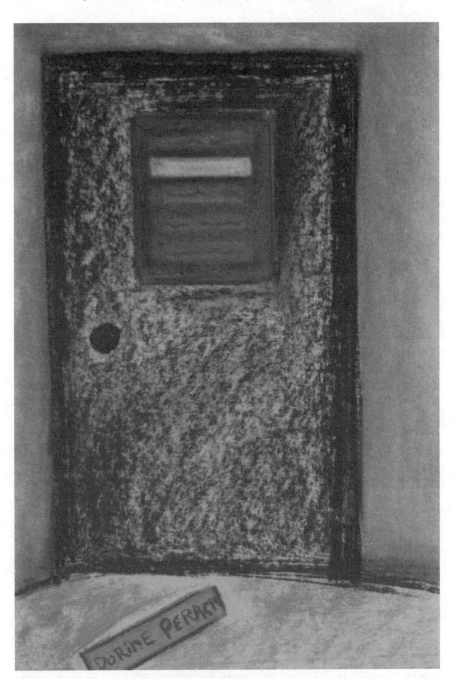

Figure 20.7. Dorine's name card, by Joanne.

nical skills. I had always felt rather powerless and insignificant since my personal presence seemed to have little impact on most of my supervisors. This had been especially painful since they were the ones I had most looked up to for role modeling in my struggle to form a professional identity.

Dorine and I had struggled successfully with the discomfort of becoming intimate within professional limitations and utilized our relational struggles as a core aspect of her learning. This had been a different form of learning than I had experienced—not merely didactic or theoretical, but experiential—emphasizing the interpersonal dimension we face continually as therapists. I shared these thoughts with Dorine and she agreed that much of the learning she had applied to her work with clients had evolved from the learning that took place within our relationship.

Dorine

With the onset of my termination class (see Chapter 21) during spring quarter, I knew I officially entered this stage. I began the phase reviewing the places I had reached with my individual clients and groups, decided how I wanted to terminate with them, and explored what unfinished goals I could still realistically meet. Though sad at moments, I felt very ''up'' and excited to be nearing graduation. Emotionally I began feeling less connected. I wrote,

> Somehow the bonds are stretching . . . and with me looking onward I question my level of commitment at this time or should I say investment. With those whom I have worked closely, I will do my best to bring our work to a comfortable closing point for both of us . . . but with newcomers, I can barely learn their names. I feel myself fading away. . . . And the members ask when my last day will be. Their eyes say, ''you're leaving us too.'' In a way they challenge each of us to stay on forever, to not be another abandoning force in their lives. Though I comfort myself knowing it's not my fault I must go. . . . I know that I too would leave them willingly some day and this fact leaves me very uncomfortable.

I trusted I would find the words to say good-bye to those wonderful and colorful people who felt like old friends by now. I found it much easier to place focus on finishing loose ends with the members than with Joanne. I could not accept the possibility that a relationship so meaningful to me would, in many ways, be coming to an end. I played with the idea of seeing Joanne privately for supervision, imagined us leading workshops together and checking in with each other as usual. For Joanne I could not find any words resembling good-bye.

Joanne once drew her personal hope for herself as a supervisor; she was a light, a presence in a picture where I was a plant, able to grow in any direction. I decided to respond to that image, wanting to let Joanne know that she had successfully achieved that goal. In Figure 20.8 I drew Joanne amidst a bright aura of energy and creativity, near fresh, blossoming flowers.

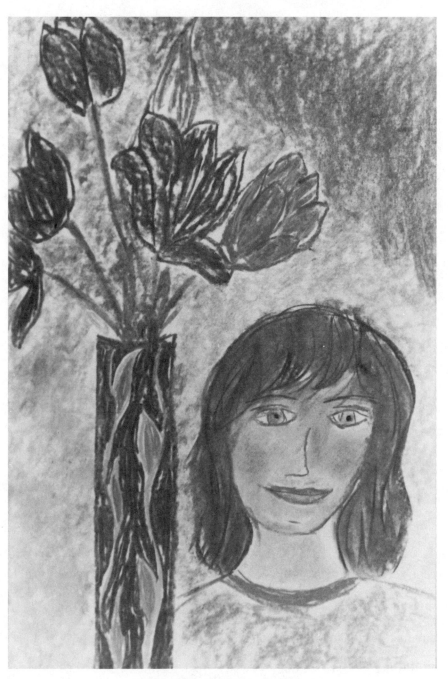

Figure 20.8. Joanne, by Dorine.

In the picture I am attracted to Joanne's eyes, which symbolize her openness, alertness, and curiosity. Yet her eyes are receptive as well; she allowed me into her world, grew from me, and permitted our relationship to be a mutual exchange. Perhaps I am the flowers, unfolding at her side, at my own pace. In Joanne's presence my professional identity as an art therapist emerged.

Joanne

During Dorine's supervision we drew "termination" pictures that facilitated that process for both of us. Figure 20.9 is my last picture about Dorine, showing her holding the "papoose blanket" high, getting ready to discard it. The blanket is bright, colorful, and warm—the way I had viewed our relationship—but it no longer restricts her or holds her back.

As Dorine's internship came to an end we began collaborating on this chapter, which further facilitated the termination process. By the time she actually terminated I was able to accept the end of our relationship but I knew I would miss her presence at New Images. Fortunately, our chapter, artwork, and journals would be there to look back upon over time as a way to remember the sharing of a special journey. My consolations in saying good-bye were the knowledge that I'd continue utilizing the supervision model we had discovered together and the hope that I would experience the richness of our relationship with future interns.

Dorine

An image that grew in importance for me was a "termination" picture that Joanne created of me (Fig. 20.9) during final weeks of my internship. About this picture I wrote,

> I look at myself, standing naked before the sun as if reborn . . . standing grounded for the first time. My arms are strong as they raise the blanket to the sky. I think of all that Joanne has helped me shed besides the binding quality I once experienced from the blanket. I look at the blanket and I think how I no longer hide inside it, amidst my fears and insecurities. The blanket now robes me with life experiences that have prepared me to continue on my way.

As I learned to accept myself, my limitations and abilities, I also learned to accept and appreciate Joanne and my clients better. I found other relationships in my life less frustrating and more satisfying as well. I knew Joanne had helped me to be transformed, to grow more comfortable with myself both personally and professionally.

As my final piece of artwork, I decided to make an actual blanket (Fig. 20.10). It emerged as a quilt on which I painted the cycle of change in life represented by seasonal imagery and tides. Central to the quilt is an image of a woman touching and nurturing the fetus within the sun, which represented both Joanne promoting my growth and me being able to accept the

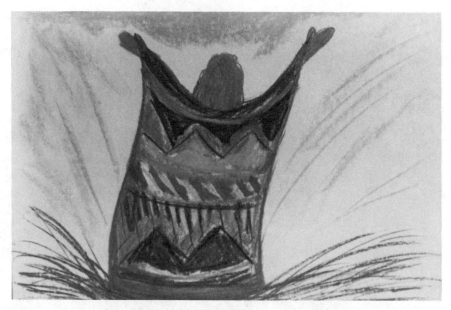

Figure 20.9. Dorine's Blanket, by Joanne.

unformed or newly forming parts of myself. I realized how uncomfortable the experience of being new and unformed could be when desiring the knowledge and confidence that can only come with time. Having only begun to build a base for my professional identity, I could now clearly recognize and accept my inexperience and the very early stage I had achieved thus far in becoming a professional.

The large drops on each side of the central image represent rain (nurturance) and tears (my sadness at leaving studenthood behind). Once it was completed, wrapping the blanket around my shoulders felt wonderful . . . a security blanket of sorts that I could carry on my way, to wear and reflect upon when needed. What I had learned with Joanne I would bring to my future wanderings.

In a world where so many supervisory relationships fail, I believe I know why ours succeeded. Besides the art and journal writing facilitating our discussions of difficult topics, Joanne was willing to grow *with* me. Not only did she share her many wonderful talents and gifts with me, she helped me discover my own. In my last entry I wrote,

> Away from the bustle of school, I learned to be a therapist, an artist, a curious human being. Seeds of learning had time to incubate . . . to bear fruit. But it's almost time to go. . . . I hesitate . . . my work is not quite done here. Can I ever return to this place of security? Once more I stand alone, the last to leave, to say good-bye. I like this time alone. Time I need to explore my full appreciation of these experiences and to acknowledge how they have transformed my life. I now walk with eyes open.

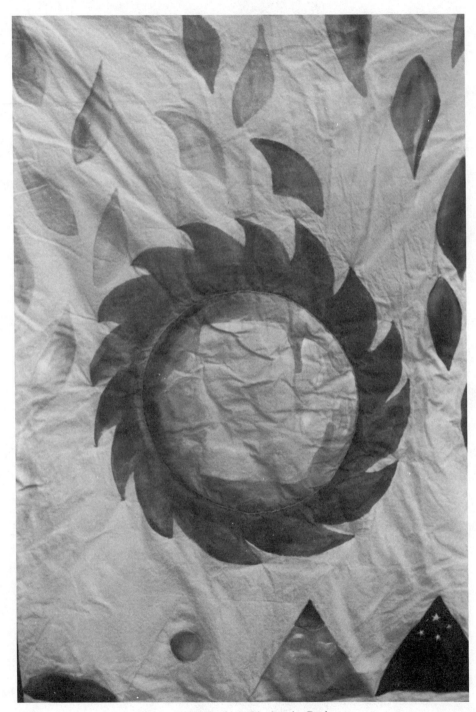

Figure 20.10. Dorine's Blanket, by Dorine.

DYAD B: ELLEN SONTAG, M.S.W., M.A., SUPERVISOR, AND JEAN DURKIN, STUDENT

Background Information

Illinois State Psychiatric Institute (ISPI) is an inpatient, short-term psychiatric hospital in addition to being a teaching institute where Ellen and Jean worked together for 9 months. It houses four adult, four adolescent, and two research units. The unit on which they worked had 28 to 38 adults with varied diagnoses. Many are chronic and have had numerous admissions, with the hospital population being constantly in flux. Reevaluation of diagnosis, regulation of psychotropic drugs, and careful placement into the community is the common treatment. There is a multidisciplined team approach. Art therapy is seen as an extension of the activity therapy department.

Formal supervision took place for 1¼ hours per week with snatches of conversation throughout the week. During that hour, hospital orientation, regulations, politics, logistics, planning, and other pragmatic needs were addressed, and there was an exchange of information regarding the art therapy Jean was practicing. Occasionally, journal entries or pictures were shared when they seemed appropriate. A complete exchange of journals never took place since this dyad found it more comfortable to read passages or excerpts of their work to each other. They did have three art-making and journal-writing exchanges, one at the beginning, one in the middle, and one at termination. They agreed to write in their journals and make art according to their needs, noting if and when they created.

Beginning Phase

Ellen

When Jean asked me to try an experiment in September, I heartily agreed. By the time November rolled around, I wondered why I had gotten myself into a project that demanded additional work, emotional involvement, and a good deal of commitment.

I questioned whether this tool would enhance supervision. With a master's degree in social work and art therapy, I had supervised one social work student but still was a neophyte when it came to supervising. Jean was my first art therapy student. In the relative safety of the traditional supervisory relationship, I could have hidden out and distanced myself in a multitude of ways; now I was vulnerable in all my insecurities. At the end of the first week I wrote,

> There is so much that I want to give to you, and there is the constant worry that I'm not giving enough; we have already touched on one of my main fears— having to be perfect. You have assured me that I don't have to be—I have assured you that you don't have to be.

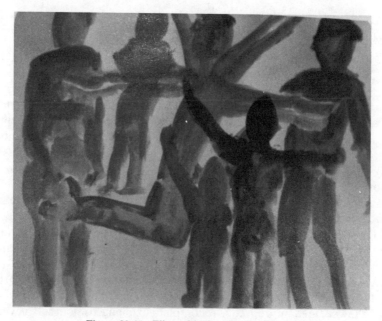

Figure 20.11. Ellen with six arms, by Ellen.

In Figure 20.11, I have depicted myself as the central figure with six arms going out in all directions. The arms are trying to give enough to my husband, children, and friends as well as to Jean. Giving enough means meeting all needs at all times—in other words, being perfect. This picture allowed us to approach, discuss, and come to the resolution that neither of us could expect or should want to be perfect. The theme had a lot of potential danger for both of us as we are people who strive for perfection.

In this way, journal writing and sharing artwork hastened some of the work that was crucial to the beginning phase of the supervisory relationship. We were able, more clearly and honestly, to reveal our expectations as we entered into this new relationship with each other. We were able to set up a model of self-reflection and questioning in supervision that would be a useful model in Jean's work with patients.

Jean

When Dorine and I discussed journal writing, our respect for the process was similar to our growing understanding of art making. When I explained it to Ellen, I found myself agreeing that sharing "secrets" was scary. We adjusted it to fit our needs. We maintained our need for control over self-disclosure. Ellen was concerned that her self-disclosure would alter the supervision process. Planned sharing did seem to create a safe area to explore ourselves and our relationship.

When I began working at ISPI, I was concerned about making a good impression and doing things right. I wrote, "Ellen is an assurance—I'll be observing the next week and a half. I still get confused. Sometimes I feel like I know what I'm doing, then I'm a sponge, then I'm trying to be cool until I figure out what I don't know enough to ask."

In the beginning phase, I drew Ellen in soft pastels with warm eyes (Fig. 20.12). I blended rose and peach colors for her face to show her warmth and gentleness. I felt grateful to have a sensitive, concerned supervisor who refused to compromise her work in this tough setting. At times I felt protective of her; other times I was like her shadow, next to her and similar to her. She varied, sharing confidences sometimes and pulling back other times.

Ellen

An issue that was important to the beginning phase of supervision was to set up an environment that would be conducive to learning. I wanted Jean to feel free to work in an atmosphere where growth was expected—where it was okay to make mistakes. The self-revealing nature of our sharing artwork about the supervision facilitated a nonjudgmental atmosphere where questioning, doubt, and discussion were permissible.

In sharing artwork, there was another understanding about the supervisory relationship that occurred to us early on. It was apparent that Jean and I would teach and learn from each other. At the end of October I wrote, "Some of the issues that I am struggling with in my parenting have surfaced, that is, feeling overprotective, trying to balance giving enough and letting go enough." This is a personal issue that I have learned more about with Jean's help. Also, being able to identify and separate personal issues was very helpful, as there was less of a tendency to act them out via the supervisory relationship.

The artwork and journal writing were instrumental in the beginning phase of supervision in "setting the stage." The sharing of artwork hastened and facilitated the clarification of expectations, goals, and norms (both personal and professional), creating an atmosphere that was conducive to learning.

Toward the end of October there seemed to be a shift in the supervisory relationship that was reflected in my artwork and journal entries. Jean had become more integrated into the daily life of the hospital unit. She was working competently with her own art therapy group and several individuals. I wrote,

I am experiencing feelings of satisfaction, relief, pride. The initial weeks are over—I am getting to know Jean and feel lucky to have her. She's smart, sensitive, willing and able to contribute to the general well-being of life on the unit. She's also mature and aware of things—knows how to get on with people, and enough about the politics here but doesn't compromise too much. It feels like we're starting to catch each other's signals and are working a lot easier together.

Most of the basics were now established and supervision became more

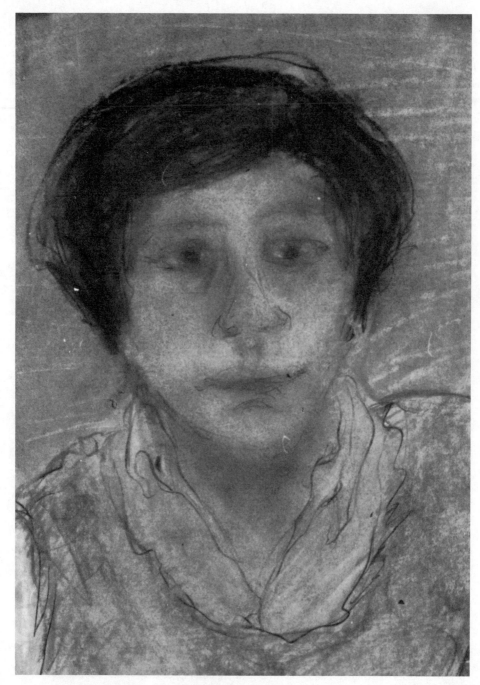

Figure 20.12. Ellen, by Jean.

complicated and sometimes difficult. I was grateful to have the artwork to help us to understand and discuss issues that were harder for me to confront.

In early November, I made a picture of three boxes, rendered carefully in colored pencil, with boundaries punctuated by dark borders (Fig. 20.13). On that day I wrote,

> There are other aspects emerging that seem to be a darker side of myself. Control issues. It may be hard for me to give up control at times. I am experiencing some resistance to doing the journaling and artwork which might relate to not wanting to reveal myself this much. I can't be the perfect supervisor. Jean knows too much about me.

I also wrote, "The other emerging ugly head is giving up control over more literal things, that is, my space and patients that I would like to work with, becoming generative rather than competitive. I can see there is a lot of work here."

This drawing allowed me to reflect on some of my feelings. Jean was accompanying me to almost everything. She was an observer of me at group, worked with me at all unit activities, and even attended the supervision that I received on the community group meeting that I led. In addition to this, she shared my art room—her desk was next to mine. I wanted Jean to have as many varied, rich experiences as possible. I now realized that I also needed more separateness.

I decided after much soul-searching that these feelings were affecting my supervision and I had to address them. I decided that I needed to do some things without Jean. I chose to attend the community meeting supervision without her. I struggled with this as I felt on the one hand, Jean would benefit from the experience. My artwork, however, was indicating that I had to consider my needs also. In reflecting on this situation further, I realized that one of the reasons that I didn't want Jean to attend the lower-functioning art therapy group that I ran two times each week was that it wasn't going very well. This group was new, too new to me, and I was struggling with it. It was a difficult and often frustrating group. I drew a picture of a particularly terrible day when the group couldn't even stay in their seats.

When I was finally able to recognize that my own need for adequate performance in front of Jean was the thing that was really bothering me, I was able to take that realization back into supervision with Jean. I shared my feelings about "messing up" in front of her. I hoped it would reinforce the idea that it's not always going to go well and give her more confidence in her own work with patients. I decided that Jean should remain an observer of that art therapy group. I felt that it was important to demonstrate to both of us that one could learn from failures and to have the courage and confidence to try other ideas.

This was probably the hardest thing for me to do. Without the artwork as a guide I might have asked Jean not to participate in that group, never

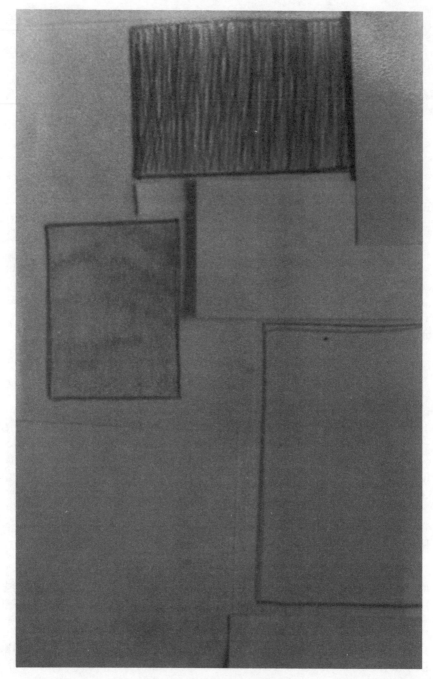

Figure 20.13. Boxes, by Ellen.

really recognizing my underlying feelings. It was time now to give Jean a gentle nudge to encourage more autonomy. This seemed to be one more part of the process—the process of Jean's becoming and my letting go. Out of necessity we did most things together at the beginning, as Jean "learned the ropes." My emerging need for separateness led next to my desire for Jean to have more responsibility. I also wanted her to move away from working so closely with me alone, toward working closely with other professional staff. I introduced the idea that she have the responsibility of being on a multidisciplinary team. The team consisted of a primary therapist, a social worker, a nurse, an activity therapist, a rehabilitation counselor, and possibly other doctors or interns. Jean seemed resistant to this idea. She also seemed angry with me. This was a time of loss, change, and regrouping for both of us, as well as a time for increased autonomy, competence, and growth.

Middle Phase

Jean

Ellen began to push me into my own sphere. She and I recognized my ambivalence and my wanting to remain in the safety of the "home" shop we had established. Intellectually, I understood the need to become independent, but it took a little push from Ellen, which I think I asked for, to enact the independence with actions.

My ambivalence around becoming more independent became confused for me with attitudes I developed about other staff. I reasoned with myself that I chose to distance myself from the other staff because of them. It took some time for me to see that it had more to do with my fear of becoming an independent professional.

My independent presence on Friday's treatment team began my next phase. I intellectualized my unwillingness by complaining about the staff rifts and infighting I observed. I used artwork to convey to Ellen just how torn I felt about the staff hurting each other.

In Figure 20.14, I drew myself as the bottom figure swirling in anger, concern, and confusion as I, though detached from the action, witness two other staff angrily shouting and fighting.

I drew using Ellen's rendered boxes to show her visually how I saw different parts of the unit as separate and divided with much strife (Fig. 20.15). The top three rectangles are labeled Team, Nursing, and Dayroom. The bottom three are our desks and the art table. I kept each separate, divided by angry scribbles both inside and outside each rectangle. I visually showed how we paralleled the strife on the unit. Ellen sympathized with me, yet remained somewhat nonjudgmental. She had earlier advised me not to side with anyone. I wrote in December,

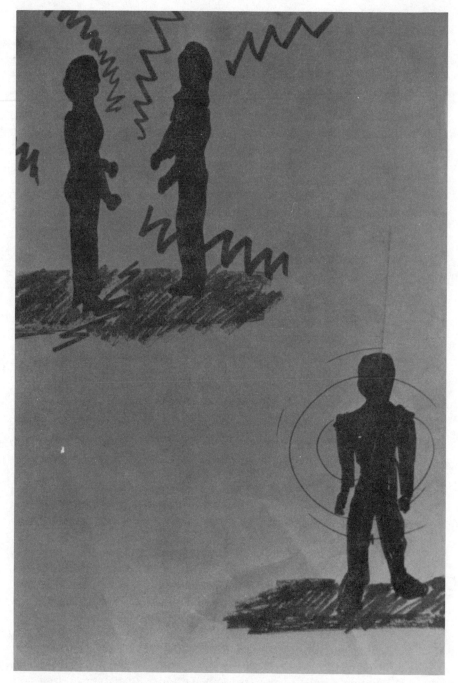

Figure 20.14. Jean (bottom) with fighting staff, by Jean.

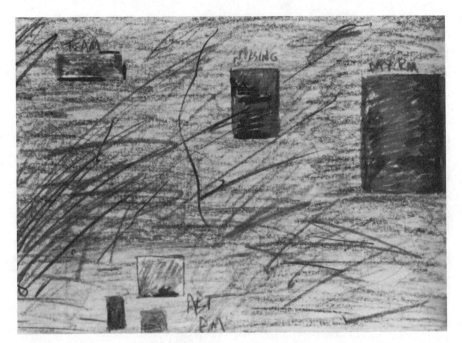

Figure 20.15. Boxes, by Jean.

There's Ellen in the middle of it doing her innocent and positive routine. There's conflict all over the place. To do my job would require me to put my feelings aside and work with these people, but their bitterness and manipulation make me exhausted. Talking to Ellen validates my feelings.

After a 2-week Christmas break, I joined the team and began voicing my opinions at staff meetings freely. As I began to see myself as a professional, so did the rest of the staff on our unit. Being able to voice my unhappiness to Ellen gave me the opportunity to make a shift and use Ellen's modeling and rejoin the unit on a more professional level.

Ellen

In January I did a picture of Jean and myself as skiers—having come so far on the trail together. The picture was of Jean as a younger sister, gaining steadily in ability and strength. Jean is the skier in the front. At that point, I felt the satisfaction of coming over the mountain ridge with her. In Figure 20.16 the figures are drawn close together as I felt a growing sense of closeness. I am positioned ready to give Jean a nudge as I still felt she needed to be pushed toward more autonomy.

In Figure 20.17, Jean drew two chicks emerging, depicting a similar theme. She saw the nest like the art room acting as a nurturing environment for the chicks to develop, poking their heads out of the broken shells with mouths

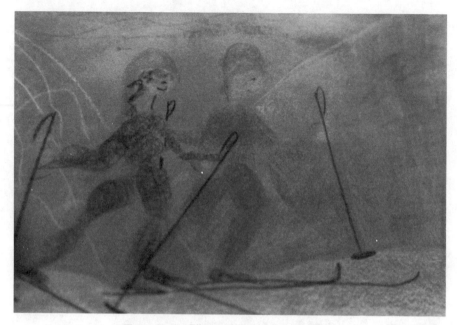

Figure 20.16. Ellen and Jean skiing, by Ellen.

open, chirping to each other. The chicks depict us equally beginning and developing in this new phase of our relationship.

After Jean assumed increased responsibility, she was reinforced by an expanded role on the unit. The increased respect and status she received from others and her own success on the unit brought a change in our supervisory relationship. I experienced this change as exciting and satisfying. I felt that Jean was confident, willing to risk, and ready for new challenges. There was more give and take in our relationship—Jean was more apt to question and challenge some of my work and assumptions.

Jean

In late January I began to question my relationship with Ellen. We were both "perfect" in a tense way. This "niceness" began to get on my nerves. I also began to see her shift from colleague to teacher, which made me confused and angry. With the help of my supervisor at school, I realized that when Ellen shifted to becoming my teacher, I missed her. I missed her because I enjoyed her when she was loose and we learned from each other in experiential ways. I remembered Ellen telling me how important separation was in the growth process and how her social work supervisor introduced it into her own supervision. Without separation I would not have the chance to become a professional. At the same time, I felt it was an ill-fitting imposed element Ellen needed more than I. It required objectivity to see its

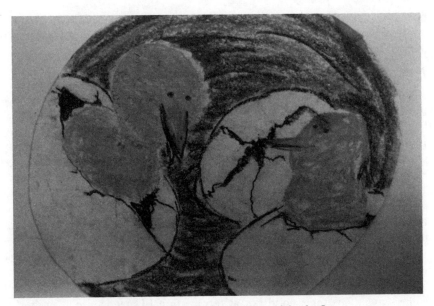

Figure 20.17. Ellen and Jean as two chicks, by Jean.

importance. When I worked it out by myself in my artwork, I informed Ellen. My missing her seemed to be a strange tribute to the importance of our relationship.

Termination

Ellen

At the end of February we began discussing our plans to write up our experiences formally for this chapter. Doing this heightened my awareness that the school year was coming to an end. Shortly after that, I made a picture about a difficult community meeting and was surprised to find myself all choked up. I realized that what I was feeling was the sadness of losing Jean. In late February I wrote:

> Loss has always been a hard thing for me. Giving up someone whom I really like has brought back past terminations. My hope as we begin this new time together is to emerge as friends, colleagues, fellow survivors, and authors.

With less than 2 months left, I had done very minimal pictures and no journal writing for a month. By my lack of pictures I was acutely aware of work that needed to be done. I had not brought up termination in our supervision. Because of the pain involved, my guess is that both Jean and I had colluded in avoiding termination work. Again, the artwork made it difficult to avoid the issue at hand. In this case, the most minimal efforts at doing artwork and the lack of investment in the artwork were a signal to me. There was more work to be done.

Jean

Ellen noticed that many of my drawings had begun to utilize boundaries as the talk of termination began. These boundaries reflected my need to establish limits as graduate school and life in general became too overwhelming. In the last month many special events were planned, marking my final days with Ellen as supervisor. I wrote in April, "We were bound to say goodbye, yet I'm trying desperately to fill this last month chock full of events."

I inquired about possible employment at ISPI yet remained inactive in following through with the application process. Through my lack of action, I realized the ambivalence I felt. I seemed to need to terminate fully before beginning another attachment.

With 2 months left, Ellen and I were able to joke about termination, but were not able to talk seriously. After helping her at a conference, I wrote, "Ellen and I are more and more equal. She sees me as a mentor for her in some ways. This feels good but at termination I'll need to lean on her." I was not ready to verbalize this. Instead, laughing and creating private jokes was my way to establish our bond firmly.

Ellen

As the termination phase of supervision progressed, I felt that we were able to complement each other, each adding to the whole.

For almost a month I felt that I wasn't doing any work at all. I knew that Jean would be leaving the hospital in early June and that, theoretically, Jean's termination ought to have been a theme coming up in my journal writing and artwork. Instead, I saw myself doing what I viewed as minimal artwork with little meaning. I wrote almost nothing in my journal during that period.

In mid-April I was consciously ready to do the necessary termination work and to bring it doggedly into supervision. I found Jean not ready or willing to deal directly with termination at that point. I knew, however, that by design and sometimes unconsciously we were working hard on termination. We communicated about it through humor, acknowledging the issue but keeping it light and safe.

Consciously, I was handing over more responsibility and freedom. I asked Jean to conduct a workshop with me, teach patients and myself painting and drawing skills, and organize a hospital-wide art show.

Sharing the artwork and journal writing was particularly helpful to me during termination. Jean expressed her perception of me as the one who was going to have the most trouble over termination. I think that she projected on me many feelings that were difficult for her to acknowledge. At the same time, she let me know that she needed me to be strong during this period for her to "lean on." The sharing helped me plan for the termination in a broader way. I was focused on helping Jean to feel more and more autonomous, thus handing over more responsibility. Jean let me know that she needed more than this.

I painted two pictures in mid-April about termination. Figure 20.18 is called "Jean the Juggler" and depicts Jean handling it all. Figure 20.19 shows a depressed, regressed-looking figure. This was the part of Jean's termination that had gone unrecognized, and we both were able to view and discuss it.

Jean

In my last month, I painted a number of pictures of the ground breaking with new growth. In March the ground was rich black earth, full of energy under the surface. By May the ground broke, the seedling popped itself out with the activity from underground, filling the air (Fig. 20.20).

Like many pictures in this series, this began unconsciously, as a playful, meditative way to start the day. Only in the last few minutes of painting was the image determined. I gradually understood these to be self-portraits, depicting me breaking the ground that was the security I needed to root. With only a few weeks left I shared with Ellen this entry:

> I've said a lot of good-byes, I wonder if she has—I feel that she's going to cry when I leave and I'll just help her and forgo my own feelings. It would be important if I went beyond this stereotypical safety and touched my feelings.

The act of saying this released my emotion, which was just under the surface. We discussed how termination is a dance with each of us leading at different times. I felt relief when I heard Ellen say that she heard me. I think it was the safety of the relationship that allowed me to risk looking at my old patterns of behavior and considering adjusting them in an important way.

At our termination sharing, Ellen focused on my feelings of leaving. This enriched my attempt to forge a new process to leave important people in my life, like Ellen, in a connected rather than cold way. Her honesty about me was blunt. It was hard to admit to the "me" she saw in her blue figure (Fig. 20.19). My own depression, I thought, had been successfully masked by the exaggerated smile of the juggler.

As Ellen focused on my needs, she seemed to minimize her own, saying her pictures had little meaning. One of these included two telephones connected by a single cord. Though simply drawn, the message of Ellen's desire for us to remain connected was very strong.

A few days after she completed her work on the chapter, she called and told me that she had left an important part out of her termination section; the part about her feelings concerning my leaving. This phone conversation surprised me. Speaking about our feelings embarrassed me, but at the same

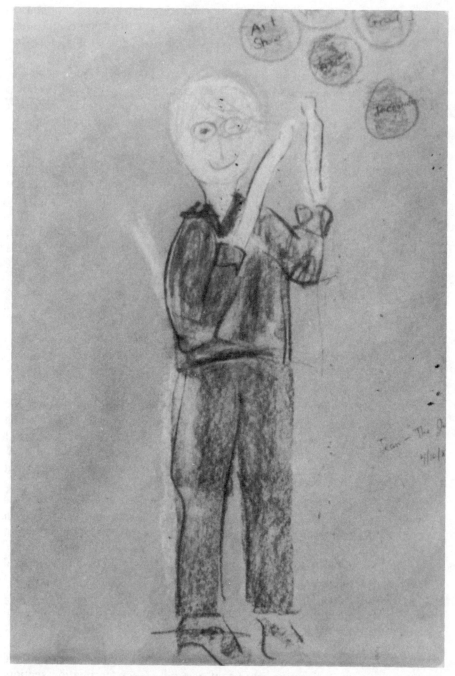

Figure 20.18. Jean the juggler, by Ellen.

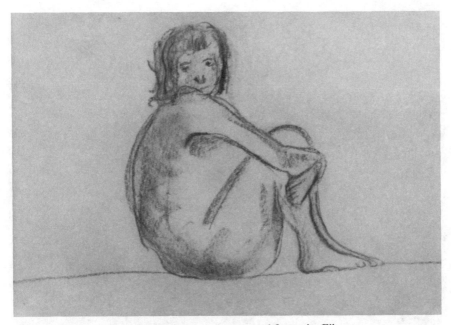

Figure 20.19. Depressed, regressed figure, by Ellen.

time it bridged our needs. I was able to leave Ellen in a more connected way and Ellen found that she did not have to shift to her teacher role as she had before to distance herself, in order to leave me.

DISCUSSION

The foregoing experiences have sketched two supervisory relationships in which the rich processes of art making and journal writing became an integral part of the supervisory process. The value of these tools in the supervisory relationship and their usefulness in forming a more appropriate model of supervision will be discussed.

The four authors share a similar art therapy education from the University of Illinois at Chicago where the experiential component of art making was utilized to process clinical and theoretical learning throughout the 2-year master's program. It was a natural extension for these two dyads to continue using their tools to process their experiences.

Having the choice of three communicative avenues, verbal, written, and visual arts, we afforded ourselves options in choosing how best to communicate or reflect an idea at any given time. As communication was enhanced significantly within the dyad, a framework for a more generative relationship formed in which professional growth and learning took place.

The self-processing tool so valuable to art therapists was particularly

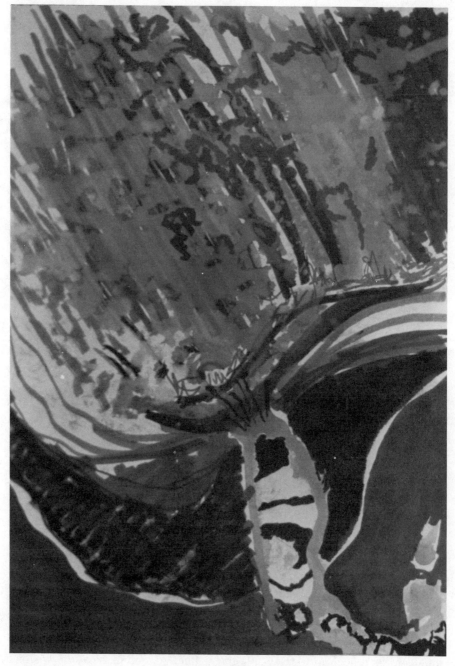

Figure 20.20. Seedling, by Jean.

beneficial in many ways. It zeroed in on issues before they were consciously identified. It became a means of self-supervision for the students by providing time and distance for self-reflection, time for the integration of ideas, and time for objectivity when emotionally charged issues surfaced. Due to the nature of making and sharing artwork and journal entries, the agendas of both student and supervisor were replaced by the more immediate needs that emerged through these self-processing tools. This was especially helpful for the supervisor as it pointed more clearly to the specific training needs of the student.

In using this experiential model of supervision, which accessed feelings and integrated cognitive learning on a more emotional level, we found our supervisory relationships providing a useful role model that paralleled the therapeutic relationship. This afforded the student and supervisor necessary experiences similar to that of their patients who utilize self-processing skills through art making.

As we had hoped, this engaging process bridged what is often an interpersonal gap between students and supervisors. Although this involved more risk taking, it also created more intimacy. It proved more difficult for the supervisors to distance themselves from the students, yet provided many opportunities to work through this distancing issue. We found that atmospheres were created in which students and supervisors were less locked into their roles. In these environments where mutual learning took place, we were more free to be ourselves and demonstrate a healthy level of professionalism where the human factor was intact rather than modeling artificial behavior. We discovered that we had given ourselves the opportunity to know each other as people rather than in the limited way traditional roles afford. This process allowed us to affect and empower each other in a generative way where learning became a mutual process.

Inviting this emotional component into our relationships often exposed more of our vulnerabilities. Yet in our sensitive handling of such areas a rich interpersonal and professional exchange emerged. The two dyads grew at different rates and in different directions. In similar ways we struggled with universal issues present in all types of relationships. Our shared willingness to discuss openly such topics as honeymoons, boundaries, competitiveness and conflict, ambivalence, and dependency issues, and the use of tools that dramatically brought these topics to a forefront, fostered growth in our professional relationships.

As our profession grows, we need to look more closely at the role supervisors play in art therapy interns' learning and training. The importance of the supervisor in shaping the student's professional identity is often overlooked. The supervisor is a significant person in students' lives, ushering them from the academic world into the professional, clinical world. The supervisor does not merely present technical skills and didactic theories, nor is the student simply a passive recipient. Rather the relationship has the power to have a significant impact upon the student's learning and professional identity. We must ask, Where can students better practice the theoretical and clinical information they learn than in the safety of a trusting supervisory relationship, and what more appropriate way to process their learning than through expressive arts tools?

Students may also be influential in the life of supervisors, who are generally the only art therapists on staff at their settings. The companionship of a student sharing a similar therapeutic orientation may be very welcoming and stimulating. Students may challenge supervisors to fine-tune their theoretical beliefs and bring a wealth of new information to their placement from their own background experiences. Thus the two afford each other unlimited growth simply by opening themselves to each other's experiences.

CONCLUSION

The development of a new model of supervision that is more conducive to our particular type of psychotherapy and healing as art therapists is a timely addition to our growing field. The experiences of both dyads illustrate mutual intensive learning for both student and supervisor on educational, professional, and interpersonal levels. It is a natural progression to include art making and other self-expressive tools to process our experiences as art therapists in more depth. In the two relationships presented, the sharing of these expressions proved to be a powerful, enriching learning experience.

As this is a beginning step, modifications to integrate the model of supervision to particular settings are expected and welcomed. It is recommended that this model be used by those who are willing to cross the limiting boundaries of traditional supervision and take personal risks with one another. In order to create supervision that is meaningful to art therapists we need to continue utilizing our best tools.

REFERENCES

Marion, P., & Felix, M. (1979). The relationship of art therapy interns and supervisors. *Arts in Psychotherapy, 6,* 37–40.

Wadeson, H. (1987). *The dynamics of art psychotherapy.* New York: Wiley.

Wilson, L., Riley, S., & Wadeson, H. (1984). Art therapy supervision. *Art Therapy, 1*(3), 100–105.

Yalom, I., & Elkin, G. (1974). *Every day gets a little closer.* New York: Basic.

CHAPTER 21

The Art Therapy Termination Process Group

HARRIET WADESON

Viewed from a certain perspective, in termination time appears to flow backward. We are accustomed to beginnings setting the stage for what will follow. But in a sense endings also set the stage for what has gone before. For example, pleasant journeys, good marriages, exhilarating love affairs come to be looked upon as failures through the lens of an unpleasant, painful or even disasterous ending. Similarly, therapy that has progressed well may reverse course as ending nears:

> The manner in which the therapeutic relationship is brought to a close is crucial to the outcome of treatment; it has a major influence on the degree to which the gains that occurred are maintained. . . . Failure to adequately explore and work out these feelings during the ending period may result in a weakening or undoing of the completed therapeutic work. (Levinson, 1977, p. 481)

For this and other reasons, termination becomes a significant component in treatment. Nevertheless, few therapist training programs give adequate attention to the difficult task of effecting a positive separation. It was for this reason that I developed a course for graduating art therapy master's degree students to study the crucial process of termination.

The objectives of the course I have developed, Art Therapy Termination Process Group, are twofold and reflect the parallel processes between client and therapist and student and teacher. The first objective applies to the clinical arena in which students develop awareness of the importance of termination for their clients, the issues paramount in this phase of treatment, and the ways termination can be handled most productively. The second objective applies to the parallel process of the student's own termination from training, to review and integrate further the many aspects of training, and thereby to understand termination issues more deeply through one's own experience, and to effect a successful transition from student to professional.

The difficulties encountered in separations are reflected in the dearth of literature on termination. Where writing on termination does occur, it usually applies to long-term psychoanalysis or to premature termination. There is very little in the art therapy literature specific to termination. The only sources I know have been written by myself. One example deals with the ending phase of supervision (see Wilson, Riley, & Wadeson, 1984). Another example can be found in a chapter on mid-phase and ending art therapy treatment in *The Dynamics of Art Psychotherapy* (Wadeson, 1987). The materials I have found most useful for readings in the course are listed in the reference section at the end of this chapter.

There is one passage from the literature, however, that captures termination issues so well that I read it to the students to open discussion in the first class:

Separation is one of life's central experiences. Particular attempts to meet this challenge constitute significant expressions of an individual personality.

Separation is inextricably bound up with that which in life we value most: growth, achievement, anticipation, the joyful sense of purposeful ongoingness. Yet each choice, each accomplishment, is a commitment, and further limits the possibilities of what can be.

It is as if each achievement, each further organization of self, that defines more irrevocably what one is, implies the death of all the selves that could have been. At each graduation, in the midst of celebration, there is mourning for the potentialities, the renounced, the varied selves, that are forever lost. Every step forward . . . implies a painful loss: the desires and gratifications of yesterday have to die that today can be fully lived.

There is no joy that is not shadowed by its transience. There is no contact with another human being, no alleviation of loneliness, without the aching certainty no matter how we try to hold it back that loneliness will come again. No matter how desirable what is to come, it is yet unknown; and what is is sweet and terrible to lose.

In the pain of separation, man is confronted by the impermanence of his condition. Being and feeling are transient, in an indifferent universe, in which pain and loss are inevitable, in which change occurs without regard to one's own will or desire.

In our time we are faced not only by the inexorable catastrophes of nature that disrupt our lives with one pitiless disaster after another, by the meaningless accidents that mock us, and by the biological inevitability that dooms us to live in the shadow of continuous endings and final ending. But society, the structure by which man seeks to hold back change, to retain what is dear, to contain violence, and to give a semblance of order, permanence, and meaning no matter how illusory to the life he leads, is itself rent by cruelty, destructiveness, and upheaval. Human relationships, more and more, in a time of social chaos and dizzy acceleration have a now, but a past that is brief, and a future that is unclear. (Edelson, 1963, p. 20)

   This passage from *The Termination of Intensive Psychotherapy* describes the importance of working with separation more poignantly than any discussion of termination I have encountered in the literature. It is with this quotation that my students' last quarter of master's degree art therapy training begins.

   In their second year of full-time training in the program I direct, students concentrate on practicum and thesis work and take electives from other departments and colleges within the university. Therefore, the termination course serves as a sort of reunion, bringing them together again as a full group for the first time since their intensive experiences together in the required art therapy courses of the first year. Part-time students who have been taking the same required courses, but at a different pace, terminate in this course as part of an identified class.

   It is deliberate that the word *group* is used in the course title. Group process and art therapy's reflection and advancement of that process (Wadeson, 1987, chap. 6) have been an important part of the students' training, and the ending of the life of this particular group is a significant event from which much learning can be derived. Students come to recognize that, as in work with clients, there may be a resurgence of old issues that had seemed to be resolved.

   When old angers and frustrations with faculty and supervisors emerge and competitive problems with classmates resurface, students are encouraged to see the relationship of these problems to termination. Throughout the course, in this way, the parallel process between clients' and students' termination experience is drawn so that the students come to grasp its issues both cognitively and experientially. The result is that the emotional impact of the students' own ending process gives life to the intellectual comprehension of termination.

   One aspect of preparing for an ending is the realization that there is still time left before the final separation. Dealing with termination necessarily calls into focus the best use of that time. For students in the termination course that time is spent in several ways. Study includes handling termination with clients; a review and integration of the entire training; the transition from student to professional; and a determination of what further training is needed. The last issue I call "Fill in the Gaps."

FILL IN THE GAPS

It is not expected that a 2-year full-time training program teach students everything they need to know. It provides a basis from which they must continue their own professional growth throughout their professional lives. Further, the training program cannot provide for every specialization. Nevertheless, students are asked to reflect on areas where they feel weak. Each student comes up with a list, and the class determines the subjects relevant to most of them. Generally, the areas have been of a practical nature, such as dealing with resistance, patient aggression, sexual overtures, working with staff, three-dimensional media, interpretation, and establishing a new art therapy treatment program.

Since students will have to be responsible for their own further training after graduation, part of their preparation for that transition begins with "Fill in the Gaps." They must be responsible for their "gap-filling" education: Each student is assigned to present to the class one of the subjects the class has selected to study further. Sometimes they work in pairs. The presentation can take the form that the student thinks will best fit the assignment, for example, a didactic presentation, leading class discussion, an experiential workshop. A student who presented on setting up a new art therapy program distributed to the class an outline her field supervisor had developed. Two students led a workshop on using clay. Another student presented a literature review on countertransference.

REVIEW AND INTEGRATION: PARALLEL PROCESS

To highlight the parallel process between clients' termination with their student therapists and students' termination from their training, a parallel termination review is assigned. At the beginning of the course, students select a client with whom they have been working for some period of time and with whom the work has been particularly meaningful. They review this client's art therapy describing the initial phase of treatment, mid-phase, and entering their termination phase, according to the stages of therapy discussed by Levinson (1977). They must also develop a termination plan for the client. The assignment for the next week is to complete a similar review for their own trajectory through art therapy training, once again noting the characteristics of the beginning phase, mid-phase, and entering the termination phase. In doing so, they review the journal they have kept throughout the program and the abundance of artwork they have created in classwork of the program's many experiential courses as well as course final projects, which are often art projects illustrating learning. They also make a termination plan for themselves, recognizing the issues they need to face and the methods they might develop for doing so.

For the first few years the course was offered, the parallel process assignment took the form of written reports. More recently, however, written processing has been replaced by art assignments. This change has resulted as a part of my continuing development of new methods for understanding, recognition, awareness, and integration through the art-making process (see Wadeson & Allen, 1983). Therefore, instead of writing about the client's initial phase of treatment, for example, the student makes a picture of it. The pictures of each phase and the termination plan are then presented to the class. Both the creation of the art representations and their presentation with the ensuing class discussion provide a much richer experience than written reports. The comparison of pictures is particularly illuminating. The imagery often highlights the student's feeling state in relation to the client as it changes over the course of treatment.

This sort of review evokes many existential questions, sometimes poignantly expressing the essential cruelty of therapy for chronic patients in training facilities who are left time and again as their student therapists move on. Also well illustrated in the client review is the student's learning of how to effect therapy, often moving from a need to *do* something for the client to understanding the importance of simply *being* with the client over time. Just what constitutes the therapeutic relationship becomes manifested in the students' art expressions of their work with the client they have chosen to present. Finally, the students' feelings about the progress the client has made or lack of it are readily expressed in the art. For some, there is the exhilaration of having helped another human being to lead a better life. For others, there is the frustration imposed by the treatment facility, the conditions of work, or the limitations of the client. Awareness of these reactions is essential in understanding the process of therapy and developing into an effective therapist.

In presenting illustrations of the phases of their own training process, students may also show particularly meaningful art projects they have made as a part of their training. The phases are often demarked differently by different students. For some the beginning phase ends after the first 10-week quarter. For others, the mid-phase is inaugurated with the practicum placement that begins in the third quarter of the first year. Initial expectations and anxieties are seen to have given way to a more integrated understanding of art therapy. Early confusion and adjustment to graduate school move into a mid-phase of settling down to the work and the life of an art therapist in training. The final phase is usually marked by a greater confidence and readiness to move on, sometimes accompanied by fear in becoming a professional and anxiety around finding a job.

The making of art to integrate this process, as well as to review a case, uses the art therapy modality itself to explore both an art therapy process (with the client) and one's own art therapy training.

The follow-through of the parallel process assignment occurs at the end of the course. At this point students present an art rendition of the actual termination in both their work with the client and their own termination from training. They note how they followed and/or modified their termination plans. This presentation also takes the form of an art project. In presenting the client's termination, students bring the client's artwork from art therapy sessions during the ending phase to show the actual process. With the focus on termination that this course encourages, it is expected that students will be dealing with termination quite actively with their clients and that client artwork will reflect separation issues.

Often there are interesting parallels between the client's work and the student's rendition of the client's termination (see case examples). In addition to the learning each student derives through the review and integration of his or her own work, much learning is achieved from viewing and discussing the varied experiences of other classmates working in different settings with different populations.

FINAL PROJECT

The final project for the course is to say good-bye in whatever way feels most fitting. This is a completely open-ended assignment. Some students have developed art project rituals involving the others in the class. One student gave a masked dance performance. Another brought her guitar and a songbook for each member of the class to sing along with her the eight songs she had written tracing the journey through art therapy training. Many projects have included personalized art gifts for everyone. And of course many have made pictures and sculptures to express their feelings about leaving.

EXAMPLE OF CLIENT AND STUDENT TERMINATION

To give an idea of how some of the art therapy termination process group work actually goes on, the following example shows Elizabeth Day's illustrations of her work with a client and her own termination from training and her practicum work.

Elizabeth's practicum placement was a child life program at a children's hospital. She worked with children hospitalized for various medical disorders. For the termination class she chose to review Torrance, an 11-year-old boy injured in a fight with a friend. Torrance's broken leg was suspended above him in traction, leaving him immobile, bored, and isolated in the hospital. Elizabeth described him as a slow learner with few social skills. The staff did not like him as much as the more engaging children. In addition, Torrance's poverty-level family visited him rarely.

Elizabeth drew Figure 21.1 to portray the beginning phase of her work with Torrance. She portrayed him in the style of his drawing of a "transformer" robot toy, experiencing him as a "pretty uninviting kid." In her picture she holds a mirror up to him to reflect himself back to him. Her goal was to be with him and help him in his isolation and boredom.

Figures 21.2 and 21.3 are two portraits Elizabeth drew of Torrance, Figure 21.2 showing how his leg was suspended and Figure 21.3 highlighting the importance of the telephone to Torrance. This was his link with home and with his father who was in prison. Torrance was very excited about Eliza-

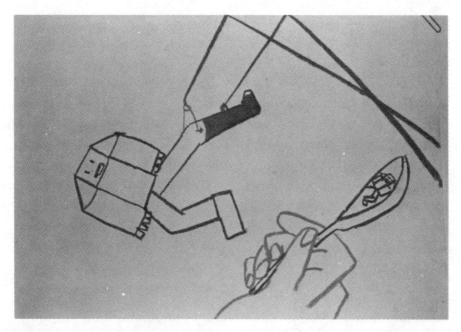

Figure 21.1. Elizabeth's beginning work with Torrance, portraying him as a "transformer" robot toy.

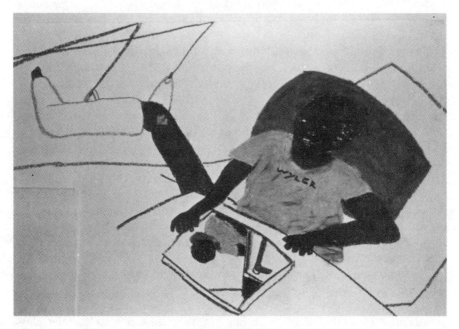

Figure 21.2. Torrance's leg in traction.

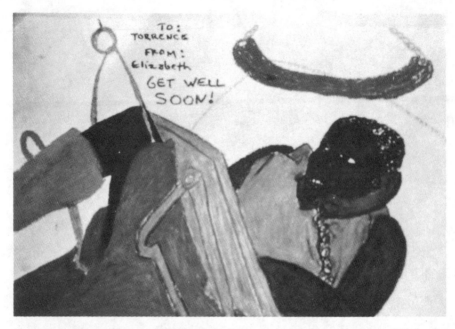

Figure 21.3. The importance of the telephone to Torrance and the tray propped on his leg for drawing.

beth's drawings of him, and this marked the beginning of his engagement with her. (Fig. 21.3 shows the tray propped on his leg that he used for drawing.)

To represent the mid-phase of treatment, Elizabeth drew Torrance saying, "Let's play art," as he then began to do, Figure 21.4. He started making art on his own and used it to relate to other hospital staff as well. Also in mid-phase Torrance began sending his art to his father and photographing it with Elizabeth's camera. In Figure 21.5 Elizabeth has drawn herself giving him stamp and envelope and providing a camera for him to shoot pictures of his art and the hospital.

In Figure 21.6 Elizabeth depicts the way Torrance enjoyed practicing script by writing his name and Elizabeth's over and over again. Also shown in this mid-phase picture are issues Torrance began to explore: his father's being in jail and the anger he felt for the boy who had beaten him up and caused his injury and hospitalization, expressed by the fist in the picture. Prior to this time he had denied any anger toward the other boy, claiming that he hadn't meant to hurt Torrance.

The importance of the patient review is to help the student plan his or her termination. Figure 21.7 is Elizabeth's termination plan for Torrance. In it Torrance is now out of traction, and Elizabeth is preparing him for greater mobility. Here she is wheeling him in a "banana cart" to the playroom where his artwork is hanging. In actuality Elizabeth drew a picture of

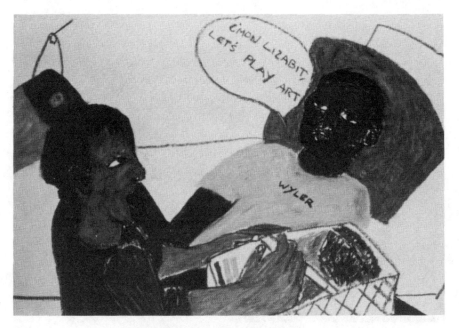

Figure 21.4. Mid-phase: "Let's play art."

the hospital playroom for Torrance to prepare him for it, and together they drew the hospital ward showing some of the children Torrance had befriended by now. The photographs and artwork were to provide a history that Torrance could take home and show his friends and family of his hospital experience, helping to effect a positive transition between hospital and home. He and Elizabeth reviewed the pictures together, noting Torrance's bravery in the face of his injury.

Figure 21.8 is Elizabeth's good-bye picture to Torrance that she gave him. In it he is a magical "transformer" flying out of the hospital. (The helicoptor is one he heard landing frequently at the hospital.)

One of the important termination lessons that students learn by sharing their work in class is that even the best-conceived termination plans sometimes misfire. In Torrance's case, the anticipated 6 weeks of traction extended to 8 weeks because he was lazy about practicing walking. Most likely he had some ambivalence about leaving the hospital. Up to this time he had been very meticulous in making sure his genitals were covered by his sheets in the awkward position the traction imposed. But during Torrance's 7th week Elizabeth walked into his room to find him fully exposed, seemingly unconcerned. This may have been regressive on his part, and Elizabeth felt very uncomfortable with him at this time.

The case review and termination plan are made early in the course to help students become aware of termination issues and plan for a positive termination. At the end of the course they present the actual termination as

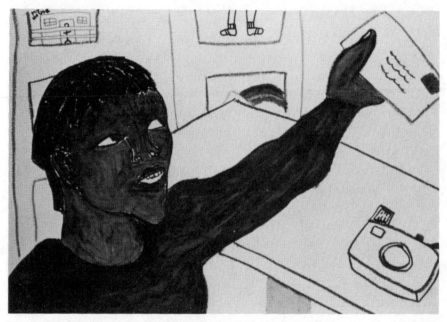

Figure 21.5. Elizabeth giving Torrance stamp and envelope to mail his art to his father and providing a camera to shoot it.

it happened, including the patient's termination pictures. Figure 21.9 is Elizabeth's depiction of the ending of her work with Torrance. Torrance stayed on after the good-byes had been completed. A new boy was moved into the room next door and Torrance began to develop a friendship with him. But he was afraid the new boy would replace him in Elizabeth's affections. He asked, "Who's going to be your best friend after I've gone?" Elizabeth has drawn herself partly turning away from Torrance, and the zigzag marks are the struggle with separation. Torrance's home is below as he had drawn it previously. The actual termination with Torrance was not as smooth as Elizabeth had planned it to be, but was accompanied by some discomfort and ambivalence on both their parts.

Elizabeth felt good about her work with Torrance despite discomfort in ending. She had helped him move from isolation and boredom to active engagement with her and others in the hospital. Her art was an important connection with Torrance. His art and hers became their meeting ground. Her art also served her well in helping her to process the development of their relationship and the important issues in treatment. The visual images made manifest the experience of conducting therapy including the important termination process.

Possibly Elizabeth chose Torrance to present to the class because he was one of the more hopeful patients with whom she worked. Many of the children at the hospital were seriously ill and dying. In reviewing her own

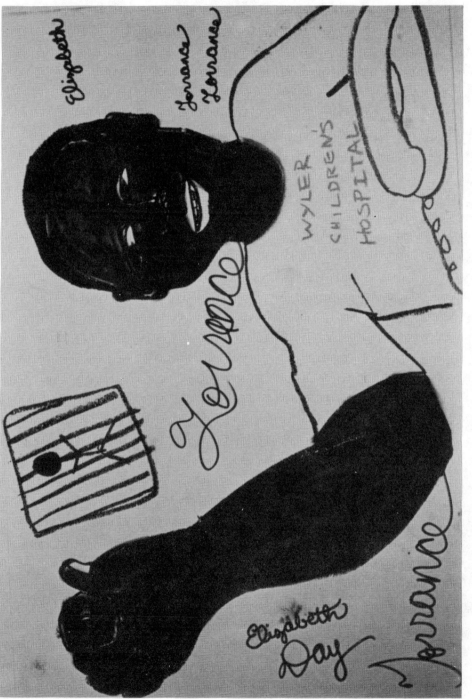

Figure 21.6. Mid-phase: Torrance practicing script and exploring issues of his father in jail and his anger at the boy who injured him.

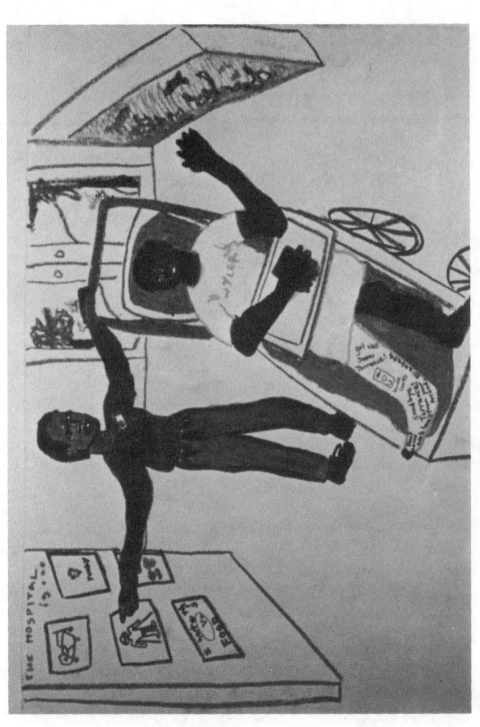

Figure 21.7. Termination plan for Torrance: wheeling him to the art room.

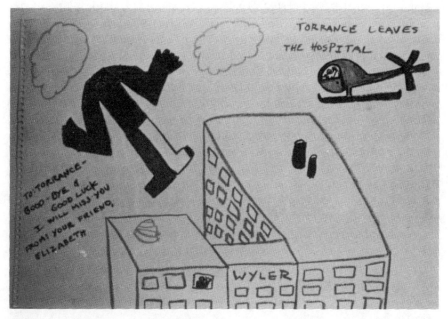

Figure 21.8. Elizabeth's good-bye picture to Torrance: "transformer" toy flying out of the hospital.

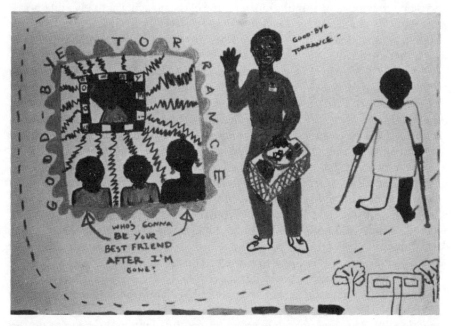

Figure 21.9. Elizabeth's picture of her actual ending with Torrance showing discomfort and ambivalence.

training in visual form parallel to her case review, Elizabeth explored this painful part of her work. Students' final projects could be whatever they wished. In hers, Elizabeth brought together both strands, her client work and her own processing. She created the doll she is holding in Figure 21.10. It reminded her of another patient, a 7-year-old child who had numerous liver transplants. For a while he did well, but then there was massive internal bleeding and he died. In making the doll, Elizabeth used fabric that she described as looking like "kids' play dough, scary, macabre." She ripped it open above the red abdominal wound and stitched it up in what was a very painful process for her. The wound is her own, accompanied by her question: "Why am I here?" She described the doll as not only all the terminally ill hospitalized children with whom she worked, but also the hurting child within herself that was touched by them. Indeed, the doll's crying face is that of an adult.

THE TEACHER

And what about the teacher's experience in such a class? For me there are many sources of satisfaction. I find myself having to *teach* less. The students have learned much, and class discussions with reactions to the art they present are lively and stimulating, with the class engaging actively and knowledgeably in contributing their observations. It's satisfying, indeed, to see how far the students have come as I review along with them the process of each one's training.

In many ways, in this course I am more of a facilitator than one who imparts knowledge. I construct a structure for review and further integration. The students flesh it out. I like being in this sort of position because it inevitably provides me with more learning than I derive from dishing out information I have thought about time and again. Each experience where students give the input is a fresh one.

Even for the teacher (or perhaps especially for the teacher), not all goodbyes are positive. There was one student who was angry because she felt I hadn't treated her fairly. She presented her anger in a picture in the class but then refused to deal with it. I processed my reaction in a series of paintings that I did not show her since I had invited her to share her feelings with me and she had refused. I showed my paintings to the other faculty and reflected on my feelings to myself. The student was an angry, hostile person and I was happy to see her leave.

Some years I have suggested and planned a celebration with the graduating students. Other years I haven't. I have learned to look at my own varied reactions to class endings, focusing, as I try to teach my students to do, on gains and losses, progress and disappointments.

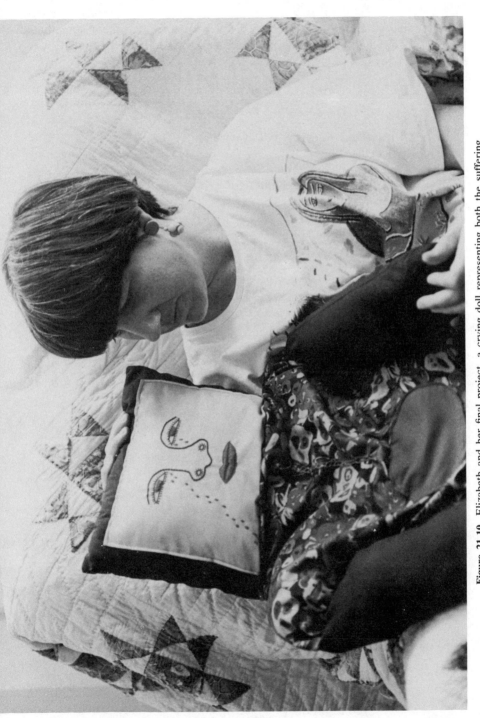

Figure 21.10. Elizabeth and her final project, a crying doll representing both the suffering children with whom she worked and her identification with them.

In saying good-bye to one class, I felt a need to give them something tangible. They had had a rough time and had worked hard. I brought them a cake and wrote a poem about it:

Graduation 1983

Black Forest Cake

The Black Forest is full of mystery
suspense, secrecy
filigreed layers of air
stacked in darkness and light
hope and despair.
Cherries sweet and tart,
red with passion,
dot the terrain
moisten the mouth.
Whip cream billows into the limitless puffs of clouds
above the Black Forest—an unbounded future
swirling beyond the darkness and light.

This mixing and rising,
leavening lightness into the compact batter,
this concoction of many cooks
takes time to bake
to swell
to grow.
And beyond whipped cream,
punctuations of dark bitter chocolate
and nuts,
kernels of growth,
not sweet—
meaty, generative.

The Black Forest is a part of us.
We partake of it together.

I also wrote a poem for each student, trying to capture the essence of my experience with each. I read them to the class as my "final project" and gave each one a copy after reading it. I had fun doing that. The following poem is the one I wrote for Rose Marano, our first student program assistant, who later became a teacher and supervisor in our program:

"A Rose is a Rose
is a Rose is a Rose"
full of mystery
unfolding as she grows.

No shrinking violet
this blossom with thorns—
lies and hypocrisies
are torn by her scorn.
"A Rose
by any other name"?
I think I'd call this one
a flame,
with a passionate spirit
that won't be tamed.

To you, Rose,
goes my gratitude
for your stamina, resourcefulness
and just plain fortitude.
Without your long hours
of program assistance
our beginning years may have succumbed
to bureaucratic resistance.

Rose, I wish you
as you prepare to depart
that you keep on fighting
with all of your heart.
The best we have
is often born
from the fragility of flowers
and the pricking of thorns.

For me, as well as for the students, there is the ambiguity of transition. I know that there are some students I will continue to see, some whose relationship with me will evolve into that of peers. Others I will see seldom if at all, and we will remain student and teacher to one another. Most gratifying are the occasions where I can welcome back graduates to serve as supervisors and teachers after they've gained experience in the field.

Recently a graduate from 2 years ago who had moved to another part of the country called me to enact a dream in which she was telling me how much she enjoyed being an art therapist. Another who had graduated 4 years ago and also moved far away visited me to report the exciting new position at a prestigious university she'd just obtained. Despite endings and distance, connections that have been forged aren't completely severed. This is the gainful side of endings. Important influences of the relationship are internalized and remain within us, paralleling for student and teacher the process between client and therapist.

Finally, I believe that my personal motivation for teaching a course on termination stems from my own difficulties with separation. Although each graduating class brings pride in students' learning and anticipation of the incoming class, once in a while I have a sudden choked-up feeling or need to draw a picture or write a poem to say good-bye.

CONCLUSION

Not only the content of the art therapy termination process group was important in the students' training; its methods were crucial as well. Almost all of the processing was achieved through art making and the subsequent reflection it evoked. By their own doing, students internalized the art therapy process further. Too often art therapists recognize the benefits of art expression for their clients but fail to utilize it for their own personal work. In the termination course, as well as in others in our program, students create imagery to integrate their learning (see Wadeson & Allen, 1983). The results are rich indeed, both in awareness development and in a final internalizing of the art therapy process through direct experience. The students graduate from training robed in a process that they are likely to wear for the rest of their lives.

The termination class raises for the students many existential questions. Most remain unanswered. This exploration brings them close to the awareness of the depths of their work. They come to see that nowhere more than in addressing issues of termination are the meaning of the work revealed and the nature of the therapeutic relationship and its significance to both client and therapist exposed. In learning to work with termination from their clients and with their own transition from student to professional, students come to grips with some of the fundamental dimensions of art therapy.

REFERENCES

Dewald, P. (1971). *Psychotherapy: A dynamic approach.* New York: Basic.

Easson, W. (1971). Patient and therapist after termination of psychotherapy. *American Journal of Psychotherapy, 25,* 635–642.

Edelson, M. (1963). *The termination of intensive psychotherapy.* Springfield, IL: Charles C. Thomas.

Johnson, C. (1974). Planning for termination of the group. In P. Glasser, R. Sarri, & R. Vinter (Eds.), *Individual change through small groups* (Vol. 12, pp. 258–265). New York: Free Press.

Levinson, H. L. (1977). Termination of psychotherapy: Some salient issues. *Social Casework, 58,* 480–489.

McGee, T. (1974). Therapist termination in group psychotherapy. *International Journal of Psychotherapy, 24,* 3–12.

McGee, T., Schuman, B., & Racusen, F. (1972). Termination in group psychotherapy. *American Journal of Psychotherapy, 26,* 521–532.

Wadeson, H. (1987). *The dynamics of art psychotherapy.* New York: Wiley.

Wadeson, H., & Allen, P. (1983). Art making in clinical training for conceptualization, integration, and self-awareness. *Leonardo, 16,* 241–242.

Wilson, L., Riley, S., & Wadeson, H. (1984). Art therapy supervision. *Art Therapy, 1,* 100–105.

Yalom, I. (1975). *The theory and practice of group psychotherapy.* New York: Basic.

Author Index

Subject Index